Principles for Evaluating Chemicals in the Environment

A Report of the

*Committee for the Working Conference on
Principles of Protocols for
Evaluating Chemicals in the Environment*

*Environmental Studies Board
National Academy of Sciences–
National Academy of Engineering*

and

*Committee on Toxicology
National Research Council*

NATIONAL ACADEMY OF SCIENCES
WASHINGTON, D.C. 1975

NOTICE: The project that is the subject of this report was approved by the Governing Board of the National Research Council, acting in behalf of the National Academy of Sciences. Such approval reflects the Board's judgment that the project is of national importance and appropriate with respect to both the purposes and resources of the National Research Council.

The members of the committee selected to undertake this project and prepare this report were chosen for recognized scholarly competence and with due consideration for the balance of disciplines appropriate to the project. Responsibility for the detailed aspects of this report rests with that committee.

Each report issuing from a study committee of the National Research Council is reviewed by an independent group of qualified individuals according to procedures established and monitored by the Report Review Committee of the National Academy of Sciences. Distribution of the report is approved, by the President of the Academy, upon satisfactory completion of the review process.

At the request of and funded by the
Environmental Protection Agency
Contract numbers 68-01-0132 and 68-01-0772

Library of Congress Catalog Card No. 74-31482
International Standard Book No. 0-309-02248-7

Available from
Printing and Publishing Office, National Academy of Sciences
2101 Constitution Avenue, N.W., Washington, D.C. 20418

Printed in the United States of America

Preface

The report which follows was in response to two separate contracts between the Environmental Protection Agency and the National Academy
of Sciences–National Research Council. The two contracts dealt with
complementary aspects of the safety assessment of chemicals—one relating to human health, the other to effects on other systems. Happily, they
were essentially contemporaneous, and those responsible for the separate
contracts wisely and immediately sensed the rightness of joining forces in a
single comprehensive approach. This early good judgment made possible
a most remarkable collaboration between the two components in what
is, after all, a series of problems with much interaction and in which
arbitrary boundaries would have led to serious and needless impediments
as well as duplication of effort by the scientific community.

A significant but not exclusive reason for undertaking this exercise has
been the anticipation that some form of legislation approximating one
of the versions of the "Toxic Substances Control Act" presented to the
last Congress might be passed in the present one. The various versions of
the Act all require that information on the safety and benefits of chemicals be submitted to the Administrator of EPA to guide him in making a
determination as to what restraints, if any, would be placed on the manufacture and use of specific chemicals. The sense of the several acts, present
and pending, places on the Administrator the burden of judging the ap-

propriate restrictions to be placed on manufacture and use; for this, he must have information. It is to the acquisition of this information that the present report is directed. Which questions can be usefully asked at the present state of the art and science of safety assessments? Which questions would be useless because present techniques are inadequate or because the information provided would be irrelevant? These issues stand on their own and will have a wide applicability whether or not a "Toxic Substances Control Act" is passed and put into force. This report is accordingly directed to all branches of the relevant governmental agencies involved in safety assessments and also to those industries concerned with the manufacture, distribution, and use of chemical products.

I would like to note here the extraordinary dedication and intense work that the distinguished scientists involved in the preparation of this report gave to its production. The assignment was a very large one; the time allowed was extremely short. Their work at their desks, in the pre-conference panel meetings, and finally at the Working Conference at which this report was completed, was extremely arduous. The task made a very substantial drain on their time. I thank them warmly. I should also like to thank the staff of the National Academy of Sciences–National Research Council for their able and perceptive backup; without this, satisfactory completion of the task would have been impossible. I especially wish to commend Mr. Ralph Wands of the Advisory Center on Toxicology, Dr. Charles Malone, and Dr. Charles Baummer of the Environmental Studies Board, and Mrs. A.L. Carlson and Miss Betsy Wilmoth for outstanding management of the central office during the San Antonio Working Conference, and Dr. Arthur J. Pallotta for his services as editorial consultant. Finally, I would like to thank Dr. John Buckley of the Office of Research and Monitoring of the Environmental Protection Agency for his wise advice in the scientific planning of this exercise.

> NORTON NELSON, *Chairman*
> Committee for the
> Working Conference on
> Principles of Protocols for
> Evaluating Chemicals in the Environment

February 1973

Contents

PART THREE
HUMAN HEALTH EFFECTS

APPENDIXES

WILLIAM D. RUCKELSHAUS
Administrator, Environmental Protection Agency

Message to the Working Conference

You are embarking on a task of great interest to the Environmental Protection Agency. In common with other agencies engaged in regulating chemicals, we recognize the need for a solid scientific basis for our regulatory actions. In contrast to most other regulatory agencies, our responsibilities encompass *all* aspects of effects of chemicals—effects on health, on crops and domestic animals, on fish and wildlife, and on those other less well-known but important life forms that share this planet with us.

Because of these diverse responsibilities, we need the broadest possible perspective. Because of the multiplicity of decisions to be made, it is essential that we ask the right questions—that we know "enough" to make good decisions, but that we do not seek to know everything about everything. Thus, we asked the National Academy of Sciences–National Academy of Engineering, with its access to talent in all elements of the scientific and technical communities, to consider this matter. Your Working Conference has been convened to study the principles of protocols for evaluating chemicals in the environment; to provide us with the benefit of your insight and knowledge as to the interactions and effects that take place when chemicals enter the environment; and thus to help us to test for the adverse effects that may result when chemicals enter the environment. This should be of great use to us in selecting the right issues to focus on and in applying our resources to those issues economically and effectively.

February 12, 1973

1

JOHN L. BUCKLEY
Deputy Director, Office of Research, Environmental Protection Agency

Charge
to the
Committee

A broad and penetrating assessment of what man needs to know to deal effectively with chemicals in the environment has long been necessary. Society's goal should obviously be to obtain the maximum *net social gain* from chemical substances—the problem is determining what constitutes net social gain.

The established practice has been to introduce new chemicals to accomplish a new purpose, or to accomplish an existing purpose more efficiently or economically. Concern has been with the intended result of the chemical, not with its unintended effects. For some decades now, we have been moving increasingly to more comprehensive assessments, which include not only the good effects but also the bad. Food additives, pesticides, and drugs are examples of categories of substances where there are now legal requirements for comprehensive assessments. There are, of course, other substances that enter the environment, and the several versions of a Toxic Substances Act considered by the executive and legislative branches of government are aimed at extending this technology assessment to these substances. And it goes without saying that it is important that this process result in technology assessment, not arrestment.

Given society's desire to maximize benefits and minimize risks, and the vast number of chemical substances that man can now make, it is essential to consider how we can best do this job.

3

Our problem in the Environmental Protection Agency (EPA) is deciding, in a socially optimal way, what to regulate (and what *not* to regulate), at what level to regulate, and in many cases how best to regulate—and assuring that our regulations are "right" and that they are being followed.

We need your help in how to think about the problem—to make it less intractable. EPA's charge to you is related to deciding what to regulate and at what level, and, to a lesser extent, checking to see that the decisions were right. We seek your advice in deciding what we need to learn, and in what sequence—so that we know *just enough* to make the right decisions. We seek your advice also on the most efficient and cost-effective way of proceeding. And we would value your thoughts on the best means of evaluation.

What Chemicals Are of Direct Concern to EPA?

The Environmental Protection Agency is predominantly a regulatory agency; and, as its name suggests, its preoccupation is with the environment—but, the environment *as the entire milieu in which man lives.* Thus, EPA is concerned with all chemical substances that reach the environment—including contaminants of the chemicals and degradation products that may be formed during use or in the environment. It is concerned with chemicals that are deliberately put into the environment, and those that escape to or leak into the environment.

EPA is not concerned with those chemicals that are administered directly to man, or that are deliberately added to foods. The procedures for evaluation may be very different for these substances in contrast to environmental exposures for at least two reasons: There is certainty that drugs and food additives will reach man; and, at least in the case of therapeutic drugs, there is opportunity to observe the effects directly in man. Many other chemicals in the environment will never reach man, or may be changed to other substances before they do; thus, the degree of safety assurance needed for these may be considerably less. It follows that the procedures and methods for evaluating therapeutic drugs and food additives may not be suitable or necessary for some environmental chemicals.

For those chemicals that do reach the environment, society, deliberately or by default, has assigned responsibility for generating information in distinctly different ways: For pervasive pollutants from many sources—for example, the common air and water pollutants—responsibility for acquiring the needed knowledge is allocated to the federal government. For chemicals distributed in the environment for one purpose, but which may have other effects—for example, pesticides—the federal government specifies the information required and evaluates the resulting information provided by the private sector.

The toxic substances bills of the last Congress anticipate that the private sector will be the data provider and, as with pesticides, the federal government will specify the information needed and will either evaluate the data or provide a basis by which the private sector will do the evaluating.

What Does EPA Need To Know?

Obviously, there are many things EPA needs to know:

- How much of a potential pollutant will reach the environment, where, when, and how?
- What will happen to it in the environment physically, chemically, and biologically?
- What effects will the chemical cause—to individuals, including man, to populations, to communities, to whole ecosystems, and to nonliving parts of the environment—if it reaches different parts of the environment (effects will include toxicity, stimulation, inhibition, destruction, alteration of processes)?
- How will it interact with other substances in the environment?
- What difference will it make if it causes these effects?

These are all-encompassing questions that need narrowing into operational and answerable terms. The likelihood of each event occurring needs to be considered, along with the acceptable degree of uncertainty in assessing the effect. The aim must be to attain the minimum amount of information needed to reach a suitable decision. EPA's requirement for information about an effect will be tempered by the likelihood the effect will occur.

All of the preceding questions pertain to the risk aspect of benefit-risk considerations. Similar considerations are important on the benefit side—efficacy for the intended purpose, value of the function performed, and alternative ways in which the function can be performed.

How Can the Necessary Information Be Obtained or Approximated?

This is the core of EPA's charge to you and involves consideration of such matters as the surrogate measures that may be available where direct data are not available, or cannot be acquired; the validity of extrapolations from one situation to another, or from animal to man; and the applicability of results to the "real world." The sequence in which additional information is required should also be considered in order to minimize the requirement for new information. Additional considerations include the following: Are there use categories of chemicals that can be designated that require different degrees of certainty in hazard evaluation? What factors should be considered in establishing such categories? Are there other systems of classifying chemicals that will make more manageable the assessment process?

Needs for New Knowledge

Though EPA's primary concern is making the best use of existing knowledge and methods for acquiring knowledge, the committee will undoubtedly discover important gaps in understanding while considering the foregoing matters. Are there broad areas where *better* understanding would permit better decisions, or permit decisions with less information on individual chemicals? Are there areas of ignorance that prevent EPA from making definitive judgments? We welcome your pinpointing these gaps and recommending ways in which they can be filled.

To sum up, we seek your advice on what information is needed and how it can be obtained, but not necessarily who should obtain it. If the thoughts above prove inadequate to the job, let me offer the advice a famous Arctic expert gave at the end of a 45-page description of how to build a snow house: "If this doesn't work, use common sense."

Part One

INTRODUCTION

I

Introduction

This chapter briefly outlines some guiding concepts, as well as the limitations, underlying the approaches used in defining the principles of protocols. To this end, attention is directed only to some of the major issues. This section is not a summary and should not be read as such. Each chapter, with the exception of Chapter II and the introductory chapters, has its own summary, and these should be examined for the highlights of the substantive sections of this report. Chapter II outlines the overall conclusions reached in the study as to those principles which should guide the evaluation of chemicals.

The Administrator of the Environmental Protection Agency (EPA) has asked the committee to advise on "the interactions and effects that take place when chemicals enter the environment; and thus to help us to test for the adverse effects that may result when chemicals enter the environment." The responsibilities of EPA "encompass *all* aspects of effects of chemicals—effects on health, on crops and domestic animals, on fish and wildlife, and on those other less well-known but important life forms that share this planet with us."

In arriving at the advice contained in this report, the committee has tried to keep in mind certain paramount considerations, among them that public policy is aimed at protecting the public and the environment from excessive exposure to harmful substances while also preserving

9

and increasing the great variety and utility of those products that have contributed so much to the convenience and enjoyment of our lives and to the vigor of our industry and trade.

Evaluation of Safety

Absolute safety is the goal of society in all endeavors. It is never achieved in any, whether it is in skyscraper construction or environmental management. An imperfect system is not to be condoned, but constantly improved, through experience and research, as rapidly as possible, within limitations placed on the system by society itself.

In the evaluation of the safety of chemicals, as in all other fields of human endeavor, some degree of risk must be considered acceptable to society. The alternative would be the needless prohibition of important benefits. Faced with the limitations of a finite but expanding resource, it is imperative that these efforts of safety evaluation be directed by a series of guidelines which assure the greatest return on the investment in terms of health protection.

It should be noted at this point that, although those aspects of safety assessment relevant to foods, drugs, cosmetics, and occupational exposures have not been directly dealt with, many of the sections in this report on human health will be directly applicable to chemical hazards.

The estimation of the safety (or hazard) of a chemical for particular uses can span an enormous range of complexity. At the simplest, the chemical may be a minor variant of a chemical already well understood, or the proposed new use may be almost identical to one for which experience is extensive. In such instances, the issue can be very simply decided. At the other extreme, the new chemical may be one for which there is no background understanding of its effects, its persistence, or of the likelihood of its chemical transformation, etc. In these cases, the range of possibilities is extremely large.

The objective of all safety testing is to ensure attainment of the desired benefits of use without incurring needless risks. There must, of course, be some balance between the benefit and the cost of assessment just as there needs to be a balance between benefit and acceptable risk. Thus, to subject all substances to a single rigid routine of study would be gravely off the mark and self-defeating.

In approaching this problem, the big questions should be asked first, and the more detailed ones broached sequentially as the need for more detail is demonstrated. Such a hierarchy or sequence of questions constitutes the only sensible means for dealing with what would otherwise be a counterproductive exercise. To impose unnecessary, time-consuming, and costly investigation upon a new chemical could lead needlessly to delaying or depriving society of important benefits from that chemical.

The temptation to develop a standard set of protocols for safety testing (in this context, "methods of procedure for safety testing") that could be used "across the board" has several dangers: On the one hand, such a course will often lead to the use of tests which are unnecessary; on the other, it is likely to fail to ask those questions that, in a particular case, may be of overriding importance. Therefore, it is important to keep in mind the danger of too rigid specification of protocols. Thus, in the present examination of the problem of safety testing, the committee emphasizes "principles" rather than details. In planning and conducting tests, there is no substitute for the vigilance of an inquiring and skeptical mind, which has assumed the full responsibility for making such safety assessments. If that responsibility is lessened by an exclusive dependence on a "check list" approach, the major assurance has been lost that a responsibly perceptive and efficient investigation will be conducted.

The approach taken here has been to (1) suggest how one can determine the significant adverse effects of chemicals (direct or indirect), (2) attempt to put these effects into perspective as to their relative gravity, (3) judge the probable reliability of answers to these questions, and (4) present and consider the state of the art of relevant testing procedures.

In some instances this approach has led to examining in some detail the specific tests to be conducted. In other instances, only very general principles could be stated at this time. However, where the present state of science is sufficient for useful tests to be undertaken, the associated principles of good practice are outlined. Thus, it is hoped that this report will make the safety assessment of chemicals more reliable and more efficient.

Benefits

The benefits of proposed chemical usage are dealt with somewhat less fully in this report than are the risk components because it is more difficult to suggest concrete procedures for the assessment of benefit than it is of risk. Benefits can take many forms—lifesaving, life-enhancing, economic gains, improvement of national security, and so forth.

These concepts are touched on in general terms; however, it is clear that the assessment of benefit is an even more *ad hoc* matter than is the assessment of risk.

Estimation of Exposure Levels to Target Systems

In the assessment of risk, we need to have answers to the question: "What will the effects be of the original agent and its altered forms on the various target systems, nearby or remote, now and in the future?" This means that we need to know where the agent and its altered forms will be in place and in time and in what concentration. Knowing this, we can begin to define the target systems.

The degree of exposure of the human population to the tens of thousands of different manufactured chemicals will vary from essentially zero to highly significant levels. For the most part the highest exposure will be associated with uses in consumer products, as food additives, drugs, pesticides, household and other personal products. However, the largest volume use of chemicals is directed toward products that involve minimal human exposure from normal use. Some of these uses are wallboard and other materials for building construction; automobile tires; synthetic fibers for carpets, draperies, and wearing apparel; plastics for table tops, trash bags and suitcases; paper products for newspapers, tissues, and grocery bags. Thousands of different chemicals are used in products of this nature and all of these uses involve some degree of human exposure.

It is incumbent on the scientific community and society to recognize the inherent difference in the degree of health risk associated with different uses of chemicals. This difference is a quantitative one associated with level of exposure. To require equal concern for all uses would be illogical, wasteful, and diversionary from more critical issues of public health.

Thus, among the first and most important steps to be undertaken is the examination of the patterns of usage. This must, of course, be done in parallel with an examination of the properties of the chemical. In some instances an examination of patterns of usage and disposal, taken with the available knowledge on the physical and chemical properties and available information on the biologic effects of the compound, will suffice to define the hazard without additional study or testing.

At its simplest, the estimation of exposure will involve no more than a tabulation of usage and disposal patterns of the agent and the form (or packaging) in which it is distributed. In other instances it will involve an elaborate examination of the movement of the chemical into the various environmental media, its transformation in such media by chemical or biological intervention and the dissemination and transport of the altered compounds. Such approaches, including the mathematical modeling of patterns of transport and alteration, have been considered here.

Effects on Man

The above considerations will help in defining the level and routes of exposure: In the case of man—is the chemical likely to be inhaled, is the oral route of importance (water or food), is skin penetration a possibility? Also, in the case of man, the effects on sensitive components of the population—individuals already stressed and with little reserve to withstand additional assaults (the aged, the ill, and the very young)—would be important. Although all significant effects would be of concern; obviously the gravity of the consequences of exposure must be an important consideration for the final decision as to usage and restrictions. Thus, a reversible functional effect, although undesirable, would be of vastly less consequence than the development of an irreversible fatal malignancy. A similar delayed consequence of substantial gravity is the possibility of mutagenic effects on later generations. Unfortunately, the testing methods for these grave threats generally are elaborate and involved, whereas testing procedures for many acute functional changes are much simpler.

Effects on Nonhuman Living Systems

With respect to wildlife, considerations are substantially different than they are with respect to humans. Although regrettable, the death or injury of an individual member of a wild population is obviously of much less consequence than endangerment of a species or population. Thus, it is appropriate to direct primary attention to the survival of a population as a whole, rather than single individuals. It has been found that survival of a given species is often dependent on very subtle things—behavioral or nutritional factors, for example—that alter breeding patterns; classical toxicological techniques may be very inefficient in assessing such factors.

In an attempt to develop an orderly sequence of evaluation, this report has approached these problems through examination at progressive levels of complexity; these may start in the test tube, progress through laboratory toxicity studies to limited trials perhaps leading to appropriately restricted usage. In many (perhaps most) cases there will remain some uncertainties, and follow-up observations will be essential.

Interactions

It is widely recognized that in many instances the action of a toxic agent can be modified by exposure to other agents. This modification can be additive, synergistic (more than additive), or inhibitory. In a few areas—for example—chemically induced cancer, there is now an extensive body of experimental and observational data on such interactions; in other fields, information and, indeed, good leads for testing for such interactions are lacking. The design of protocols must always recognize the possibility of interactions with other environmental agents and realistically include appropriate tests where this is practicable. Although no single section has dealt exclusively with interaction, it has received attention in a number of chapters.

Inanimate Systems

The atmosphere has been given special attention as a target system since it is the universally unavoidable medium for mankind. Thus, it has been dealt with as a target system in itself as well as a transport medium for the conveyance of chemicals from the point of release to other target systems.

Inanimate systems of a variety of kinds represent targets for unintended adverse effects of chemicals. This report has not been able to deal with all such effects but has examined systematically the means for assessing the effects of chemical agents on metals, glass, masonry, surface coatings, textiles, and some other materials.

Impurities

Of key importance is the issue of impurities in commercial chemicals. Sometimes it is a contaminant of the chemical rather than the chemical itself which is of importance: Thus, the presence of a few parts per million of the very toxic chemical, dioxin, in 2,4,5-T markedly increased the toxicity of this herbicide. Such occurrences require studies of the material as actually manufactured and distributed, rather than as a chemically pure reagent. Changes in manufacturing practices may result in alteration in kind and quantity of impurities and must be kept in mind.

Alterations

Another problem which frequently arises is alteration of the basic chemical; in some instances chemical alteration will lead to a loss of toxicity and in others it will produce more toxic forms. An example of the latter is the methylation of mercury, which converts it into what may be its most toxic form. In other instances, toxic agents are indirect byproducts of environmental reactions: Ozone is produced through a series of catalytic reactions involving sunlight and nitrogen dioxide working on the substrate of atmospheric hydrocarbons from auto exhaust; the ozone is much more toxic to plants and man than are the initial hydrocarbons. Thus, it is important to examine in some detail the environmental alteration of chemicals. On the other hand, there are practical limitations in the reliability or completeness with which such assessments can be made. In the examples given above, ozone and mercury, the processes by which such reactions occurred were unknown prior to their actual detection in the environment. Accordingly, predictions of hazard must always be presented with a certain amount of caution and humility. Nevertheless, in most instances useful predictions will be possible.

Accelerated Testing Procedures

Unfortunately, many of the test schemes available at the present time are cumbersome, elaborate, time-consuming, and costly. There is accordingly a continuing eagerness to find "quickie" tests, short cuts that would save both time and money. This is as it should be, and some progress has been made in a number of areas. These will be dealt with in relation to the specific tests examined. Unfortunately, the reliability of most such short cuts is at this time limited to very restricted groups of homologous chemicals. Used within such a restricted framework, they are an extremely valuable tool. In a few instances, they may have more general usage. Nevertheless, given the present state of knowledge the dangers of overreliance on such short-cut procedures need to be kept constantly in mind.

On the other hand, the potential advantage through increased sensitivity and timesaving is so great that a major research effort is justified to develop and validate such systems.

Monitoring and Analysis

Where entry of a chemical into one or several of the environmental media is likely, it will be essential to develop monitoring methods to ensure that the chemical does not reach undesirable levels. For this reason, an adequate analytical technique needs to be available at the time the material goes into use, not later. This report deals with those considerations relevant to measurement of the extent of entry of chemicals into the environmental systems, including both analytical techniques and monitoring strategies.

Statistical Aspects

In nearly every instance, statistical considerations are of vital importance both in setting up the test systems and in evaluating their applicability to the target populations, whether human or otherwise. On this basis, the Panel on Statistics has interacted with essentially every panel engaged in this study.

Follow-Up

In each instance, and at almost every stage, potential gaps and errors in the assessment of the hazard can be found. When the final stage is reached and it is possible to move on to production and distribution, reasonable and proper assurance of reliability should be present. Nevertheless, as there will remain a degree of uncertainty, it will be not only prudent but essential that appropriate follow-up schemes be maintained to detect possible errors in prediction of safety. This will require epidemiological alerts watching for unanticipated human effects and a similar systematic monitoring for unanticipated effects on wildlife.

Episodic Environmental Exposures

This report has not been primarily directed to the consideration of episodic pollutant discharges (accidental spills, "week-end" dumping, etc.). However, significant parts of the report will directly or indirectly provide guidance for some aspects of the problems created by such dumping and spills, and a short discussion of the relevance to this topic is included.

Research Needs

Inevitably the present exercise revealed many gaps and inadequacies in methods now available for assessment of safety and benefits. Where concrete suggestions for research to meet these needs could be made, appropriate recommendations have been developed. These recommendations represent an extremely important product of the work of the experts producing this report; research along the lines proposed is the major hope of developing the desperately needed improvements in the methods presently available.

II

Summary of Principles for Evaluating Chemicals in the Environment

Some of the effects of environmental chemicals and some of the test systems available for measuring certain of their effects are examined in this report. It will be apparent from a careful reading that the behavior and effects of chemicals in the environment are extraordinarily varied and that our ability to predict and measure these phenomena, although growing rapidly, is fragmentary and uneven.

The effects can in fact be classified according to their degree of conspicuousness, that is, the ratio between the magnitude of the effect to be measured (the *signal*) to the natural variability in the environment (the *noise*). At one end of the scale are local and unmistakable effects with clear end-points and relatively clear causes—such as dead trees around smelters, dead fish in creeks near chemical plants, and lung cancer in cigarette smokers. At the other end of the scale are the possible occurrences of wide-scale, subtle effects, which are difficult to discern among the natural variability in the environment—such as small changes in behavior of human populations, changes in fertility in animal populations, or changes in the productivity or stability of ecosystems or modifications to the climate of the earth. In close correspondence to this range in signal-to-noise ratio of the effects is a range of comprehensiveness and precision of test procedures: We have relatively good tests for toxicity and carcinogenicity, for example, but relatively poor and insensitive tests for effects on ecosystems.

However, our ability to measure effects precisely should not be confused with our estimate of their importance. The primary concern of the conference was not to evaluate specific test systems, but to formulate principles for evaluating chemicals in the environment and the social risks and benefits associated with their use. The ecologists at the conference argued strongly that effects on ecosystem functioning would not necessarily be of less social consequence than the more easily measured effects on other biological parameters. Indeed, the pervasive and subtle nature of these effects may make them of special concern: If they occur, they are unlikely to be noticed and measured until they are already relatively large. For this reason, a set of procedures for evaluating the potential impact of environmental chemicals should take these effects fully into account, even if standardized test protocols are not yet available.

HOW MUCH TESTING SHOULD BE REQUIRED?

Chapters III and VI–XIX summarize a very wide range of methods for evaluating and testing the potential impact of chemicals in the environment. For certain very widespread, persistent, mobile, and toxic chemicals (for example, mercury), almost the entire range of procedures would be necessary to define the full social risk. The costs involved would be so large that they could preclude development of any but the most valuable chemicals in this class. In general, however, it would be neither practicable nor prudent to demand full testing of all new chemicals. A point will be reached in the evaluation procedure—rather early in the case of most chemicals—at which further testing would provide diminishing returns. The additional knowledge of potential social risks that could be gained from further testing will be offset by the cost of the tests and by the risk of foreclosing development of a socially beneficial product. An important goal in designing a sequence of evaluative procedures is to permit the testing to end at this point of diminishing returns. An ideal test sequence would utilize quick and inexpensive tests to identify at an early stage those chemicals with a very high or a very low risk–benefit ratio. The resources of the regulatory agency and the industry are best devoted to thorough investigation of the marginal cases.

In formulating these principles, it has been assumed that most or all of the cost of testing will be borne by the manufacturer. Thus, as in the case of drugs, for example, the cost of evaluating the potential risk of a new product would form part of the cost of developing it. If the requirements for testing are judiciously adapted to the degree of risk identifiable in advance, the development of the more harmful products would be discouraged through the mechanism of the marketplace. To demand too much testing would prevent the development of some socially and technologically beneficial chemicals; to demand too little would permit the development of certain products whose net impact on society is harmful. The problem in devising an evaluative procedure is to maximize the net social gain by balancing the costs of testing against the benefits.

GENERAL PRINCIPLES

The conference participants reached a consensus on a number of general principles that should underlie the planning of any scheme for evaluating chemicals: Some of the following principles are stated explicitly in one form or another in individual chapters; others were found to underlie the discussion in several chapters or emerged in interpanel discussions.

Fallibility

With our present incomplete knowledge, we cannot expect to predict all the potential hazards of each new chemical. Even with a reasonably elaborate evaluation scheme, some hazardous chemicals with peculiar properties could well go unrecognized. It is unrealistic to expect that any system of premarket evaluation will ensure absolute safety. A more reasonable goal is to minimize the hazard within the limitations imposed by our knowledge and resources, with periodic review if manufacturing processes or uses change significantly.

Need for Flexibility

Our understanding of the effects of chemicals is increasing very rapidly. Hence, it would be very unwise to establish a rigid evaluation scheme at this time. Any testing sequence designed now should be provisional and flexible enough to permit continuous updating as scientific understanding advances and new procedures become available.

Wise Use of Resources

In the regulatory context, resources should not be wasted on lengthy testing of chemicals which are considered unlikely to create problems, nor on chemicals that clearly are too hazardous to release. Resources should be concentrated on thorough investigation of marginal cases.

Imprecision of Tests

No test procedure provides an exact measure of all the potential effects that need to be identified; toxicological tests on laboratory animals must be extrapolated to predict potential effects on man at much lower doses, with considerable resulting uncertainty. Even after a chemical has been released into the environment in quantity, only a limited number of its effects on possibly non-representative species and materials can be measured. All tests are thus models in some sense and, as predictive tools, are subject to error: They may give both false positive and false negative results.

Multiple Basis for Decisions

Accordingly, it would be unwise and probably dangerous to attempt to base a decision procedure on dichotomous tests. No single test should be the basis of a "go" or "no-go" decision. Each decision as to whether to test a chemical further should depend on clues provided by several previous steps in the evaluation scheme.

Need for Feedback Within the Test Scheme

In view of the variety of effects and patterns of dispersal of environmental chemicals and the consequent variety in their potential receptors, any efficient testing scheme will, in general, be complex. It would be unwise to specify in advance a standardized sequence of tests; some tests may be of high priority for one class of chemicals, but give little useful information for another. In some cases, simple tests made early in the sequence of evaluation may need to be repeated with greater depth or precision if a subsequent test gives rise to doubt about the original result. Ideally, each case should be treated on its own merits (although in practice many chemicals may fall into natural groups that present similar problems and will demand similar sequences of testing).

Cost Effectiveness of Tests

An important consideration in selection of tests is cost effectiveness. At each stage in the process of evaluation the value of the information likely to be obtained by further testing should be weighed against its costs (including costs in time and human resources). In some cases, the results of three or four simple but relatively imprecise tests may be more valuable than the result of one more elaborate but precise test, especially if the latter also requires more time to conduct. As pointed out in Chapter IV, similar considerations apply to the development of models for estimating exposure levels: The trade-off between the effectiveness of the model and the costs of developing it must therefore be weighed against the importance of the information that a model system can provide.

Value of Short-Term Tests

Short-term tests are of special interest in the context of this study, especially in cases where both the social risks and benefits are relatively small (as will be the case for many new industrial chemicals). Short-term tests are discussed briefly in several chapters and in detail in Appendix A. They appear to be useful predictive tools in some contexts, less useful in others. However, they are under rapid development and they are likely to become progressively more important in the future. At least in marginal cases, they can already be valuable in setting priorities for further testing (Chapter IX).

Structure–Activity Relations

Many important decisions, at least about the sequence of testing, can be made without testing at all on the basis of analogies with other known chemicals. Structure–activity relations are reasonably well understood for some groups of chemicals and some toxic effects, less well known for others. However, many new industrial chemicals differ only trivially from other known materials and relatively few fall into genuinely unknown groups. Those that do will require correspondingly more complex testing.

Need for a Multidisciplinary Approach

All decisions will necessarily be based on incomplete information. Accordingly, the most important element in the process of evaluating chemicals will be *the mature judgment of experienced professionals.* At each stage in the evaluation, it will be necessary to weigh information by several different areas of scientific specialization. Accordingly, there is a need for a multidisciplinary approach: Evaluations should be made by a team of professionals working together; applications should not be passed from department to department for independent comment.

Need for a Dialogue

It follows from the above principles that information on each new chemical must be repeatedly evaluated in order to guide the sequence of testing. It will be impossible to make reasonable decisions on the basis of a single submission of test results, unless the data demanded are prohibitively extensive. A much more efficient procedure would be to establish a dialogue between the manufacturer and the regulatory agency at an early stage in the process of development of a new chemical, so that the agency can guide the testing procedure and advise the manufacturer at an early stage if the risk–benefit ratio of the chemical appears likely to prove unfavorable. Of course, if such a procedure were established, adequate precautions would need to be taken to ensure confidentiality, at least in the early stages of development. Once a decision to permit release had been made, however, the underlying data should be made available for independent review.

Provisional Licensing and Periodic Review

New chemicals cannot be evaluated for benefit and risk at the time of their initial release into the environment and then forgotten. The evaluation of both benefit and risk will change with time due to factors such as changes in quantities or patterns of use, the appearance of alternative chemicals, the acquisition of new scientific information, the development of new test procedures, or the discovery of damage that only becomes apparent with widespread use. In addition, society's standards for acceptable risk will also be changing; therefore, all evaluations of a chemical must be in some sense provisional, and any regulatory scheme should include provisions for regular reporting of quantities and patterns of use, periodic re-evaluation of risks and benefits, and appropriate changes in regulations.

Importance of Formulation and Use Patterns

Many examples quoted in this report show that knowledge of the uses to which a chemical is put, the patterns of its disposal after use, and the way in which it is formulated or packaged are at least as important in predicting its environmental impact as knowledge of its inherent toxicity. Accordingly, any regulatory scheme must classify chemicals according to uses and expected patterns of disposal and must make separate evaluations of risk and benefit for each major category of uses. As pointed out in Chapter IV, uses and formulations are determined as much by secondary manufacturers as by the original manufacturer. The responsibility for reporting and testing should be distributed accordingly.

Liaison With Other Regulatory Agencies

Responsibility for evaluating certain aspects of the safety of new chemicals is already assigned to other agencies, including the Occupational Safety and Health Administration (OSHA) in the U.S. Department of Labor, the Food and Drug Administration (FDA) in the U.S. Department of Health, Education and Welfare, and the U.S. Department of Transportation. To avoid wasteful duplication of effort, it will be very desirable to establish close liaison with these agencies and to develop common standards and protocols so that the same tests will satisfy the requirements of all the agencies where jurisdictions overlap.

RISK-BENEFIT ANALYSIS

The bulk of this report is concerned with methods for evaluating the risks resulting from production and use of chemicals. Benefits are treated briefly in Chapter III, where there is a section summarizing and listing questions to be asked in weighing potential benefits against potential risk.

This report, however, contains no specific recommendations for principles to be adopted in seeking answers to these questions. Estimating benefits and estimating risks are procedures that clearly require the professional expertise of economists, engineers, and scientists. The primary task of this conference was to review the tools available for making these estimates and to recommend principles for selecting the best tools in individual cases.

Weighing risks against benefits, however, is a procedure which requires an additional type of professional expertise, not fully represented at the conference. At best, the estimation of risks and benefits provides a set of statements about probabilities. Prediction of the effects of changes in the use patterns of chemicals is a very inexact science, and in many cases the range of uncertainty in the predictions will be wide. In addition, few of the costs and not all of the benefits can be expressed adequately in economic terms: The decision-maker is faced with the necessity of weighing incommensurables. Decisions of this kind must primarily reflect the underlying social values, including their evolution under the pressure of experience, and require representation of those affected as well as technical experts. Scientists and engineers have the professional expertise to make technical assessments of risk and benefit, and those who have specialized in the study of individual aspects of the environment have the social responsibility to argue for adequate consideration of these aspects in the decision-making process. However, the decisions themselves require the weighing of these arguments and should involve others.

GENERAL SEQUENCE OF AN EVALUATION SCHEME

The study recommends the following general sequence for the step-wise evaluation of new chemicals:

1. preliminary evaluation of benefits;
2. preliminary estimation of exposure levels and identification and probable response of receptors;
3. review of basic toxicity data;
4. decision whether to require additional toxicity testing;
5. detailed estimation of exposure levels and extent of involvement of the above receptors;
6. sequential testing for effects appropriate to predicted receptors;
7. evaluation of risks associated with production and with individual use;
8. detailed evaluation of benefits and risk–benefit ratio;
9. provisional clearance for manufacture, with restrictions on uses if justified;
10. retesting of technical products and by-products;
11. survey of workers occupationally exposed;
12. periodic reports on quantities used;
13. monitoring of releases into the environment and, in appropriate cases, of exposure to predicted receptors; and
14. periodic review of licensing and restrictions.

Several aspects of this proposed sequence require explanation. Although the sequence is linear as presented, in some cases the results of testing or monitoring would require return to an earlier step in the sequence. Many chemicals produced in limited quantities would not need to be subjected to each stage in the sequence.

The need for provisional licensing and periodic review has been summarized earlier in this chapter. Some hazardous chemicals are expected to slip through the evaluative net, and their effects will be detected only by subsequent monitoring or epidemiological studies (Chapter VIII). Indeed, the proposals for field studies made in Chapters XV and XVI are predicated on this assumption.

There is an argument for making a preliminary evaluation of benefits before the assessment of risks so that EPA can advise the manufacturer at an early stage if the risk–benefit ratio appears likely to prove unfavorable.

The recommendation for testing the technical product is intended to ensure early detection of cases where toxic impurities are significant (Chapter XX). The committee suggests that, in such cases, the technical product should be regarded for regulatory purposes as a mixture of chemicals, and that the important impurities should be subjected to a separate evaluation and licensing procedure. Toxic by-products and cogeners are also important at the stage of commercial production. They can generally be regulated under existing pollution control laws if they are regarded as waste products; however, if new uses are devised for them, they may not be covered by such laws.

The committee suggests that each substantially new use for a chemical should be subjected to a new evaluation procedure (analogous to registering different formulations of a pesticide). In many cases, only steps 1–4 would be required, but if the new use involved a substantially new type of human exposure (e.g., packaging in spray cans) or a substantially new pattern of release (e.g., general use of a chemical previously used in closed systems), more extensive testing would generally be required. In such cases, the responsibility for providing the requisite data should fall on the secondary manufacturer proposing the use.

The recommendation for periodic reporting of production and periodic review of effects would cover cases in which a chemical that was safe when first produced in small quantities starts to cause adverse effects when uses increase substantially (road application of salt to melt ice is a classic example). Although some cases could be controlled by regulation of effluents, dispersed uses would be difficult to control without authority to regulate production or use patterns.

OUTLINE OF A PROPOSED TESTING SCHEME

The following is an outline of the way in which the general principles put forward above might be utilized in setting up a decision web for selecting the depth and sequence of toxicological tests to be carried out for each individual chemical. Because of the complexity of the proposed scheme, no attempt has been made to specify all the criteria for choice at each point in the sequence.

Stage 1. Initial Submission of Data by Manufacturer

In the first phase, only limited data (chemical formula, a few chemical and physical properties, proposed uses and rough estimates of volume) would be required. This would be sufficient (1) to screen out some non-problems (e.g., compounds with known properties), (2) to identify chemicals for exclusively in-plant use (which would be covered by existing regulatory authority for occupational safety, effluents, and transportation), and (3) to provide information for EPA to indicate to the manufacturer the likely extent of testing to be required.

Stage 2. Second Submission of Data

Sufficient data for estimating losses to the environment and ultimate fate should be included in this phase (Chapter IV, Preliminary Estimates of Exposure Levels). Basic data required for analysis and monitoring should also be included (Chaper XX), along with some additional data necessary for predicting atmospheric effects (Chapter XVIII, Conclusions) and effects on specified materials (Chapter XIX). The basic toxicological data required at this stage would be those required in any case for regulation of occupational exposure: acute, subchronic and chronic toxicity, and dermal and inhalation toxicity where appropriate (Chapters VII and VIII). It would be appropriate at this stage to require that behavioral observations be included in the test protocols (Chapter XI) and to require a preliminary screen for mutagenicity (Chapters IX and X). Where a water route of discharge is expected, static bioassay data for two or three representative organisms would be required (Chapter XIII) along with oxygen demand data for the larger volume materials (Chapter XVI).

This list of requirements may appear long for a preliminary screening, but most of the tests are comparatively simple and straightforward; further, the list is scarcely longer than is already required by existing regulations or is routinely carried out by responsible manufacturers. The only ill-defined and difficult area is the requirement for data on persistence and on products of metabolism and combustion (Chapter IV). Detailed protocols need to be devised to provide sufficient information at reasonable cost*.

---

* For persistence, several tests would be desirable (using clean water, soil, visible and ultra-violet light irradiation, etc.). At least some of these tests should be in closed systems and should be designed to separate losses by volatilization from losses by metabolism or degradation. Since the toxicity of metabolites and breakdown products is of more importance than their precise identity, indications of delayed or cumulative toxicity are of major significance and should be sought in the test protocol. Where preliminary testing indicates moderate or high persistence, a test in a multispecies microcosm (Chapter XIV) is indicated for Stage 4 in the testing. These tests for persistence presuppose either an analytical method for measuring levels in substrates or capability for radiolabeling. To identify products of complete and incomplete combustion may be a major research task, but the likelihood of production of known hazardous chemicals

Stage 3. Detailed Estimation of Exposure Levels

Detailed estimation of exposure levels by the methods discussed in Chapter IV should use appropriate physical and chemical properties of the materials and analogies with similar chemicals. The primary aim should be to classify chemicals into categories according to the type of exposure expected and the predicted receptors.

For human exposure, the criteria to be considered include the population incidence of exposure, the anticipated dose, and the anticipated duration; the depth of testing required will depend on all three of these criteria. Another important criterion would be the intermittency of the exposure, that is, whether occasional high doses or continuous low doses are expected. Here, the most important criterion to consider is the method of exposure: Chemicals could be classified into categories of direct contact (fabric flameproofers, volatile solvents, glues, paints, artists' materials, etc.), or indirect contact (many domestic products of low volatility, persistent chemicals entering food chains, or general air pollutants, etc.). A major consideration in classifying chemicals for testing would be the route of exposure; whether dietary, through inhalation, or by dermal absorption. A final consideration would be the likelihood of exposure to potentially sensitive groups—for example, the chronically ill, babies, pregnant women, or those exposed to other major pollutants.

For ecological exposure, Chapter XIII has proposed a classification into 12 exposure categories on the basis of predicted biological impact and chemical dispersal.

Stage 4. Choice of Toxicity Tests

The most important decisions in the evaluation procedure will take place at this stage. It is at this time that the chemicals should be reviewed by a multidisciplinary team and priorities set for additional testing according to the general principles listed earlier. By this stage, the chemicals will have been categorized according to ecological exposure, human exposure, and inherent toxicity. Breakdown products and possible effects on materials and the atmosphere will also be considered. In addition, analogies with other known chemicals will be an important guide. There are so many possible combinations of circumstances that it is impossible to specify in advance how the priorities would be set in an in-

---

(HCN, HF, NO_x, H_2SO_4) could be evaluated in advance. Since the toxicity rather than the identity of the combustion products is again of primary interest, bioassay techniques would probably be appropriate. The development of satisfactory protocols for these evaluations is an urgent research need.

dividual case. However, two extreme categories can be identified. At one extreme, many chemicals would need no further testing (chemicals with low volume production, short persistence, little predicted human exposure and/or low toxicity). At the other extreme, the most persistent toxic chemicals would need very extensive testing*. The important cases are the marginal chemicals.

Several panels have proposed decision webs, screening schemes, or generalized protocols for effects falling within their purviews (Chapters VII, IX, XI, XIII, and XVIII); other panels have considered that specific recommendations cannot be made at this stage (Chapters VIII, XIV, and XVI). However, our general recommendation is that these sequences of tests should not be run independently but should be integrated so that the results of tests for one type of effect should be used to guide the choice of tests for others.

Stage 5. Testing of Technical Products and By-products

Simple short-term tests for acute toxicity, mutagenicity, and other end points may be of special value in detecting variations in the commercial products. The advantage of selecting short-term tests at an early stage is that they can be used efficiently for periodic checking of batch-to-batch variability of commercial products in cases where problems are suspected.

Stage 6. Monitoring

The need for monitoring and for continuing field studies, and the principles for designing monitoring schemes, are discussed in some detail in Chapters XV, XVI, and XX.

SPECIAL CONSIDERATIONS

Chemicals Already Manufactured and in the Environment

Many potentially hazardous chemicals are already being manufactured and released into the environment. (Indeed, it seems likely that such chemicals are likely to be of more general concern than new chemicals developed in the future because of the increase in awareness and understanding of environmental hazards.) In general, the methods available

---

* As pointed out above, the requirement for extensive testing (or the prospect for restricted uses of chemicals of this type) may make the continued development of the chemical uneconomic.

for evaluating their impact and risk–benefit ratio are the same as those for new chemicals, with the important difference that the estimates can be more precise because some effects actually can be measured. The important regulatory questions—who should be responsible for providing data and whether authority exists to regulate production and uses—fall outside the scope of this report.

Two or More Manufacturers

A proposal by one manufacturer to produce a chemical already licensed for production by another raises several problems. The question of sharing test data or the cost of testing falls outside the scope of this report. Where the total production of the two manufacturers is predicted to result in increased hazards, additional testing and/or limitations on production or discharge might be required. The allocation of the resulting costs among the two manufacturers needs consideration, but there are regulatory precedents for this situation (e.g., the regulation of oxygen-demanding effluents into rivers). In allocating the costs, it will be necessary to consider the relative contribution of different uses to the total environmental hazard. For example, if manufacturer A produces a toxic chemical for use in essentially closed systems, it would be unreasonable to impose restrictions on his production simply because manufacturer B subsequently proposes to introduce the same chemical for a more leaky application. The burden of additional testing and of appropriate restrictions should in this case fall largely on manufacturer B.

Additions to Levels of Natural Chemicals

Many natural chemicals (especially heavy metals) are potentially hazardous if their levels are artificially increased by discharge into sensitive areas. In principle, the mere presence of a chemical in natural form should not relieve in any way the requirement for providing data from which the environmental impact of an addition can be assessed adequately.

Transformations

Some serious environmental problems in the past have resulted from unpredicted transformations of chemicals into more persistent and/or toxic forms. Photochemical smog, methylmercury, and the DDT degradation product DDE are classical examples. Optimism about the possibility of predicting some of these transformations on the basis of present and prospective chemical knowledge is expressed in Chapter IV, but we should nevertheless be prepared for further surprises. Of course, the discovery of a hazardous transformation product would require a re-evaluation of the risk–benefit ratio of the parent chemical.

Interactions and Activation

Interactions have been discussed at many points in this report and were shown to play an important role in the assessment of at least two types of effects: chemical carcinogenesis and effects on the atmosphere (Chapters IX and XVIII). Interactions between chemicals raise two different types of problems, scientific and regulatory. The scientific problems are prediction and detection. Although certain types of interaction—such as enzyme induction or inhibition—are beginning to be understood, there are so many different possibilities for potential interactions that it is unrealistic to demand that all of them be tested in advance. The committee suggests that the primary responsibility for investigating general rather than specific and reasonably predictable interactions, both at the level of research on mechanisms and at the level of monitoring for effects, should rest with government agencies. Again, the finding of significant effects will justify review of the parent chemical and raise the regulatory problem: If two chemicals have joint effects in the environment, how should the costs of the necessary restrictions be assigned?

Transportation and Spills

Large spills are most likely to result from accidents during storage and transportation. The special problems raised by spills are discussed in Chapter XVII.

Part Two

GENERAL CONSIDERATIONS

III

Benefits

INTRODUCTION

In formulating regulations and test protocols for controlling and evaluating toxic substances such as chemicals, their by-products, and wastes, consideration must be given to the benefits that society can realize from such materials so that judgments on the social utility of a chemical can be balanced against undesirable consequences of its commercial use. Knowledge of benefits is necessary also in order to determine the amount of testing and the degree of certainty that may be justified for a particular compound. For example, highly useful materials may warrant considerable testing to reveal unwanted side effects, if the nature of the chemical or preliminary experience suggests such possibilities. And, of course, highly beneficial substances may be acceptable to society at greater risk to health and the environment than less useful chemicals.

Although there are regulations to govern the use and discharge of some materials (e.g., food additives, drugs, cosmetics, pesticides, and radioactive materials) to the environment, many substances are unregulated and, until recently, the practice has been to permit their unrestricted use and dispersion until significant adverse effects on human health or the environment had been substantiated. There was little systematic effort to foresee potential harmful effects, and undesirable consequences were found by accident or indirectly through basic research. Thus, where benefits were obvious and the use of a product resulted in an economic profit, it was presumed that substances were safe and that risk of harm was small.

These values are now changing, and the recent history of commercial chemical development in the United States shows the primary motivation to be an attempt to meet or develop new market demands (as contrasted with previous emphasis on exploitation of raw materials or manufacturing techniques). That is, the wants and needs of society are continually analyzed by the chemical industry for opportunities for profitable, beneficial, attractive, and innovative applications. The ability to "tailor-make" chemical compounds and formulations to perform to design has established this pattern. Therefore, the identification of benefits is a natural and strongly supported function of the private sector.

There are and will continue to be an increasing number of questions about the net social utility of introducing new chemicals into the environment, and new regulatory measures will emerge. The goal to be achieved in regulating chemicals is to provide society maximum protection from adverse effects while at the same time not denying it access to beneficial products because of testing procedures that are prohibitive in terms of economic, scientific, or other resources. Optimum achievement of this goal will depend in large part upon a clear understanding of the kind and extent of the benefits to be derived from a substance.

The importance of assessing benefits cannot be overemphasized, especially since there is an increasing tendency on the part of many to look only at the risks involved with chemicals in the environment. This section thus focuses upon "benefits" and reviews some of the considerations and questions important in weighing benefits against risk.

PRACTICAL SOCIAL BENEFITS OF CHEMICALS

The benefits to society from an existing chemical or class of chemicals might be evaluated by determining what society would have to forego if the chemical were not available. For a new chemical, the determination might be of the gain society would realize from making the chemical available. A look at several examples of existing needs and chemical products will illustrate some of the kinds of benefits gained in the past and that can be expected in the future from new or existing chemicals.

New materials often create new uses and benefits. For example, polyurethane foam, introduced originally as a substitute for latex foam in mattresses and cushions, soon found diverse uses as a protective packing material, in life preservers, as padding on automobile dashboards, and as a flexible thermal insulator in clothing.

Another example of benefits realized is the development of water-based paints. These paints have made painting less of a chore (requiring less time for application and cleanup), are less flammable, and can yield a more durable finish. The savings in time and effort as well as in extended useful life of the painted article would make it difficult for the average homeowner to go back solely to oil-based paints and finishes. Indeed, the recent development of synthetic coatings has provided finishes that in many ways are superior to those based on natural pigments and oils.

An example of an item that is often more convenient than vital is the polyethylene bag. Such bags are inexpensive, light, waterproof, and transparent or opaque, and can be made in any size, of almost any desired strength, and shaped to meet almost any purpose. Table 1 describes use patterns for low density polyethelyne. Yet, use of the bag does consume a valuable resource (ethylene from petroleum), recycling is not presently feasible, discarded bags are a source of visual pollution, and large bags in the hands of small children are a suffocation hazard. However, few people at this time would choose to stop the manufacture of polyethylene bags—the benefits are large, the risks are small.

In fact, even campers have come to depend on polyethylene and other synthetic polymers for polyethylene canteens, polyethylene bags and ground sheets, emergency shelters and blankets, nylon rope, nylon garments insulated with dacron, and nylon zippers. Table 2 describes use

TABLE 1 Approximate Use Patterns for Low Density Polyethylene (LDPE)

Density Category	Use Designation	Quantity Used (million lb) and Percent of Total	Description of Use
LDPE	Film	2,805 (54%)	Packaging, trash and water bags, industrial cover sheets; about 70% used by individuals; short use-life, ultimate disposal through municipal refuse systems
	Injection molding	600 (11%)	Molded objects such as housewares and toys; most are consumer items with short lifetimes
	Wire cable	460 (9%)	Major use in telephone cable; very long use-time
	Extrusion coating	460 (9%)	About 90% used in coated milk cartons and other paperboard containers
	Roto and blow molding	130 (3%)	About half is used in large industrial vessels and household squeeze bottles
	Miscellaneous and export	595 (14%)	

TABLE 2   Approximate Use Patterns for High Density Polyethylene (HDPE)

Density Category	Use Designation	Quantity Used (million lb) and Percent of Total	Description of Use
HDPE	Blow molding	800 (35%)	Rigid containers (e.g., milk and detergent bottles); short-lived consumer items
	Injection molding	480 (20%)	About half used as consumer items (e.g., tops on aerosol cans, pails, toys); about half used in durable industrial products
	Pipe	110 (5%)	Sewer gas, water, and irrigation piping used in permanent installations
	Miscellaneous and export	920 (40%)	

patterns for high density polyethelyne. The U.S. Forest Service now requires that canoeists and backpackers carry their supplies only in reusable containers that are taken out of as well as into wilderness areas. These containers are usually fabricated from polyethylene.

It is apparent from these few examples that benefits to many facets of society can come from chemicals developed to meet specific needs and that benefits perhaps unanticipated are often eventually realized. At the same time, it is clear that the use of chemical products carries some degree of risk or unpleasant consequence. Once the public becomes accustomed to enjoying the rewards of a technological advance, returning to the state of affairs prior to the advance becomes difficult, often almost impossible. This adds to the urgency of making the initial assessment of risk–benefit as sound as possible. An informed public can often determine whether a product's benefits outweigh its liabilities, but the public will seldom have the knowledge and expertise to compare substances or products in terms of (1) relative safety, (2) relative efficiency in the use of natural resources and energy during manufacture, or (3) relative impact on the environment at various stages of manufacture or use. Thus, industry has the responsibility for offering the public the highest utility (greatest benefit) at the lowest risk. Both industry and other institutions have the responsibility for defining the risks and informing the public as to what is known and what is not known about these risks. Unfortunately, the prediction of both risks and benefits is still an imperfect science and must be recognized and acknowledged as such.

RISK-BENEFIT ANALYSIS

Benefits are the advantages that accrue to society as a whole or to individuals through the use of a chemical in the process of living. They may be entirely utilitarian or aesthetic, or a combination of both. Risks are the disadvantages, liabilities, or harmful effects that accrue to man directly or through adverse effects on his environment and thus eventually to man himself, either individually or to society. Three major categories for both benefits and risks can be listed.

Benefits	Risks

1. Value to the consumer
  a. Practical utility
  b. Aesthetic value
	1. Adverse effect on health
	  a. Well-being and general health
	  b. Death

2. Conservation of natural
   resources and energy
	2. Environmental damage
	  a. Air, water, and land pollution
	  b. Wildlife
	  c. Vegetation
	  d. Aesthetic
	  e. Property damage

3. Economic
  a. Employment
  b. Regional development
  c. Balance of trade
	3. Misuse of natural resources
	  and energy sources.

While most chemicals, and especially those under consideration for production and utilization by man, offer some degree of benefits, the ultimate evaluation of their practical and social benefit must be decided in a trade-off of benefits and risk. The factors involved are usually very complex.

What may be beneficial and even essential (lifesaving) to society in the context of a given time and social, economic, and political situation, may subsequently be viewed as unneeded, undesirable, or an unnecessary liability. New knowledge may demonstrate hazards in the use of a long-used substance or point the way to new uses of it. Once society deliberately directs itself to assessing benefits and risks in order to decide on the use or nonuse of a substance, it has the difficult task of exercising a judgment as to whether benefit outweighs risk. There is no established model or procedure for assessing benefits or risks in terms of an objective measure, and the final judgmental decision must be made by society or its delegated agents. The wrong decision either way can be costly. However, in evaluating the impact of abandonment of the production of specific chemicals on the economy and the labor force, it should be recognized that substitute agents will probably replace them, so that any effects would be temporary rather than permanent.

DDT is a prime example of a substance whose benefits have been assessed differently in the context of changing time and by different societies. Its use is no longer considered beneficial in the United States, where it is now essentially banned. We have no major malaria threat, and the possible effects of this insecticide on wildlife as well as the possible long-term toxicity of DDT to man himself has caused U.S. society to change its assessment of DDT's value. In some other societies of the world—for example, in Africa and the Far East—millions of lives are dependent on its continued use to control malaria.

The petroleum industry is an excellent example of an industry whose chemical products from research and development have found extensive and even unanticipated use—while providing employment and economic gain. This phenomenon has changed the very character of our society, although the transformation has not been achieved without certain liabilities.

Petroleum, as a source of liquid energy, has resulted in the development of the internal combustion engine, which, in turn, has provided mobile power plants for automobiles, trucks, farm machines, construction equipment, power and heating plants, and airplanes. The resultant effect in the development and expansion of our industrial society has been tremendous. Great benefits and serious liabilities have accompanied this development. The automobile has provided convenient, cheap, and rapid transportation, which has made possible a society able to move quickly, live at considerable distance from employment, and know and enjoy the diverse advantages of its country. The industrial expansion has caused a shift in population from rural communities to cities that offered employment opportunities. Mores and family lifestyles have thus changed. These changes have been accompanied by certain liabilities: atmospheric pollution; increased crime; use of great amounts of land for roads, with resulting erosion; disruption of living space; and the deaths and injuries due to automobile accidents.

The state of the art in risk–benefit analysis and recent references are summarized in *Perspectives on Benefit–Risk Decision Making: Report of a Colloquium* (National Academy of Engineering, 1972).

CRITERIA FOR ASSESSING BENEFITS

In weighing the necessity or advisability of establishing sanctions against the use of certain chemicals, or of imposing certain limitations on their use, the following criteria should be considered:

1. What needs of society are met by the chemical or the class of chemicals in question? In other words, what specific benefit does the chemical or class of chemicals supply?

The usefulness of a chemical may range from the merely aesthetic to the highly utilitarian: For example, a chemical may be used to make a fiber which is supplied for practical use. A plastic film used to package a product may have a dual purpose; that is, to make the product more appealing, and to keep it in better condition on the way to market (as in the packaging of lettuce). A polymer used in a paint may supply a more attractive gloss without necessarily providing greater protection.

If the threat of toxicity is significant, merely aesthetic values may not be sufficient for retention. But aesthetic properties have very important values to the public and are thus significant considerations in marketing.

2. If a chemical should be proscribed or limited in any significant way, are there adequate alternatives for meeting the need and providing the benefits it would have furnished? Are the alternatives likely to be more or less safe, expensive, or difficult to use, or require significant time spans for adjustment?

3. What is the extent of public use established by the substance or likely to be established, in volume or in dollars?

4. What level of employment is or will be involved in making, distributing, and marketing the substance? Could displaced employees be fairly quickly assimilated through other employment? Does the chemical in question have an impact on employment by creating business in other products by making them more useful or more attractive? Would restrictions on the use of the chemical cause unemployment?

5. If changes or substitutions affect the end-use applications of the substances, how will these alter the cost picture and the utility of the product to the public?

6. How do any manpower or economic dislocations measure up in magnitude against the overall impact on the economy, either locally or on a broader scale?

7. Does the production of the chemical have other significant effects on the economics of the particular region where it is produced or consumed? What would be the effect of proscription on local revenues?

8. Is the chemical proposed for regulation one that is manufactured only in a small region of the country?

Will alterations in such an industry contribute to other significant social effects, such as the crime rate, water and sanitation factors, poverty, housing requirements?

9. If the threat of toxicity seems too great to permit continued use

of a chemical in one or more applications, how can the effects of proscription be moderated to minimize impact on the public, such as unemployment and essential services? Developing and producing large volumes of alternative materials can sometimes take considerable time, effort, and investment (or, in other instances, fully absorb the released labor force).

10.   How do other critical social problems impinge upon the problem of securing adequate benefits from alternative materials? The current energy crisis, for example, severely limits the options among petrochemicals and some of the correlative materials used in end products of the petroleum industry.

11.   How would proscription or less severe limitations on the manufacture and distribution of a particular chemical affect the export market to those countries which have no such restrictions, either for the chemical itself or for other chemicals which might be offered as part of a complete line of products including the specific chemical?

THE CHEMICAL INDUSTRY

Although decisions to restrict the use of any particular chemical or class of chemicals for one or more uses must take into account the benefits and the liabilities conferred, these decisions in many cases must be considered against the background of the complex socioeconomic picture as a whole. Among the factors having particular relevance are the size and scope of the industry in the United States, its impact on the national income and the gross national product, its impact on employment, its effect upon such national problems as balance of trade, the preservation of natural resources, environmental cleanup and its impact on related industries.

Scope of the Chemical Industry

The U.S. chemical industry is now producing and selling upwards of $68 billion worth of materials per year. About half is accounted for by basic chemicals. To illustrate a typical overall production and use pattern, the case of polyethylene is discussed below.

In 1972, 7.5 billion pounds of polyethylene were sold in the United States at about 13¢ per pound ($975 million), an increase of nearly 500 percent from 1961 when the total sales were 1.56 billion pounds. The forecast for 1977 is 13.4 billion pounds. The 1972 production was divided into two main types: low density polyethylene (LDPE), 5.2

billion pounds; and high density polyethylene (HDPE), 2.3 billion
pounds.

The end uses for polyethylene are approximately as shown in Tables 1
and 2. The total U.S. export of both classes of polyethylene amounted
to about 610 million pounds in 1972, while only about 20 million were
imported. On a per capita basis, each person in the U.S. uses about 37.5
pounds of polyethylene each year. Uses are divided as follows:

end-use	U.S. per capita consumption (lb/yr)
bottles, industrial tanks	4.5
toys, pails, bottle caps	5.3
piping	1.0
cable insulation	3.6
coated paperboard and milk bottles	2.6
wrapping film, garbage bags, etc.	13.0
miscellaneous	4.5
export	3.0
total	37.5

Interdependence

The interrelations of chemical products and processes are very complex,
and much of the economy of the chemical industry depends upon successfully putting by-products of each process to use, either as end
products themselves or as the intermediates for some other process.
Other efforts are directed at eliminating by-products by improving
yields. Not only does an improved yield improve process economies, but
elimination of by-products reduces waste disposal problems and lessens
the load on environmental pollution.

In the ceaseless search for lower costs, increased efficiency, and optimum use of resources, the chemical industry constantly alters and adjusts its major processes. New restrictions or limitations on chemicals
now in use may lead to dislocations in the complex patterns, perhaps
felt economically at points far removed from the immediate end use of
these chemicals and impacting the public in unexpected ways. Almost
every phase of chemical manufacturing provides examples of this principle: One is the role of styrene.

Styrene is an organic intermediate, made in more than 30 countries
and used in such products as packaging, appliances, automobiles, toys,

furniture, paints, and tires. All U.S. styrene is made by catalytic dehydro-genation of another intermediate, ethylbenzene, made readily and cheaply by reacting ethylene with benzene separated from refinery streams. Process improvements and economies of scale have reduced the price of styrene to the point that producers have found it economically advantageous to build very large plants and to make, not only the styrene, but its raw materials and polymers as well.

An example of interdependence is found in recent uncertainties in styrene production costs, which have been created by the anticipated removal of lead from automotive gasoline. In the efficient styrene process, the single most important factor in the price of the intermediate, ethylbenzene, is the cost of the benzene. The major source of benzene is catalytic reforming of petroleum. If refiners use these fractions to counteract the effects of removing lead, they will also directly affect the demand–supply–price structure for benzene, and thus affect the total economics of the styrene industry.

Impact on Total U.S. Economy

As a capital intensive industry, the manufacture of chemicals requires only 5 percent of the U.S. manufacturing force. The value of its ship-ments, however, is nearly 8 percent of the value of all manufacturing. Its capital expenditures yearly run to more than 10 percent of the total for all U.S. manufacturing, and its total assets are more than 6 per-cent of assets for all manufacturing. Its research and development ex-penditures are about 15 percent of R & D outlays by U.S. manufacturers.

Because the products of the chemical industry largely go to other in-dustries, however, their impact is best read, and their benefits best understood, by examining their significance to those industries. Again, one example may suffice: the role of synthetic fibers such as nylon, acrylic, and polyester, in the textile industry. In 1960 only 39 percent of U.S. mill consumption was provided by man-made fibers, whereas in 1970 man-made fibers accounted for 64 percent of U.S. mill con-sumption. Consumption passed 3 billion pounds in 1970 and is ex-pected to reach four billion pounds in the near future.

Behind the production of the fibers themselves is a large production force required to produce the chemical intermediates from which the polymers are formed and spun. A 1-billion pound output of nylon for example, requires about 1.8 billion pounds of intermediates.

Once again, the element of interdependence is of paramount im-portance. The large-volume consumption of intermediates has led to economies of scale that have, in turn, made the intermediates attractive building blocks for other products, inlcuding polyester films, synthetic rubbers, plastic products, disposable soft-drink bottles.

Employment and Balance of Trade

The U.S. chemical industry employed somewhat more than 1 million people in 1972 and thus provided employment for about 5 percent of the total manufacturing force. The industry employs about 100,000 technically trained professionals such as chemists, engineers, and many other scientists. It is also an important employer of research people, and in 1971 these totaled approximately 43,000—about 22,700 of which were in basic chemicals research.

The chemical industry has always been an important factor to a trade balance in the United States, and in 1971 the industry contributed a positive trade balance of $2.2 billion. However, it should be noted that the U.S. share of the world chemical market declined rather steadily from 1961, when it stood at 28.2 percent, to 21.4 percent in 1971.

SUMMARY

The goal in regulating chemicals is to provide society maximum protection from adverse effects while not denying it access to beneficial products because of testing procedures that are prohibitive in terms of economic, scientific, or other resources. Optimum achievement of the goal will depend, in large part, upon a clear understanding of the kind and extent of the benefits to be derived from a substance.

The value of chemicals to the consumer ranges from trivial (e.g., silly putty) to essential (e.g., lifesaving drugs). Although such practical benefits are difficult to quantify, they might be evaluated by determining what society would have to forego if the chemical in question were not available.

The economic benefits of chemicals include effects on employment, regional development, gross national product, balance of trade, conservation of natural resources, and environmental quality. The assessment of economic benefits from chemicals is made difficult by the complex interdependence of chemical products and process that exists within the industry.

REFERENCES

National Academy of Engineering. 1972. *Perspectives on Benefit–Risk Decision Making: Report of a Colloquium.* Committee on Public Engineering Policy, National Academy of Engineering, Washington, D.C. 157 pp.

SUGGESTED READINGS

Calabresi, G. 1970. *The Costs of Accidents: A Legal and Economic Analysis.* Yale University Press, New Haven, Conn. 340 pp.

National Academy of Engineering. Committee on Public Engineering Policy. 1969. *A Study of Technology Assessment.* U.S. Government Printing Office, Washington, D.C. 208 pp.

National Academy of Engineering. 1970. *Public Safety: A Growing Factor in Modern Design.* National Academy of Sciences, Washington, D.C. 115 pp.

National Academy of Sciences. Committee on Science and Public Policy. 1969. *Technology: Processes of Assessment and Choice.* U.S. Government Printing Office, Washington, D.C. 163 pp.

Starr, C. 1969. Social benefit versus technological risk. *Science* 165:1232–1238.

IV

Estimation of Exposure Levels to Target Systems

INTRODUCTION

The task of the Panel on Estimation of Exposure Levels has been to assess current ability to determine the rates, routes, and reservoirs of chemical substances moving through the environment, and to estimate the resulting level of exposure to susceptible targets, both living and nonliving.

A rough estimate of exposure would be a logical early step in the evaluation of a chemical, for it would serve to identify the kinds of tests necessary to determine the risks associated with use and indicate the need for more refined estimates of exposure.

Four kinds of information are required to make these estimates: (1) data on the quantities of the chemical released to the environment as a result of production, use, and disposal; (2) data on physical and chemical properties; (3) the expected environmental transformations of the chemical; and (4) the likelihood of bioaccumulation.

A few features of the present state of the art should be emphasized at the outset:

1. Until a few years ago there was very little interest in following

the path of chemicals through the environment and, as a consequence, very little work has been done.

2. The processes of movement of materials through the environment are very complex and include time delays that may sometimes be long but are largely unknown.

3. The physical and chemical properties of these substances, together with biological activity, greatly affect their movement, destinations, and effects.

4. Our knowledge of transformations that change substances from harmless to hazardous, and vice versa, is sparse.

5. There have been very few efforts to determine what pollutants are where and in what amounts, or to monitor changes in these baseline levels.

6. The number of different substances that are dispersed in the environment through use and disposal is probably in the hundreds of thousands. Presumably most of these are not injuring man or other organisms; however, recent discoveries that certain substances are harmful and are widespread makes it necessary to identify any that should be restricted or banned and to avoid the introduction of new substances that promise unaceptable exposure risks for man, other organisms, and the environment.

Given this state of affairs, the panel has endeavored to evaluate existing methods (referred to here as *models*) for studying the movement of substances, from the site of production to the ultimate sink or degradation products, and for estimating the exposures along the way.

The panel has concluded that the development of predictive models for estimating exposure levels of target systems to toxic substances is in a very primitive state. No established and proved detailed procedures can be put forward for developing these models. In the absence of more fully matured procedural approaches, examples and principles will be outlined in the following discussion, with reference to work on the topics. These can serve as a starting point from which to undertake the development of specific models.

PRODUCTION, USE, AND DISPOSAL

A consideration of production, use, and disposal is helpful—first, because these factors represent the major stages in the fate of a chemical with respect to the ways in which it enters the environment and, second, because they identify different sectors of society in which selected controls can be effected in order to minimize releases to the environment. In general, releases associated with production are amenable to controls on manufacturers; those associated with use, to controls on users or consumers; those associated with disposal, to controls at the municipal level. Production, use, and disposal are considered here as representing the major stages in the fate of a chemical.

Production

The production process is not only the first stage in the flow of a chemical through the environment; it is also sometimes a source of emissions into the environment. Quantities of the manufactured chemical, its by-products, and other chemicals associated with the process are often discharged at the point of production. While many of the effects of these discharges are considered in existing legislation dealing with occupational health and environmental quality, proposed legislation on the control of toxic substances raises the need for new methods of estimating exposure to important targets.

Data on production and production losses must be obtained from manufacturers of chemicals and from manufacturers of products containing chemicals to allow an estimation of direct injection of chemicals into the environment at the production site. These data are not generally available now. Thus, if the evaluation is to be effective, the information must be explicitly requested and required by the regulatory agency.

The quantities of the manufactured chemical or product must be known, as well as all industrial clients who intend to use the chemical in their products. The latter would then be required to provide the production data for their respective products. Inventory statistics and data on methods of transportation to major clients will also be important in determining exposure levels in the environment. All data should be for commercial grade products because, in some cases, impurities may be more harmful than the chemical itself.

Data on the leakiness of the production and transportation processes are of critical importance. Important considerations include the geographical distribution of sources, the media receiving the discharge, the quantity and chemical content of the discharge, and the temporal characteristics of continuous or intermittent emissions. Some of these data are required or relate to processes regulated under existing laws, but the information will generally be difficult to obtain because of the proprietary nature of industrial processes and the liabilities that might be incurred from such disclosures. Provisions will have to be made by the government to protect the confidential nature of these data.

Uses

Data on uses and use patterns are required to determine exposure levels resulting from normal use and to follow the chemical through its next stage of life. Use data should be obtained from the manufacturer of a specific product or from the distributor for a specific market. The reporting procedure should be worked out to assure response by all manufacturers.

There are many dimensions that would be useful in characterizing the types of use information that should be reported. One categorization might be according to types of uses. There are many possible breakdowns from the very general (e.g., household, industrial, construction, etc.) to the fairly specific (e.g., paints, plasticizers, synthetic fabrics, etc). The panel has not systematically considered all the possibilities, but does feel that development of a categorization would be consistent with the purposes of the committee's approach to qualitative determination of exposure levels.

The panel feels that a first cut at categorization should be a division into contained and dispersive uses. Contained uses are those in which the chemical is not systematically released to the environment as a direct result of use: for example, lead in cans, plasticizers in vinyl upholstery, asbestos in fireproof clothing, and polychlorinated biphenyls (PCB's) in transformers. Dispersive uses are those in which the chemical is released to the environment as a direct consequence of use (e.g. Freon in aerosol cans, solvents in paints, lead in gasoline, and pesticides).

In general, those uses that are designated *contained* will not introduce large quantities of chemicals to the environment during the use stage, but careful attention must then be given to the disposal stage. Information on possible releases of the chemical during normal contained usage should, however, be carefully considered because these may be particularly insidious, such as the contamination of food by substances found in packaging materials. For dispersive uses, data should be given on the percentage of the chemical likely to be emitted into the air, water, or land. Data should also be required on the quantity of the product involved in each use, the geographical distribution of uses, the average lifetime of the product, and the most probable methods of disposal.

The use of consumer products can result in significant exposure to toxic chemicals. Skin contact often accompanies the use of a variety of household chemicals ranging from dishwashing detergents to paint removers, whether or not such contact is advised against by the manufacturer. Another source of dermal exposure is residues of washday products in laundered clothes, such as the fluorescent whitening agents implicated in carcinogenesis. Ingestion may result from the contamination of cooking and eating utensils, and from the failure of the user to wash his hands before eating following exposures. Exposure through inhalation is particularly important since the air within a closed house may contain aerosols or gaseous chemicals introduced by the use of fuels, household cleaners, paints, solvents, products packaged in spray cans, and the like. It may be possible to determine the level of such exposures experimentally with existing analytical techniques. Exposures may, in principle, be estimated from the release rate of chemicals and ventilation rates in homes. However, the wide variation in human behavior, use of household chemicals, and house construction complicate such modeling activities.

Disposal

The flow of discarded products can be traced from records on the disposal of wastes. Statistics are available on national and, to a lesser extent, regional levels of the amount of solid waste disposed of by incineration, open-burning, dumping into waterways and lakes, and landfill. The fractions of the solid waste disposed of by each method roughly approximate the disposal pattern of individual consumer solid products. Similar statistics for sewage include the amounts undergoing primary, secondary, and tertiary treatment, and the fraction of the sewage sludge that is disposed of by incineration, wet oxidation, landfill, discharge at sea, or in soil conditioning.

The amount of a given chemical that is discharged depends on its production rate and product life. For products with a short life, disposal rates are approximately equal to production rates. For products with a longer life and rapidly growing consumption rate, the rate of disposal will be considerably smaller than the rate of production and may be estimated from the service life of the product and the historical record of production. It is thus possible to generate an approximate profile of the disposal pattern of a chemical from information on production rate, use, approximate service life, and regional and national statistics on solid waste and sewage disposal.

The fate of the chemicals that have been discarded by the different routes is not as easily established. Compounds incinerated are often converted essentially to the products of complete combustion. The incineration of halogenated and nitrogenated compounds will result in emissions of the corresponding halogen acids and oxides of nitrogen, generally in concentrations that may be estimated. Metals and metallic compounds will be emitted as the metal oxide in amounts that depend on their vapor pressure, the incineration conditions, and the efficiency of air pollution control devices. Some estimates are available on the fraction of different metals that escape from existing units and a "worst case" estimate of emissions may always be obtained by assuming all the metal is in the stack effluent.

Open-burning can lead to emissions of significant quantities of products of partial combustion or pyrolysis, including carbon monoxide, polynuclear aromatics, and possibly hydrogen cyanide, ammonia, and nitric oxide; however, burning dumps are being eliminated rapidly. The fate of chemicals in landfills and in sewage treatment plants depends on their physical, chemical, and biochemical properties as discussed later in this chapter. Examination of these properties is necessary in order to determine the extent of possible contamination of the groundwaters surrounding dumps, and those subject to the effluents and sludge from sewage treatment plants. It is extremely difficult to predict the fate of chemicals used in such products as packaging materials since the rate of release is often unknown.

Although industry is not responsible for the ultimate disposal of most of its consumer products, it appears reasonable to request data from industry regarding the most probable methods of disposal. This information, coupled with quantitative and geographic use statistics, will provide a picture of entry to the environment in the disposal stage. The discussion above suggests that from this picture an estimation of flows from points of disposal could be developed.

INFLUENCE OF PHYSICAL AND CHEMICAL PROPERTIES ON MOBILITY: CHEMODYNAMICS

Chemodynamics is the study of the relationship of physical and chemical properties to the behavior of chemicals in the environment. In this section those properties will be discussed that can be used to generate a qualitative estimate of the level of exposure. Although many of the examples presented here deal with pesticides, the principles involved could be applied to other organic compounds as well.

When a chemical is released into the environment, it is distributed to the atmosphere, soil, and water. The concentration in any geosphere will be a function of the properties of both the chemical and the geosphere.

Behavior in Atmosphere: Vapor Transport

Once a chemical is introduced into the environment, its entry into and transport through the atmosphere will depend on such factors as its vapor pressure and heat of vaporization, the partition coefficient between atmosphere and any other phase, and the air flow mass that will transport the chemical through the atmosphere.

The vapor pressure of the chemical plays a major role in determining the exchange of chemicals between the atmosphere and other geospheres. The vapor pressures (Hamaker and Kerlinger, 1969) of chemicals and pesticides vary widely from those of gases, such as CO, CO_2, SO_2, to those of volatile organophosphates and carbamates (parathion 0.03 mm Hg, Sevin 0.005 mm Hg), to those of the less volatile materials such as triazines, DDT, aldrin, and dieldrin (10^{-6} to 10^{-9} mm Hg), to those of materials with negligible vapor pressures.

The presence of suspended dust or aerosol particles may result in adsorption of some of the vapors, which will consequently increase the partition function of the chemical between atmospheric and condensed phases of the environment. The rate of vaporization of a chemical from a surface is related to its diffusion in the air and, hence, can be affected by air currents (Hartley, 1969).

Many chemicals in aqueous solution will evaporate simultaneously with the water, i.e., they co-distill. It has been shown that DDT (Acree *et al.*, 1963) and other chemicals whose solubility in aqueous solution is in the parts per billion range, co-distill with water into the atmospheric phase. Vapor loss of a chemical from a soil system is accelerated by the presence of moisture (Freed *et al.*, 1962; Freed and Witt, 1969; Frost, 1969).

Although vapor pressure of a chemical to a great extent determines the entry of the chemical in the atmosphere, caution must be exercised in interpreting the data. The vapor pressure of a chemical can give a good estimate of volatility as long as the chemical is in free state or is deposited on an inert surface. However, when the chemical is bound to soil, the vapor pressure cannot be used as a measure of volatility. Factors affecting the vaporization rate from soils include temperature, moisture, and pH.

[*See also* Chapter XVIII, Some Criteria for the Classification of Atmospheric Pollutants.]

Behavior in the Aquatic Environment

The major factors contributing to the partitioning of a chemical into the aquatic environment are its water solubility and the latent heat of solution. Many organic compounds are hydrophobic, having water solubilities in the parts per million (ppm) or even parts per billion (ppb) range. Consequently, an exact determination of their solubility is quite difficult. Reported values of DDT solubility (Bowman *et al.*, 1960) range from 1 to 1000 ppb, depending on the worker and the technique, with the lower values (1.2 ppb at 25°C) being presently accepted. Many of these compounds have a tendency to accumulate at the air–water interface and to form clusters of varying particle size (Bowman *et al.*, 1959; Biggar *et al.*, 1967).

The pH of a solution may influence the stability and solubility of a chemical. Thus, the solubility of triazine molecules usually increases with lowering pH and is attributed to protonation of nitrogen with the formation of cationic species (Ward and Weber, 1968). The presence of salts in an aqueous solution of pesticide may cause ion-complex formation, as has been reported for the quaternary pyridinium cation type pesticides diquat and paraquat (Haque *et al.*, 1969).

Changes in temperature significantly influence the behavior of chemicals in aqueous solution. Solubility usually increases with temperature. The latent heat of solution, which may be obtained by substituting the solubility of a compound at two different temperatures into the van't Hoff equation, may be used as an approximate index of the tendency of a chemical to dissolve.

Interaction with the Soil Surface

The two major processes controlling the behavior of chemicals in soils are adsorption and leaching-diffusion, both of which are affected by temperature and the moisture content of the soil–chemical system.

In general, the mot convenient way of representing the adsorption data for a soil–chemical system is with the Freundlich isotherm,

$$\frac{x}{m} = KC^n;$$

where x/m is the amount of chemical sorbed per weight of the adsorbent, C the equilibrium concentration of the chemical, and K and n are constants. The constant n throws much light on the nature of the adsorption, whereas K represents the extent of adsorption and is related to the free energy changes in the adsorption. A direct relationship between K and the parachor of pesticides has been reported by Lambert (1967). The constant K is also highly dependent on the nature of the soil–surface (Haque and Sexton, 1968). For a sandy soil, K is very small, while a soil rich in organic matter gives a high value (Sherburne and Freed, 1954; Haque and Sexton, 1968).

Usually, inorganic salts or organic cations adsorb on the clay portion of the soil through an exchange reaction (Weber *et al.*, 1965), whereas the adsorption of neutral organic molecules from aqueous solution is a

physical process. As a result, solubility of the adsorbate is often an indication of the extent of binding. With the neutral organic molecules, the
amount of chemical sorbed is inversely proportional to the solubility
(Leopold *et al.*, 1960).

Adsorption of pesticides from aqueous solution is, in most instances,
an exothermic process. Usually, a decrease in temperature means an increase in adsorption. However, the temperature effects are more complex and results have been reported where the amount of adsorption
appears to be independent of temperature. The heat of adsorption can
give some indication about the nature of adsorption.

Adsorption processes usually require only a few hours to attain 70–80
percent of the equilibrium distributions of a substance between liquid
and solid phase; however, it may take several days to attain the final
equilibrium. Simple first-order kinetics are usually not applicable. Several
models have been proposed to explain the kinetics of adsorption (Weber
and Gould, 1966; Lindstrom *et al.*, 1970).

Spectroscopic techniques can provide insight to the structure of the
adsorbed species and, thus, often indicate the type of interaction between adsorbate and adsorbant. Infrared spectroscopy has been widely
used in the study of adsorbed pesticides (Mortland *et al.*, 1963; Farmer
and Mortland, 1966; Mortland, 1966, 1968; Mortland and Meggitt,
1968; Russell *et al.*, 1968a, b; Haque *et al.*, 1970; Haque and Lilley,
1972).

Another important process that controls the transport of a chemical
in soil is its movement with water. Although downward movement is
most common, lateral and even upward movement are sometimes significant. The upward movement, which is a result of evaporation from the
surface, is effective in removing chemicals from the root zone.

Where water percolation is rapid, the downward movement of the
chemical in the direction of the water flow predominates, but as percolation becomes slower and slower, diffusion into the pores of soil particles
becomes important in determining the distribution of the chemical. As a
chemical is carried through the soil by water movement, a localized
equilibrium exists between the dissolved phase and the adsorbed phase.
As a consequence, a chemical that is tightly adsorbed will be leached
slowly.

Leaching may be considered analogous to chromatography. Consequently, we should expect a maximum at some point in the concentration profile of the chemical in the soil following the release of a pulse
or slug of contaminants. The theoretical treatment of leaching has led to
development of several models (Gardner and Brooks, 1957; Nielson and
Biggar, 1961, 1962a, b, 1963a, b; Lindstrom *et al.*, 1967).

The intensity and frequency of rainfall will markedly influence the distribution of a chemical. Since the adsorption process depends on the nature of the soil, the type of the soil will also affect the rate of leaching.

Biological Interaction and Mobility

The binding of small organic compounds—such as drugs, dyes, detergents, and steroids—with proteins and related compounds has been studied extensively. A quantitative approach to the structure of organic compounds with respect to their biological activity has been treated by Hansch (1969) with a semi-empirical equation. Since chemicals contact organisms, knowledge of the partition coefficient in various biological systems is needed. Many examples of the effect of pesticides on natural enzymatic process have been reported. The binding of pesticides with proteins and phospholipids has also been reported (Brian and Rideal, 1952; Aldrich and McLane, 1957; Freed et al., 1961; Tinsley et al., 1971; Haque et al., 1973).

ENVIRONMENTAL ALTERATION OF CHEMICALS

Toxic substances in the environment can be divided into two groups: naturally occurring elements and compounds and wholly synthetic compounds that are not found in nature.

The danger associated with naturally occurring toxic materials arises largely from man's alteration of their distribution. For example, a substantial fraction of the mercury produced by man is lost to the environment. However, by a natural biological process, some of the mercury that enters aqueous systems is converted to methylmercury, which can accumulate in fish and other food organisms, posing a threat to public health. Man's discharge of mercury in locations where it can more readily undergo natural metabolic processes is the essence of this environmental problem.

The evolution of metabolic pathways to cope with the naturally occuring toxic compounds, both for their synthesis and degradation, provides a balance for the natural level of such compounds. Therefore, it is necessary to maintain an awareness of the circumstances which lead to an increase in the rate of synthesis or release of toxic compounds compared to the rate of their degradation or removal. The natural poisons are undoubtedly the most difficult to study because background levels are always present in the environment. Also, small changes in an ecosystem can bring about a natural increase in the rate of synthesis of these compounds.

The behavior in the environment of totally synthetic toxic compounds is often less difficult to predict than that of natural compounds. In many cases, biological systems have not developed the genetic capacity to degrade them. Because mutation frequency is much higher under controlled laboratory conditions than under natural conditions, the transformation in the environment may be anticipated by *in vitro* studies.

Microbial Interconversions of Toxic Chemicals

Microorganisms are exceedingly versatile in the metabolism of natural products. When confronted with a toxic substance the microorganisms attempt to detoxify their environment; however, the product of this detoxification may be more toxic to higher organisms than the original chemical.

A consideration of the heavy metals indicates the complexity of biological interconversions possible. As expected, aerobes and anaerobes have developed enzymes that can both reduce and oxidize inorganic compounds to give equilibrium mixtures of the different valence states of the metal. An important corollary is that when a metal is introduced into a microbial system, all its valence states often become available for chemical or biochemical reactions.

For example, with mercury, there is the following disproportionation:

$$Hg_2{}^{2+} \rightleftharpoons Hg^{2+} + Hg^0$$

Vaporization of mercury metal (Hg^0) shifts the equilibrium to the right, but return of Hg^0 from the atmosphere to the earth's crust shifts the equilibrium to the left. Some bacteria detoxify their environment of Hg^{2+} by converting it to methylmercury and dimethylmercury. Other bacteria detoxify their environment of methylmercury by reducing it to Hg^0 and methane. Dimethylmercury is volatile, but in the atmosphere photolysis yields Hg^0, methane, and formaldehyde. These interconversions in the mercury cycle lead to steady state concentrations of methylmercury in sediments. These steady state concentrations need not reflect the rate of synthesis of methylmercury.

Since the mechanisms for the synthesis of methylmercury are well understood, it can be predicted that tin, platinum, gold, and thallium will be methylated in the environment, but that lead, cadmium, or zinc will not be methylated because mechanistically the methyl group cannot be transferred to these metals in biological systems. These predictions have been found to be correct.

Current knowledge of the properties of toxic elements permits the prediction of their behavior in the environment. For example, one can predict that a natural cycle exists for arsenic just as with mercury. Arsenic compounds are reduced and methylated to form dimethylarsine by many species of anaerobic bacteria. Dimethylarsine is volatile, and escapes to the atmosphere where it is oxidized to cacodylic acid. Cacodylic acid returning to anaerobic environments is reduced once again to give dimethylarsine. On the basis of our understanding of arsenic chemistry, similar metabolic reactions are expected for selenium, tellurium, and sulfur.

These natural biosynthetic processes are influenced by a variety of parameters. For example, the rate of synthesis of methylmercury and dimethylarsine depends on the microbial population, the pH, temperature, redox potential, availability of the inorganic species, and synergistic or antagonistic effects of other metabolic or chemical processes. Biological methylation of metals and metalloids is inhibited by some low-molecular-weight chlorinated hydrocarbons.

Alkyl lead and alkyl silicon compounds can change the equilibrium in the mercury cycle by a mechanism involving the chemical transfer of alkyl groups to Hg^{2+} and their subsequent biological conversion to methyl groups, thus increasing the concentration of methylmercury. The methylmercury which is manufactured as a fungicide, or lost in the effluent of a vinyl chloride plant, will also disturb the natural cycle. Similarly, the commercial use of cacodylic acid disturbs the arsenic cycle.

Decomposition of Chemicals

Chemicals degrade in the environment through chemical, photochemical, and microbial processes. Examples of chemical degradation include air oxidation, neutralization, and hydrolysis. Many organic compounds decompose in the presence of sunlight (Smith and Grove, 1969; Archer and Crosby, 1969).

Microorganisms are known to metabolize a wide variety of chemicals. Microbial activity is extremely important in soils (Kearney and Kaufman, 1969). Although some industrial chemicals are not rapidly degraded by microorganisms, sufficient information is generally available to predict, on the basis of chemical structure, which compounds are likely to be biodegradable.

The substitution of biodegradable compounds for persistent ones may affect microbial activity in localized areas. Increased activity could either enhance detoxification or aggravate problems akin to methylmercury formation.

On the basis of existing knowledge, it is generally possible for microbiologists, biochemists, and chemists working together to determine metabolic sequences for both natural and totally synthetic compounds and to identify those that might pose environmental problems.

BIOACCUMULATION

In this section we present a description of bioaccumulation purely with the view of the model-builder in mind. No attempt is made to present a comprehensive review of the problems associated with factors such as degradation, excretion, and food-chain magnification. Rather, emphasis has been placed on the descriptions of predictive techniques, which may give values for the accumulation of synthetic compounds useful for the preliminary evaluation of environmental impacts of new chemicals. Biological accumulation of chemical compounds occurs in four main categories of processes:

1. direct, active ("intended") transport;
2. active transport, where the compound is mistaken for one with similar properties;
3. passive complex formation, with ligands in the organism; and
4. solubility equilibrium between fat (in the organism) and water.

Natural Compounds

The direct, intended uptake and active transport of a particular compound is essentially impossible to predict. Nonetheless, a substantial body of knowledge on the identity of the substances involved and on the biochemical processes responsible for their accumulation has been compiled.

Active accumulation of a substance that resembles another chemical is frequently predictable from the properties and structures of both. A classic example is the accumulation of arsenic in marine organisms through the same process that accumulates phosphate.

Passive accumulation through complex formation with ligands in the organisms is predictable from the chemical properties of the compound and knowledge of the strength of complexes formed with ligands common to biological systems.

Biological accumulation dependent on solubility equilibria between lipids and water requires high lipid·solubility versus water solubility, high persistence in the biological system, and a low tendency for complex formation with organic ligands. It is unusual for organisms to produce and release natural products with these properties. Therefore, there are few natural compounds for which this process of bioaccumulation is expected to be of significant importance.

Totally Synthetic Compounds

Intended active transport is regarded not to occur but may develop through evolution.

Active transport "by mistake" may occur if the compound resembles a natural one that is actively accumulated. Here, predictions from this resemblance are possible.

The synthetic compounds that are most likely to accumulate through complex formation with organic ligands are the organometallic ones. This accumulation can be predicted from their tendency for complex formation with natural bases.

Accumulation in organisms dependent on equilibrium between fat and water solubility is common among persistent hydrocarbons. It can be predicted from the relation between fat and water solubility.

It is evident that it is easier to predict bioaccumulation for totally synthetic compounds than for naturally occurring ones; however, the extent of our existing knowledge on the active transport of natural compounds makes predictions less necessary here.

In most cases, knowledge of the structure of a compound, resemblance to actively accumulated compounds, tendency for complex formation with organic ligands containing sulfhydryl and amine groups, and the relation between fat and water solubility will allow us to make a reasonable prediction of the *potential* accumulation. This theoretical or equilibrium level will not usually be reached, however, because of the low concentrations of these chemicals normally encountered in the environment, and because of the continual replacement of tissues in which accumulation occurs. This replacement would lead to the excretion or metabolism of the stored compound.

PRELIMINARY ESTIMATES OF EXPOSURE LEVELS

The development of the kinds of information described above constitutes an important first step in the prediction of the possible hazard associated with the introduction of a chemical substance to the environment. From such data, it will be possible to make preliminary estimates of the level of exposure which would identify the most probable routes through the environment and give some idea of the rates of degradation or transport from source to sink. Knowing the probable routes and sinks, it is possible to identify those species or physical structures that would be exposed and that should be considered in an evaluation of possible effects. If more refined estimates of exposure are needed, there are several approaches that might be taken in selecting or developing models to provide these estimates.

The first consists of a materials balance in which all major discharges are followed through the environment. This approach is most helpful in determining the ultimate fate of a chemical in the environment.

The critical pathways approach is based on the belief that the number of routes by which a hazardous substance could ultimately result in exposure to man or some other sensitive component of the environment can be reduced to one or two that are more important than the others. These are termed the *critical pathways* (Preston and Wood, 1971). The identification of these critical pathways would not only limit the scope and the complexity of models needed for refined estimates of exposure, but also form the basis of a monitoring program.

It is expected that with our present imprecise knowledge of the transport and transformation of chemicals a few potentially hazardous substances will always escape detection. The methodologies developing for predicting the impact of chemicals are usually based on the tracing of chemicals from the source to receptor. An alternative intuitive approach that may detect a few problems undistinguished by more conventional techniques is the construction of *scenarios*. This technique (Friedlander *et al.*, 1970) would involve a few imaginative individuals charged with constructing scenarios portraying the possible effects of discharges which might be considered unusual or unconventional. For example, a scenario might be constructed to show the possible effects of releases of plutonium resulting from the cremation of individuals fitted with pacemakers containing this element. The minute quantities involved, which would not be detected in a materials balance for plutonium, could conceivably present a hazard to a few individuals.

The discussions of chemodynamics, biotransformation, and bioaccumulation have been concerned primarily with the modeling of molecular, highly localized, processes. In order to complete the evaluation of exposure levels it is also necessary to consider the convective and diffusive processes that transport chemicals. A review of our ability to simulate these processes is described in the following section.

EXAMPLES OF TRANSPORT MODELS

All mathematical transport models are simplified descriptions of natural systems, often with predictive capacity. In addition to the simplifications built into a model, the other simplifications and approximations usually necessary in using a model place restrictions on the resolution of temporal and geographical scales for the interpretation of results. There exists a fundamental trade-off between the degree of resolution and the costs of model development and simulation.

The efficient and effective use of models in predicting the flow of chemicals through the environment demands that the degree of resolution obtainable from a model be consistent with the purpose for which the model is employed. This principle seems self-evident, but it is often disregarded. The user of a particular modeling technique is not always aware of the entire set of simplifications and assumptions involved and therefore of the constraints on the degrees of resolution. In the following discussion of models, this principle should be borne in mind.

A useful classification on the basis of scale, illustrated in Figure 1, is based upon a liberal interpretation and extension of the meteorological classification proposed by Monin (1972). It will be used where appropriate, but primarily with respect to atmospheric transport.

Such a classification will be valuable, first, in an initial categorization of a substance based upon its persistence and volatility, and, second, in the selection of transport models for estimating exposure levels.

For example, a potentially toxic substance that is only moderately volatile and highly reactive might fall within the micro- or mesoscale class. On the other hand, a mildly toxic substance, which is highly persistent and volatile, should be associated with one of the global classifications. Its long-term persistence would determine the specific global class applicable.

Global Classes

The global dispersion of materials introduced from the continents to the atmosphere or to the oceans (usually via rivers or estuaries) may be described or predicted by models, usually involving a limited number of reservoirs, with the transfers of materials among them governed by first-order rate constants. The use of such models makes global distribution problems tractable. Although the state of the model-making art is primitive, these models have described in consistent, although often approximate, ways the global distribution of elements in the major sedimentary cycle (Garrels and Mackenzie, 1971), of DDT (Woodwell *et al.*, 1971), of CO_2 (Machta, 1971) and of radioactive nuclides (National Research Council, Committee on Oceanography, 1971). Global models usually include some of the reservoirs and transport paths shown in Figure 2.

The residence times within the atmosphere are of the order of weeks

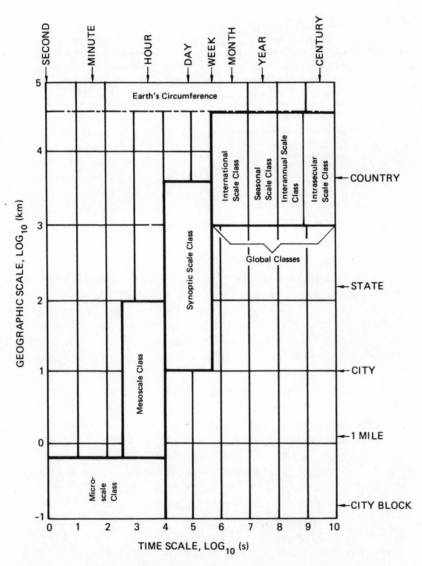

FIGURE 1   A proposed nomenclature for protocol scale classes for atmospheric transport models, based upon authors' interpretation of meteorological terminology.

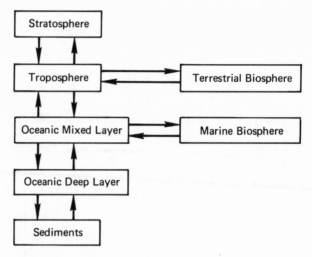

FIGURE 2   Diagram of reservoirs and pathways of chemicals in the environment.

for liquids or solid particles small enough (usually under 10 μm in diameter) for transcontinental or transoceanic movements. Gases can remain in the atmosphere for periods of years, the times being governed by their water solubility and their interactions with the biosphere. Transport in the troposphere usually takes place latitudinally. It takes 2–4 weeks for particles to circumnavigate the earth in midlatitudes, 3–6 weeks in the equatorial regions.

In the oceans, residence times vary from a century (iron, aluminum, or titanium particles) to hundreds of millions of years (sodium). The times are determined by the chemical nature of the substance. Refractory organic materials appear to have oceanic half-lives of the order of thousands of years. Oceanic mixing times range between several hundred years in the Atlantic to a thousand years in the Pacific for materials introduced into the deep layers. Passage through the mixed layer usually takes from several years to a decade for most dissolved substances.

The terms *equilibrium, kinetic, steady state,* and *time dependent* (transient state) have been used to describe global models. Equilibrium models have been applied in particular to the distribution of ionic, molecular, and gaseous species within single large global reservoirs. Sillen (1961), for example, proposed a multiphase equilibrium model for the ocean in which the composition of seawater was determined by choice of temperature, chlorinity, and seven solid phases that are found in marine sediments. Equilibrium models are used principally for describing an idealized state of a system. Their strength lies in their use to evaluate quantitatively departures from equilibrium. Computational methods are now available for calculation of equilibrium distributions in multicomponent homogeneous and heterogeneous systems. Mass transfer involved as a system tends toward equilibrium.

Steady-state models assume that the flux of a particular constituent into a reservoir is equal to the flux out of the reservoir. For multireservoir systems in which each reservoir is in steady state, the system as a whole is in steady state. Examples of these models include that proposed by Garrels and Mackenzie (1973), and that proposed by Kellogg *et al.* (1972) for the global distribution of natural and pollutant sulfur compounds. Steady-state models are limited by the fact that they cannot be used for time-dependent phenomena; however, when rate constants are not known, they can provide a baseline against which departures can be evaluated. For example, knowledge of the prehistoric steady-state chemical cycle of CO_2 can be used to assess the impact of CO_2 derived from the burning of fossil fuels.

Kinetic models consider the distribution of a particular substance within a reservoir as being controlled by rate factors. These models may either be steady state or time dependent. Kinetic models have been used by Broecker (1971) to evaluate factors controlling nutrient distributions in seawater, and by Berner (in press) to determine the distribution of dissolved carbon, nitrogen, sulfur, and silicon species in interstitial waters of marine sediments. This latter model has direct application to pollution problems involving the bacterial degradation of sewage discharged into an aqueous environment and to the remobilization of heavy metals in sediment pore waters.

Time-dependent models have the greatest potential for predicting the consequences of pollutant injection into the global environment. It is true, however, that these models have been little used to date, although the mathematics of time-dependent systems and computational techniques for solving the array of equations are available for multireservoir, cyclic systems. Transient state models have been used by Lerman (1971, 1972) and Lerman and Childs (1973) to describe transport of conservative chemical species in two- and three-layer lakes, transport through a chain of lakes, transport of oxygen and radium-226 in the oceanic water column, and transport and concentration of ^{90}Sr in the Great Lakes. Time-dependent models should have general application to prediction of the rates of transport and concentrations in sinks for a pollutant injected into the global environment. The one limitation at present is that linear rate constants are used in the flux equations.

Keeling and Bolin (1967) demonstrate the theoretical link of global models to the continuity equation. They are concerned with ocean models, but their conclusions can be extrapolated to atmospheric models. Multibox models have the advantage that boxes representing other abiotic and biotic reservoirs can be added easily. This aspect has already been exploited by many authors (Eriksson and Welander, 1956; Young et al., 1971; and Crews, 1973).

Other, potentially more accurate methods are at a more speculative stage. Dwyer and Petersen (1973) have studied control volume procedures. Bolin and Keeling (1963) have made the first contribution to the study of the global continuity equation by eigenfunction expansion.

Models of transport at the air–sea interface are rudimentary due in large measure to ignorance of the processes operating. For example, there is little information available on the chemistry of the sea surface microlayer and on the influence of surface slicks on particle and gaseous exchange.

Models have been developed for the effect of bursting bubbles on the transport of sea salt particles into the atmosphere and for gas exchange across the air–sea interface. Gases may be transferred from the atmosphere to the sea by diffusion or by bubble formation caused by breaking waves; however, the relative importance of these mechanisms is unknown.

[See also Appendix F, Sources and Dispersal of Atmospheric Pollution.]

Hydrologic Transport Models

In this section, models of the hydrologic transport of materials are discussed, starting with the raindrop and proceeding downstream as far as the mouth of the estuary. Included are stream basin models, reservoir models, lake models, and estuary models. These models are relatively specific, and purport to compute quantitative concentration distributions in a given system. Most of the models presently in use have been developed over approximately the past 5 years. Broadly speaking, the purpose of all these models is to trace the progress of a chemical constituent through the hydrologic system. Thus, as sketched in Figure 3, a tracer particle entering the catchment basin at its uppermost end can be followed downstream by a series of connected models describing transport in the free-running stream, through any lakes or reservoirs, and finally through the estuary into the coastal zone.

The basin hydrology and the contribution of materials that are washed from the land surface by rainfall and overland flow must be considered in modeling a river basin. A series of models is available to consider such

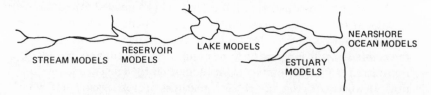

FIGURE 3 Connected hydrologic transport models.

factors as the distribution of rainfall in the basin, infiltration, soil moisture, and the velocity and duration of overland flow. These models,
when properly calibrated for an individual basin, are capable of giving a
reasonably accurate estimate of the quantities of water and dissolved
material entering a stream.

Many of the earlier models of stream, reservoirs, and estuaries use a
"box" concept. A stream, for instance, may be considered as a series of
reaches represented by boxes, in each of which equations are written to
express the conservation of water flux and of dissolved mass flux. In a
similar box division for deep reservoirs (Figure 4), the reservoir is divided
into a series of layers, and also possibly into segments along the reservoir
axis. The conservation equations are written for each layer and each segment. Vertical mixing and meteorological inputs are included. The
scheme can be used to predict such variables as the vertical distribution
of temperature and dissolved oxygen. Box models of this sort are currently in use for the prediction of outflow temperatures from a number
of existing reservoirs.

In estuaries, flow conditions are much more complex than in rivers or
reservoirs, but box models are also widely used. The *dynamic estuary
model*, which is presently being applied to a number of estuaries through-

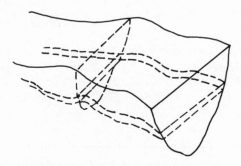

FIGURE 4 Box model of a deep reservoir.

out the country, assumes that the estuary can be divided into a number of compartments. Flow between the compartments is computed by the usual hydraulic equations for unsteady flow in open channels. Each of the compartments is assumed to be completely mixed, and material is transferred from one compartment to another by being carried with the flow. In operation, the model has sometimes proven unsatisfactory because the assumption of complete mixing in the compartments sometimes yields an unacceptable degree of numerical overmixing.

Finally, recently developed models have tried to incorporate a more exact description of fluid mechanics. These models take several forms. In deep reservoirs, attempts have been made to model the effects of stratified flow, including the mechanics of selective inflow and withdrawal (Water Resources Engineers, 1969). Significant recent progress has been made in computing circulation in lakes. Figure 5 shows the distribution of current velocities computed in Lake Erie by Gedney and Lick (1971). Incorporation of the effects of computed current distributions of this sort would seem to be the next logical step in the development of constituent models for lakes. Similarly, estuary models are be-

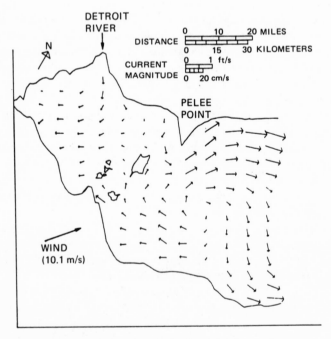

FIGURE 5   Computed horizontal velocities, 4.5 m from surface, west end of Lake Erie (Gedney and Lick, 1971).

ing developed to compute the detailed distribution of the tidal currents, and to incorporate these details into a finite difference model of constituent transport (Leendertse, 1970; Fischer, 1970).

At the outset, the scope of hydrologic transport models was limited to landward of the mouth of the estuary. There is substantial interest in coastal processes, but these are much more difficult to model because of the complexity of the current structure. Models can be used for specific applications, such as the siting of ocean diffusers for sewage (Fischer and Brooks, 1970), and deposition of sludge particles on the ocean floor (Koh, 1971; Chen and Orlob, 1972). The dilution in the initial plume can be computed with reasonable accuracy as a result of a substantial body of empirical data. Field studies at the site can estimate travel times from the outfall to the coast, and bacterial die-off rates can be estimated. Hence, for a specific site, concentrations of coliform bacteria at the shore can be estimated with reasonable accuracy. However, a complete numerical simulation of coastal diffusion processes is not yet within the state of the art; indeed, observations of diffusion rates near the coast have often led to conflicting results. At the present time, models for diffusion in open seas cannot be said to have been accurately validated for predicting local diffusion patterns near the coast.

An alternate for estuary diffusion studies is the use of physical hydraulic models, which exist for many of the world's estuaries. These models, however, are distorted in scale, and hence local diffusion processes are distorted (Crickmore, 1972). Nevertheless, the models do, when correctly adjusted, reproduce the large-scale circulation. In some applications, hydraulic models may be the most accurate tools for predicting constituent transports. Figure 6 shows the correspondence between a model and a prototype test of dispersion of a slug of dye injected into South San Francisco Bay. As can be seen, after five tidal cycles the distributions of a dye in the model and the prototype were not greatly different. Hydraulic models appear to give accurate results in those cases where the primary transport of constituents is by the bulk motion of the water and where turbulent diffusion is not important.

Less satisfactory models are available for single particle reactions in flowing systems, for example, suspended sediment transport and reaction in rivers. Lerman and Lal (in press), however, have modeled transport and reaction of single particles in the ocean.

One major limitation of existing current models is the degree to which the flow is properly represented and understood. Virtually all models include some sort of "ignorance coefficient," i.e., one or more coefficients which represent the effects of mechanisms which are not themselves well understood. For instance, we do not really understand what causes ver-

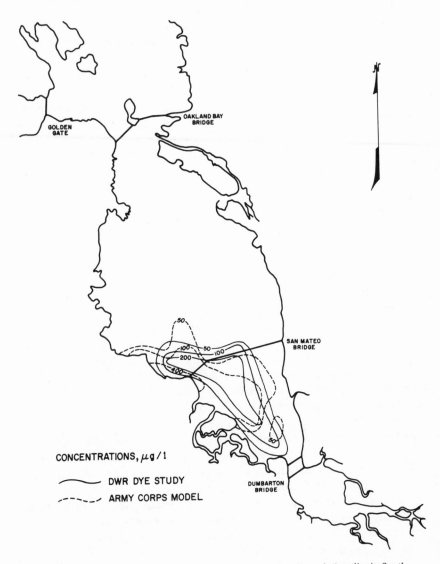

FIGURE 6 Comparison of results of model and prototype dye dispersion studies in South San Francisco Bay, 5 tidal cycles after dye injection. Replotted from results given by Nelson and Lerseth (1972).

tical mixing in stratified reservoirs, so our models include a coefficient of vertical eddy diffusivity whose magnitude can, at best, be measured *in situ*. Similarly, in estuaries, few firm data exist on the rate of transverse turbulent mixing. We do not understand the details of circulations induced by density gradients. In fact, no present model can adequately describe in three dimensions the distribution of material in a partially stratified estuary.

Another major limitation is that present transport models can express only in a relatively rudimentary way the chemical and biological reactions that occur in streams, and the effects of water–sediment interactions.

Mesoscale: Atmospheric Modeling for Urban Basins

Urban and industrial basins represent hot spots of pollution production and, as a result, community exposure to pollutants. Thus, it is especially important to be able to estimate exposure of humans and ecosystems over the ranges of time and space corresponding to such basins. Four classes of air pollutants can be considered:

1. inert (non-reactive) gases;
2. reactive gases;
3. interacting aerosol–gas systems; and
4. inert aerosols.

The simplest case to handle in urban basin modeling is the inert gas. The problem is then one of turbulent diffusion in the atmosphere and an extensive literature exists (Pasquill, 1961a, b). The usual example is CO, which, for its passage time through an urban basin, is believed to undergo little chemical change. The principal urban source of CO is the automobile. Hence, CO measurements or theoretical models for CO diffusion (Lamb and Neilburger, 1971) can be used to scale the concentrations of all conservative gaseous species emitted from the tail pipe of the automobile in a given region if the ratio to CO in the tail pipe exhaust is known. Industrial sources of inert gases have also received much attention, and approximate estimates of exposure levels downwind from these sources can be made, based on a variety of plume dispersion models. The problem of short time exposures to high levels of pollutants is difficult to handle.

When mixtures of reactive gases are considered, the problem becomes much more difficult. The most thoroughly treated reactive gas problem is that of photochemical smog in Los Angeles (Leighton, 1961; Hecht and Seinfeld, 1972). The gases involved are primarily nitrogen oxides and hydrocarbons which react in the atmosphere to form ozone and many new organic species. The reaction products include eye irritants and phytotoxicants. Estimating exposures to the products of such reactions requires detailed information on chemical kinetics as well as on the aerodynamics of the basin; however, even in the case of Los Angeles smog, the identity of some of the noxious products of the atmospheric reactions remains unknown. Attempts to model the behavior of previously unstudied reactive gaseous pollutants face great difficulty because of the complexity of atmospheric chemical reactions. [See Appendix F, Photochemical Reactions in the Atmosphere.]

Interacting aerosol–gas systems are among the most complex and important in air pollution. Perhaps the best known example is the atmospheric conversion of SO_2 to sulfate and sulfuric acid. This problem has been with us much longer than photochemical smog, but it is still not well enough understood to permit reliable estimates of concentrations of products downwind from a source. A model for the conversion process in cloud drops has been proposed by Scott and Hobbs (1967) and measurements in plumes have been made by Weber (1970) and others. The formation of particulate sulfate has important public health implications, as shown in recent epidemiological studies reported by Shy and Finklea (1973). Other chemical species involved in the aerosol–gas interactions are NO_2, NH_3, and a variety of hydrocarbons (Junge, 1963). Although the extent to which airborne metallic species participate in atmospheric reactions is not known, experiments with guinea pigs indicate that metallic sulfate salts have a significant effect on pulmonary resistance (Lewis et al., 1972).

For a nonreactive component of the aerosol or a conserved chemical element such as a metallic species, it is possible to estimate atmospheric fallout and the fraction of particulates which remain airborne, provided the size distribution of the particulates at the source is known. Such calculations, based in part on new measurements, have been carried out for particulate lead emitted by the automobile. Huntzicker and Friedlander (1973) used two different approaches. The first was made by comparing measured size spectra for tail pipe emissions with atmospheric aerosol spectra for the lead portion of the particulates. For all ambient distributions, the greater than 9 μm fraction is less than 1 percent. Since such particles settle out quite rapidly, particles with equivalent diameters greater than 9 μm were assumed to fall out in the vicinity of the roadway. This fraction was designated "near fallout." Values for far fallout (distant from the source) were obtained by assuming that the emitted lead in the smaller than 0.3 μm range remains permanently airborne. The exhaust spectrum (with the greater than 9 μm fraction removed) was normalized to the ambient spectrum by allowing particles in the 0.3–9 μm range of the exhaust spectrum to fall out until the less than 0.3 μm fractions were equal for both spectra.

An independent set of calculations was made, based on the lead content of atmospheric fallout measured at several sites in the Los Angeles basin. The amount of lead that remains airborne was estimated from the measured relationship between lead and carbon monoxide concentrations in the atmosphere and estimated values of CO emissions. Figure 7 is a summary diagram showing the flow of automotive lead through the Los Angeles basin. The numbers in the brackets refer to average values calculated from the site distribution data, and the numbers in parentheses are based on field data. About 20 percent of the lead in gasoline remains in the lubricating oil and the engine and exhaust system. The 80 percent exhausted to the atmosphere is made up of the following components: 43 percent fallout in the vicinity of the roadway and 16 percent fallout over the land and coastal waters. The remainder, about 13 percent of the total, remains airborne and is transported out of the basin by the wind. The primary sink for lead is fallout on the land. If the lead content of gasoline is reduced to zero, the air will be rapidly

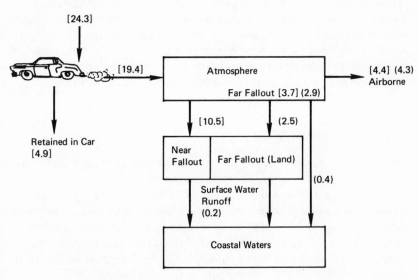

[ ] Size Distribution Data, tons/d
( ) Field Data, tons/d

FIGURE 7 Flow diagram of automotive lead in the Los Angeles basin.

cleansed of lead and lead fallout reduced to a small value. Because of the immobility of the lead on the land, soil concentrations of lead will remain elevated for some time until mobilized by winds and by human activity. The lead concentration of surface water runoff will probably taper off slowly.

The approaches adopted in this analysis are sufficiently general to apply to other particulate atmospheric pollutants. Although the lead problem is traceable because of the large volume of available data, size distributions for other pollutant sources are only now becoming available, and in general, the data for other trace metals are more scarce.

Crews and Truffer (1973) are investigating the combined use of a box model with an aggregated reservoir of human physiology to develop estimates of the public health hazard from lead in the atmosphere. Early results are encouraging.

To sum up, urban basin modeling, and the estimation of community exposure to pollutants that do not react in the atmosphere, are often difficult but feasible. Corresponding calculations from first principles for the products of chemical reactions in the atmosphere are at present beyond our capability for gases and particulates, except for some aspects of photochemical smog. Unfortunately, it is the secondary conversion products that are usually most troublesome. Needed are studies of the chemical and physicochemical changes which gaseous and metallic species undergo in polluted atmospheres. Such studies should be carried out both in the field and laboratory. Since pollutants emitted to the urban atmosphere are eventually transported to both the soil and water, it is necessary to consider the entire urban environment in dealing with non- or slowly degradable species such as metals and insecticides.

[*See also* Chapter XVIII, Atmospheric Processes.]

Microscale: Sediment–Water System

Pollutants are often found associated with particulate matter suspended in rivers, lakes, and oceans. Heavy metal ions, for example, are sorbed to suspended organic particulates or bound to inorganic matter owing to solubility and ion-exchange equilibria. Exchange of pollutants between solid phases and water will depend on such factors as the oxygen content, ionic strength, and composition of the water. Much of this suspended material, along with attached pollutants, will be deposited in lacustrine and marine sediments or ephemerally in river sediments.

Reactions occurring in these deposits may recycle pollutants back into the water body. Bacterial degradation of organic matter in anaerobic sediments, for example, may result in the release of heavy metals to interstitial water and their subsequent diffusion into the overlying water mass. Also, certain of these metals may redistribute themselves in anoxic sediments from the organic to the sulfide phase. Metal oxides precipitated from oxygenated environments may be reduced in anoxic sediments and release soluble metal compounds to interstitial waters. These, along with dissolved carbon, nitrogen, and phosphorus compounds formed by bacterial degradation of sedimentary organic matter, may diffuse or advect into overlying water. Thus, sediments are both a source and a sink, although not necessarily the ultimate sink, for ionic and molecular species.

Steady-state and time-dependent (transient state) models are available for sediment–water interactions and flux calculations. In general, because vertical concentration gradients are much greater than lateral gradients in pore waters, one-dimensional depth models (Berner, in press) are sufficient to describe and predict the distribution and flow of dissolved constituents in the sediment–water system. These models can account for the processes of advection, sediment deposition, diffusion, adsorption ion exchange, radioactive decay, decomposition of organic matter, and precipitation or dissolution of minerals. Steady-state mathematical solutions are simpler, and therefore have been used more frequently, than time-dependent ones.

Depending on the knowledge about the kinetic mechanisms involved, first or higher order kinetic functions can be used to describe the formation and decomposition or dissolution of a solid phase in the pore water–sediment system. First order kinetics have been used to describe the decomposition of organic matter and the concomitant reduction of sulfate and release of nitrogen and phosphorus compounds in anaerobic sediments (Berner, in press). Both surface-controlled and diffusion-controlled reactions for mineral precipitation and dissolution can be handled in the models. Also, provision can be made for incongruent reactions in which an original mineral reacts to form a new mineral plus dissolved species.

In the pore water–sediment system, transient-state or steady-state models have been used to describe

1. the distribution and flux of nitrogen, sulfur, phosphorus, and silicon in anoxic marine sediments (Berner, in press); this model has particular application to modeling of remobilization of organic compounds and heavy metals in sediments;
2. diffusional transport of ^{90}Sr into sediments of the Great Lakes (Lerman, 1972);
3. the distribution of ^{226}Ra in sediments (Lerman, 1971);
4. the distribution of dissolved carbon, nitrogen, and phosphorus

compounds in sediments, with a consideration of advection due to bio-
turbation (Thorstenson and Mackenzie, 1973);

5. diffusion of radioisotopes in interstitial waters (Duursma, 1966);
and

6. distribution of trace heavy metals in estuarine sediments (Wollast,
unpublished).

Equilibrium modeling can be used to determine partial or complete
equilibrium states of a system and to assess mass transfers where solids
and aqueous solutions interact. The principle limitation of these models
is that kinetic factors have not been integrated into the general mathematical model or computational procedures (Helgeson, 1968, 1969;
Helgeson et al., 1969; Thorstenson, 1971); however, it is true that, where
rate constants are unknown and cannot be estimated, this type of modeling can provide necessary baseline information to evaluate equilibrium
states and deviations from them. Equilibrium modeling has been employed in estimating the degree of approach to equilibrium (Helgeson
et al., 1969; Helgeson and Mackenzie, 1970) and in predicting the equilibrium distribution of small organic molecules in interstitial waters
(Thorstenson, 1971).

Major limitations in the modeling of sediment–water systems result
from insufficient knowledge of rate constants, inadequate terms in the
generalized equation for such processes as organic degradation and
mineral precipitation and dissolution, and lack of knowledge of chemical and biochemical conversion steps. A positive feature of these models
is that they are capable of providing at least order-of-magnitude estimates for fluxes of pollutants into and out of sediments.

Microscale Atmospheric Models

Turner (1969) compiled a very useful workbook which illustrates the use
of plume models. A complete derivation of these models is given by
Haltiner and Martin (1957). The required information is stability class
and wind speed. Pasquill (1961a, b) discusses more accurate models that
require wind fluctuation measurements; sampling times of about 10
minutes are appropriate for this use of these models and would provide
adequate resolution for microclass protocols. It would appear that typical, or perhaps "worst case," meteorological conditions must be hypothe-
sized to provide the most useful estimate of exposure levels. Ide (1971)
discusses the relationship between sampling time and scale resolution.
[See Appendix F, Sources and Dispersal of Atmospheric Pollutants.]

SUMMARY AND CONCLUSIONS

Data on production, use, and disposal are essential in determining the quantities and sources of a chemical released to the environment. The behavior of a chemical in the environment is influenced by its physical and chemical properties and its susceptibility to transformation and accumulation by living organisms. Models of various kinds are becoming valuable tools for study of the movement of substances through the environment and for identifying points of exposure where tests for effects and monitoring are indicated.

Existing models of transport in the water and the air were reviewed, both on a global and a local basis and across interfaces, along with models of biotransformation and bioaccumulation. The panel concluded that current understanding of the flows and transformations of chemicals in the environment is primitive. Major uncertainties arise in identifying points in the environment at which leakage may occur, predicting chemical and biochemical transformations in the environment from first principles, and predicting nonlinear interactions involving multiple causative agents. Nevertheless, models may be used to predict to a fair approximation the flow and ambient concentrations of compounds that do not undergo chemical change during transport.

The information needed for the development of detailed models of transport includes production and use patterns, emission rates, methods of disposal, the behavior in the environment as determined by physical and chemical characteristics, chemodynamics, biotransformation and bioaccumulation, and the identity of decomposition products.

Three guidelines should be followed in obtaining this information:

1. Where similarities to existing compounds can be established, maximum use should be made of the available information on these compounds.
2. Maximum use should be made of capability to derive information from existing data as an alternative to actual measurement.
3. Wherever possible, substitutions should be made using data parallel to those which are desirable but are yet to be measured: For example, Tariff Commission data might be substituted for finer geographical patterns of use when appropriate.

The panel recommends that the estimate of exposure level be developed in two stages. The first stage, a preliminary estimation of the level of exposure, would consist of an identification of the probable routes through and reservoirs in the environment, and a rough estimate of the rates of transport and degradation. From such information it would be possible to determine which organisms and inanimate objects should be considered in tests for effects. Both the preliminary estimate of exposure level and preliminary data on effects would determine the need for additional effects data and for more refined estimates of exposure.

The second stage, that of developing these more refined estimates, would logically involve mathematical transport models; however, the judicious use of models demands that we not lose sight of the simplifications and assumptions built into them. Estimation of exposure levels is not a substitute for monitoring. Modeling and monitoring are, in fact, complementary. Models must be verified by monitoring, while models can be valuable in identifying critical pathways that could serve as a basis for monitoring strategy. [*See* Chapter XX, Analysis and Monitoring.]

There is urgent need for research supported by EPA on the origin and fate of potentially toxic chemical agents emitted to the environment as a result of man's activities. Such studies should be carried out at EPA, university, and other research laboratories and should be related to technological forecasts of the production of new agents.

Such studies are essential to the development of a reliable technique, not yet available, for the assessment of hazards associated with the production of new chemicals. In the absence of such research, there is a danger that *ad hoc* assessment procedures will eventually be discredited.

REFERENCES

Acree, F., Jr., M. Beroza, and M. Bowman. 1963. Codistillation of DDT with water. *J. Agric. Food Chem.* 11:278–280.

Aldrich, F.D., and S.R. Mclane, Jr. 1957. A paper chromatographic method for the detection of 3-amino-1,2,4-triazole in plant tissues. *Plant Physiol.* 32:153.

Archer, T.E., and D.G. Crosby. 1969. The decontamination of animal feeds. *Residue Rev.* 29:13–37.

Berner, R.A. (In press.) Kinetic models for the early diagnosis of nitrogen, sulfur, phosphorus, and silicon in anoxic sediments.

Biggar, J.W., G.R. Dutt, and R.L. Riggs. 1967. Predicting and measuring the solubility of p,p'-DDT in water. *Bull. Environ. Contam. Toxicol.* 2:90–100.

Bolin, B., and C.D. Keeling. 1963. Large-scale atmospheric mixing as deduced from the seasonal and meridional variations of carbon dioxide. *J. Geophys. Res.* 68:3899–3920.

Bowman, M.C., F. Acree, Jr., and M.K. Corbett. 1960. Solubility of DDT-C^{14} in water. *J. Agric. Food Chem.* 8:406–408.

Bowman, M.C., F. Acree, Jr., C.H. Schmidt, and M. Beroza. 1959. Fate of DDT in larvicide suspensions. *J. Econ. Entomol.* 52:1038–1042.

Brian, R.C., and E.K. Rideal. 1952. Plant growth regulators. *Biochim. Biophys. Acta* 9:1–18.

Broecker, W.S. 1971. A kinetic model for the chemical composition of sea water. *Quat. Res.* 1:188–207.

Chen, C.W., and G.T. Orlob. 1972. The accumulation and significance of sludge near San Diego outfall. *J. Water Pollut. Control Fed.* 44:1362–1371.

Crews, W.B. 1973. Preliminary static and dynamic models for the global transport of lead and DDT. Master of Science thesis, Department of Mechanical Engineering, University of California, Davis.

Crews, W.B., and M.F. Truffer. 1973. Example of the transport of a toxic substance from fossil fuel use through the environment. Appendix D. In *Second Annual Report of the Interdisciplinary Systems Group. Vol. 4: Models of Global Pollution by Energy Systems.* Department of Mechanical Engineering, University of California, Davis.

Crickmore, M.J. 1972. Tracer tests of eddy diffusion in field and model. *ASCE J. Hydraul. Div.* 98:1737–1752.

Duursma, E.K. 1966. Molecular diffusion of radioisotopes in interstitial water of sediments. In *Proceedings of the Symposium on Disposal of Radioactive Wastes into Seas, Oceans, and Surface Waters.* International Atomic Energy Agency, Vienna. pp. 355–371.

Dwyer, H.A., and T. Petersen. 1973. Time-dependent global energy modeling. *J. Appl. Meteorol.* 12:36–42.

Eriksson, E., and P. Welander. 1956. On a mathematical model of the carbon cycle in nature. *Tellus* 8:155–175.

Farmer, V.C., and M.M. Mortland. 1966. An infrared study of the coordination of pyridine and water to exchangeable cations in montmorillonite and saponite. *J. Chem. Soc.* Ser. A:344–351.

Fischer, H.B. 1970. *A Method for Predicting Pollutant Transport in Tidal Waters.* Contribution 132. Water Resources Center, University of California, Los Angeles. 143 p.

Fischer, H.B., and N.H. Brooks. 1970. Technical aspects of waste disposal in the sea through submarine outlets. In *Marine Pollution and Sea Life.* Proceedings of the FAO Technical Conference on Marine Pollution and Its Effects on Living Resources and Fishing, Rome, 1970. pp. 464–471.

Freed, V.H., J.B. Vernetti, and M. Montgomery. 1962. The soil behavior of herbicides as influenced by their physical properties. In *Proceedings of the Nineteenth Western Weed Control Conference.* Iowa State University Press, Ames. pp. 21–36.

Freed, V.H., and J.M. Witt. 1969. Physiochemical principles in formulating pesticides relating to biological activities. *Adv. Chem. Ser.* 86:70–80.

Freed, V.H., F.J. Reithel, and L.F. Remmert. 1961. Some physical and chemical aspects of synthetic toxins with respect to their mode of action in plant growth regulators. In *Proceedings of the International Conference Plant Growth Regulators.* Vol. 4. Iowa State University Press, Ames. pp. 289–306.

Friedlander, S.K., H. Brown, G. Bugliarello, L.B. Dworsky, J.J. Harrington, T. Hatch, and J. Wei. 1970. Technological trends. Chap. 10. In *Man's Health and the Environment—Some Research Needs.* Report of the Task Force on Research Planning in Environmental Health Sciences, National Institute of Environmental Health Sciences. U.S. Government Printing Office, Washington, D.C.

Frost, J. 1969. Earth, air, water. *Environment.* 11:15–29, 31–33.

Gardner, W.R., and R.H. Brooks. 1957. A descriptive theory of leaching. *Soil Sci.* 83:295–304.

Garrells, R.M., and F.T. Mackenzie. 1971. *Evolution of Sedimentary Rocks.* W.W. Norton and Co., New York. 397 pp.

Garrels, R.M., and F.T. Mackenzie. 1973. A quantitative model for the sedimentary rock cycle. *Mar. Chem.* 1:27–40.

Gedney, R.T., and W. Lick. 1971. *Numerical Analysis of Steady-State, Wind-Driven Currents in Lake Erie Using Shallow Lake Model.* NASA TMX-67804. National Technical Information Service, Springfield, Va.

Haltiner, G.J., and F.L. Martin. 1957. *Dynamical and Physical Meteorology.* McGraw-Hill Book Co., New York. 470 p.

Hamaker, J.W., and H.O. Kerlinger. 1969. Vapor pressure of pesticides. *Adv. Chem. Ser.* 86:39–54.

Hansch, C. 1969. A quantitative approach to biochemical structure–activity relationships. *Acc. Chem. Res.* 2:232–239.

Haque, R., W.R. Coshow, and L.F. Johnson. 1969. Nuclear magnetic resonance studies of diquat, paraquat, and their charge-transfer complexes. *J. Am. Chem. Soc.* 91:3822–3827.

Haque, R., I.J. Tinsley, and D. Schmedding. 1973. Lipid binding and mode of action of dichlorodiphenyltrichloroethane type compounds. Proton magnetic resonance study. *Mol. Pharmacol.* 9:17–22.

Haque, R., and S. Lilley. 1972. Infrared spectroscopic studies of charge transfer complexes of diquat and paraquat. *J. Agric. Food Chem.* 20:57–58.

Haque, R., S. Lilley, and W.R. Coshow. 1970. Mechanisms of adsorption of diquat and paraquat on montmorillonite surface. *J. Colloid Interface Sci.* 33:185–188.

Haque, R., and R. Sexton. 1968. Kinetic and equilibrium study of the adsorption of (2,4-dichlorophenoxy) acetic acid on some surfaces. *J. Colloid Interface Sci.* 27:818–827.

Hartley, G.S. 1969. Evaporation of pesticides. *Adv. Chem. Ser.* 86:115–134.

Hecht, T.A., and J.H. Seinfeld. 1972. Development and validation of a generalized mechanism for photochemical smog. *Environ. Sci. Technol.* 6:47–57.

Helgeson, H.C. 1968. Evaluation of irreversible reactions in geochemical processes involving minerals and aqueous solutions: I. Thermodynamic relations. *Geochim. Cosmochim. Acta* 32:853–877.

Helgeson, H.C. 1969. Thermodynamics of hydro-thermal systems at elevated temperatures and pressures. *Am. J. Sci.* 267:729–804.

Helgeson, H.C., R.M. Garrels, and F.T. Mackenzie. 1969. Evaluation of irreversible reactions in geochemical processes involving minerals and aqueous solutions: II. Applications. *Geochim. Cosmochim. Acta* 33:455–481.

Helgeson, H.C., and F.T. Mackenzie. 1970. Silicate–sea water equilibria in the ocean system. *Deep-Sea Res.* 17:877–892.

Huntzicker, J.J., and S.K. Friedlander. 1973. A preliminary report on the flow of automobile emitted lead through the Los Angeles basin. Background report prepared for the NAS Conference on Toxic Substances. Paper presented at the American Chemical Society meeting, Chicago, August, 1973.

Ide, Y. 1971. The effect of observation time on turbulent diffusion in the atmosphere. *Water, Air, and Soil Pollut.* 1:32–41.

Junge, C.E. 1963. *Air Chemistry and Radioactivity.* Academic Press, New York. 382 pp.

Kearney, P.C., and D.D. Kaufman. 1969. *Degradation of Herbicides.* M. Dekker Press, New York. 394 pp.

Keeling, C.D., and B. Bolin. 1967. The simultaneous use of chemical tracers in oceanic studies: I. General theory of reservoir models. *Tellus* 19:566–581.

Kellogg, W.W., R.D. Cadle, E.R. Allen, A.L. Lazrus, and E.A. Martell. 1972. The sulfur cycle. *Science* 175:587–596.

Koh, R.C.Y. 1971. Ocean sludge disposal by barges. *Water Resour. Res.* 7:1647–1651.

Lamb, R.G., and M. Neilburger. 1971. An interim version of a generalized urban pollution model. *Atoms. Environ.* 5:239–264.

Lambert, S. 1967. Functional relationship between sorption in soil and chemical structure. *J. Agric. Food Chem.* 15:572–576.

Leenderste, J.J. 1970. *A Water-Quality Simulation Model for Well-Mixed Estuaries and Coastal Seas. Vol. I: Principles of Computation.* Rep. RM-6230-RC. The Rand Corp., Santa Monica. 76 pp.

Leighton, P.A. 1961. *Photochemistry of Air Pollution.* Academic Press, New York. 300 pp.

Leopold, A.C., P. Van Schaik, and M. Neal. 1960. Molecular structure and herbicide absorption. *Weeds* 8:48–54.

Lerman, A. 1971. Time to chemical steady-states in lakes and ocean. *Adv. Chem. Ser.* 106:30–76.

Lerman, A. 1972. Strontium-90 in the Great Lakes: Concentration-time model. *J. Geophys. Res.* 77:3256–3264.

Lerman, A., and C. W. Childs. 1973. Metal-organic complexes in natural waters: Control of distribution by thermodynamic, kinetic and physical factors. In P.C. Singer, ed., *Trace Metals and Metal-Organic Interactions in Natural Waters.* Proc. ACS Symp. Ann Arbor Science Publ., Ann Arbor.

Lerman, A., and D. Lal. (In press.) Dissolution and behavior of particulate biogenic matter in the ocean: Some theoretical considerations. *J. Geophys. Res.*

Lerman, A., and H. Taniguchi. 1972. Strontium-90–diffusional transport in sediments of the Great Lakes. *J. Geophys. Res.* 77:474–481.

Lewis, T.R., M.O. Amdur, M.D. Fritzhand, and K.I. Campbell. 1972. *Toxicology of Atmospheric Sulfur Dioxide Decay Products.* Rep. AP-111. U.S. Environmental Protection Agency, Washington, D.C. 47 p.

Lindstrom, F.T., R. Haque, and W.R. Coshow. 1970. Adsorption from solution. III. New model for the kinetics of adsorption–desorption processes. *J. Phys. Chem.* 74:495–502.

Lindstrom, F.T., R. Haque, V.H. Freed, and L. Boersma. 1967. Theory on the movement of some herbicides in soils. Linear diffusion and convection of chemicals in soils. *Environ. Sci. Technol.* 1:561–565.

Machta, L. 1971. The role of the oceans and biosphere in the carbon dioxide cycle. In D. Dryssen and D. Jagner, eds., *Nobel Symposium 20: The Changing Chemistry of the Oceans.* John Wiley and Sons, Inc., New York. pp. 121–145.

Monin, A.S. 1972. Chap. 1. In *Weather Forecasting as a Problem in Physics;* trans. by Paul Superak. M.I.T. Press, Cambridge.

Mortland, M.M. 1966. Urea complexes with montmorillonite: An infrared adsorption study. *Clay Miner. Bull.* 6:143–156.

Mortland, M.M. 1968. Pyridinium montmorillonite complexes with ethyl N, N-dipropylthiolcarbamate (EPTC). *J. Agric. Food Chem.* 16:708–709.

Mortland, M.M., J.J. Fripiat, J. Chaussidon, and J. Uytterhoeven. 1963. Interaction between ammonia and the expanding lattices of montmorillonite and vermiculite. *J. Phys. Chem.* 67:248–258.

Mortland, M.M., and W.F. Meggitt. 1966. Interaction of ethyl N, N-di-propylthiolcarbamate (EPTC) with montmorillonite. *J. Agric. Food Chem.* 14:126–129.

National Research Council. Committee on Oceanography. 1971. *Radioactivity in the Marine Environment.* National Academy of Sciences, Washington, D.C. 272 pp.

Nelson, A.W., and R.J. Lerseth. 1972. *Dispersion Capability of San Francisco Bay*

Delta Waters—Final Report. Publ. 45. State Water Resources Control Board, Sacramento, Calif. 89 p.

Nielsen, D.R., and J.W. Biggar. 1961. Miscible displacement in soils. *Soil Sci. Am. Proc.* 25:1–25.

Nielsen, D.R., and J.W. Biggar. 1962a. Miscible displacement: II. Behavior of tracers. *Soil Sci. Am. Proc.* 26:125–128.

Nielsen, D.R., and J.W. Biggar. 1962b. Miscible displacement: III. Theoretical considerations. *Soil Sci. Am. Proc.* 26:216–221.

Nielsen, D.R., and J.W. Biggar, 1963a. Miscible displacement: IV. Mixing in glass beads. *Soil Sci. Am. Proc.* 27:10–13.

Nielsen, D.R., and J.W. Biggar. 1963b. Miscible displacement: V. Exchange processes. *Soil Sci. Am. Proc.* 27:623–627.

Pasquill, F. 1961. The estimation of the dispersion of windborne material. *Meteorol. Mag.* 90:33–49.

Pasquill, F. 1961b. *Atmospheric Diffusion.* D. Van Nostrand Co., Ltd., New York. 297 pp.

Preston, A., and P.C. Wood. 1971. Monitoring the marine environment. *Proc. R. Soc. Lond.* 177B:451–462.

Russell, J.D., M. Cruz, and J.L. White. 1968a. The adsorption of 3-amino-triazole by montmorillonite. *J. Agric. Food Chem.* 16:21–24.

Russell, J.D., M. Cruz, J.L. White, G.W. Bailey, W.R. Payne, Jr., J.D. Pope, Jr., and J.I. Teasley. 1968b. Mode of chemical degradation of *s*-triazines by montmorillonite. *Science* 160:1340–1342.

Scott, W.D., and P.V. Hobbs. 1967. The formation of sulfate in water droplets. *J. Atmos. Sci.* 24:54–57.

Sherburne, H.R., and V.H. Freed. 1954. Adsorption of 3-(*p*-chlorophenyl)-1,1-dimethylurea as a function of soil constituents. *J. Agric. Food Chem.* 2:927–939.

Shy, C.M., and J.F. Finklea. 1973. Air pollution affects community health. *Environ. Sci. Technol.* 7:204–208.

Sillen, L.G. 1961. The physical chemistry of sea water. In M. Sears, ed., *Oceanography.* Publ. 67. American Association for the Advancement of Science, Washington, D.C. pp. 549–581.

Smith, A.E., and J. Grove. 1969. Photochemical degradation of diquat in dilute aqueous solution and on silica gel. *J. Agric. Food Chem.* 17:609–615.

Thorstenson, D.C. 1971. A chemical model for early diagenesis in Devil's Hole, Harrington Sound, Bermuda. In O.P. Bricker, ed., *Carbonate Cements.* Johns Hopkins University Study in Geology No. 19. Johns Hopkins University Press, Baltimore. pp. 285–291.

Thorstenson, D.C., and F.T. Mackenzie. 1973. Temporal variations of dissolved constituents in interstitial waters. *Geochim. Cosmochim. Acta,* in press.

Tinsley, I.J., R. Haque, and D. Schmedding. 1971. Binding of DDT to lecithin. *Science* 174:145–147.

Turner, D.B. 1969. *Workbook of Atmospheric Dispersion Estimates.* Publ. 999-AP-26. National Air Pollution Control Administration, Cincinnati, Ohio. 84 p.

Ward, T.M., and J.B. Weber. 1968. Aqueous solubility of alkylamino-*s*-triazines as a function of pH and molecular structure. *J. Agric. Food Chem.* 16:959–961.

Water Resources Engineers. 1969. *Mathematical Models for the Prediction of Thermal Energy Changes in Impoundments.* Environmental Protection Agency Rep. 16130EXT12/69. U.S. Government Printing Office, Washington, D.C. 182 pp.

Weber, E. 1970. Contribution to the residence time of sulfur dioxide in a polluted atmosphere. *J. Geophys. Res.* 75:2909–2914.

Weber, W.J., and J.P. Gould. 1966. Sorption of organic pesticides from aqueous solution. *Adv. Chem. Ser.* 60:280–304.

Weber, J.B., P.W. Perry, and P.R. Upchurch. 1965. The influence of temperature and time on the adsorption of paraquat, diquat, 2,4-D and prometone by clays, charcoal, and an anion-exchange resin. *Soil Sci. Soc. Am. Proc.* 29:678–688.

Wollast, R. (Unpublished.) Discharge of particulate pollutants in the North Sea by the Scheldt.

Woodwell, G.M., P.P. Craig, and H.A. Johnson. 1971. DDT in the biosphere: Where does it go? *Science* 174:1101–1107.

Young, J.W., J.W. Brewer, and M.M. Jameel. 1971. An engineering systems analysis of man's impact on the global carbon cycle. In *Systems and Simulation in the Service of Society*. Proc. Ser. Vol. 1, No. 2. Simulation Councils, Palo Alto, Calif. pp. 31–40.

V

Biological and Statistical Considerations in the Assessment of Risk

Applying the results of toxicological investigations conducted in the laboratory to the population of interest generally involves two kinds of extrapolations. The first, which is more difficult to deal with and more important with respect to human exposure, involves predicting the probable effects on one species from the results of experiments performed on another. The second kind of extrapolation is that of extending dose–response curves beyond the limited range of observation to determine the dose corresponding to an extremely low incidence of adverse effects on the organism tested.

ROLE OF THE TOXICOLOGIST IN THE ASSESSMENT OF RISK

This report concerns itself primarily with the task of developing objective technical information needed to make decisions on the course of action to be followed to ensure the safe use of chemicals. It does not, except for a general statement of principles, go into the sociopolitical aspects of decision-making.

Terms such as "toxicological insignificance," "safe," "zero tolerance," "no effect level," and "negligible risk" have been in rather common use. All of these contain in one way or another value judgments or technical

implications which have no place in an objective assessment of risk.
There is no substance which, under certain circumstances, could not be
dangerous and unsafe. There is no battery of tests, however elaborate,
which can prove beyond challenge the complete safety of a chemical.
For the toxicologist to apply the terms "toxicologically insignificant"
or "negligible risk" to a set of observations makes a premature judgment
in the wrong arena by the wrong person as to insignificance or acceptability. An attempt has been made to eliminate such terms from this report.

Another common term of wide usage is the "no-effect level." This is
statistically meaningless and therefore of limited value since it merely
means that no effect was observed in studies using a group of animals of
particular size. Such an observation is completely compatible with the
presence of an adverse effect, which in further studies with larger sample
sizes or with different types of observation might lead to a positive outcome. We prefer the usage of the term "no observed effect," which
should always carry with it a qualifying statement as to size of the group
in which no adverse effect was observed.

In most instances it will be imperative to develop a dose–response
relationship. Because many toxicological techniques are relatively insensitive, high doses (which produce high incidence of effects) are frequently
required. These can be and have been called "unrealistic" or "inappropriate." Such exposures may be well above, sometimes many orders of
magnitude above, likely levels of exposures to human or wildlife systems.
Nevertheless, they are often an essential part of practicable laboratory
studies which necessarily use limited numbers of animals. The underlying challenge to the toxicologist is to use these points on the dose–response curve as a means of quantifying responses, and to devise, with
suitable margins of safety, appropriate means for extrapolating to realistic, actual exposure conditions. The biological aspects of this extrapolation will be discussed first, and the statistical considerations will be
developed later.

BIOLOGICAL CONSIDERATIONS

For clarity, it will be assumed that we are concerned in the following
discussion with extrapolation from the laboratory situation to human
populations. Except in the case of lifesaving drugs, only very low risks
will normally be accepted in chemical usage. The acceptable risk will,
however, vary with the benefit anticipated. In the case of risk of death
from a chemical of trivial utility, the acceptable risk would be essentially
zero. Put in explicit terms, this might mean 1 death in 100 million persons. As noted in the section on statistics below, extrapolation to such

risk levels from experiments on small numbers of animals is extremely uncertain. Again, and as noted repeatedly in this report, the gravity of the effect is a major determinant in an overall assessment of risk. At one extreme lies a fatal outcome and, at the other, a temporary functional alteration producing no disability or discomfort and lying fully within the range of physiological compensation. The susceptibility of human populations varies widely since genetic background, age, prior or co-existent disease are all important determinants. Part of the toxicologist's task is to identify susceptible groups in the population as the basis for establishing limits of exposure.

Another and vital factor constantly facing the toxicologist is the often striking biological differences between the effects of chemicals on laboratory species and on man. It has been repeatedly shown that no one species (including nonhuman primates) has responses parallel to the human over a wide range of the effects of chemicals. The choice of species must then be based on a determination of the biological similarity in the responses to the chemical under study.

In extrapolating from animals to man, the transfer is often made on a dose per unit weight (milligram per kilogram) basis. This practice over-looks the well-demonstrated (Freireich et al., 1966) observation that dose per unit surface area (milligram per square meter) is generally a better transfer parameter.

There has been much loose talk about thresholds. The term *threshold* means "the entrance or beginning point of something." This implies (and is normally so used) a discontinuity in the slope of the dose–response curve. True discontinuities in biological phenomena are rare. However, they do occur. One example is the threshold for glucose excretion by the kidney. Most biological dose–response relationships appear to be smooth functions and, in absence of concrete evidence dose–response curves, should probably be assumed to be smooth. Many dose–response curves have an "S" shape, with a much lower slope at the low end of the curve than in the mid-range. This could be regarded as a quasi-threshold. The steepness of the dose–response curve is an important consideration for predictive purposes. A steep dose–response curve implies a sharp cut-off (again, a quasi-threshold) with decreasing dosage.

Some dose–response curves appear to be linear, especially when attention is limited to relatively low incidence rates. One example of this is cigarette smoking and lung cancer (Doll, 1967); there are many experimental situations where this appears to be the case.

Despite the above comments, there are some biological reasons for anticipating that, with some chemical agents, there may be something approximating a true threshold. The biological basis for this is twofold:

(1) the possibility of a relatively greater effectiveness of repair mechanisms at low dose levels; and (2) the possible presence of competing biochemical processes which could convert the chemical to harmless products at low dose levels. It is difficult to generalize about these mechanisms since they can be expected to depend on the chemical and the species. Unfortunately, investigation of these questions has rarely been undertaken. In the past, these complex considerations have been dealt with pragmatically by the use of arbitrary "safety factors."

STATISTICAL CONSIDERATIONS

The need for a proper consideration of statistics in the design of toxicological experiments and in the interpretation of the results cannot be overemphasized. First, before meaningful results can be obtained, attention must be given to identifying and reckoning with possible sources of error. Second, statistical techniques are available that can give meaningful estimates of the level of exposure to chemicals corresponding to the level of risk which the decision-maker considers acceptable.

Experimental Error and Sampling Error

The outcome of an experiment is normally dependent upon innumerable factors, only some of which are known and even fewer of which are controllable. In dose–response experiments with animals, for example, some identifiable factors influencing the outcome include (1) the composition of the particular batch of test preparation, which typically represents a significant source of variation in independent repetitions of the experiment; (2) animal variability; (3) technician reliability; and (4) the precision of laboratory techniques, such as dilution techniques or dose preparation. Since such factors influence the dose–response relationship, they represent sources of experimental error and, hence, independent replications that randomly sample the levels of these factors are necessary in order to estimate their contributions in the measure of experimental error. If major sources of variations are not considered in such replication, then statistical precision as reflected in the width of confidence intervals, for example, may be grossly misleading.

When several major sources of experimental error can be identified, a conceptually simple experimental design would consist of independent replicates at each target dose level randomly sampled with respect to all sources of variation. If batches from the chemical manufacturer represent a source of variation, for example, then this design might assign each animal at each dose level to a different batch of chemicals from the manufacturer. If dilution errors are important, then dilutions to target dose should be independent—not only among dose levels but also among animals within dose levels. When several such sources of errors exist, this conceptually simple, completely randomized experimental design clearly becomes impracticable, and blocking becomes a more feasible means of conducting the experiment. Thus, each batch of the chemical from the manufacturer might be administered to a group of animals at every test dose to produce, in effect, a separate dose–response curve for each batch. For any one batch, the proportion of animals responding at a given test dose is subject to sampling error due to factors such as animal differences and possible errors in dilution, that would result in each animal receiving a slightly different test dose. At any given dose level, the proportion responding also varies among batches; thus, the average proportion responding at a dose level is subject to both sources of error—namely, the sampling error within batches and the variability among batches—which together comprise experimental error. A valid statistical analysis should utilize the appropriate experimental error and not merely its sampling error component. Since standard statistical methods of bioassay often are addressed only to the analysis of sampling error, there is need for caution in applying these methods.

Estimating Low Effect Levels

Estimation of low effect levels poses a difficult problem. Direct experimental estimation of the level affecting one percent of the population may require several hundred animals to obtain adequate statistical precision. For many reasons, particularly in human populations, much lower risks than one percent are desired. A true no-effect level cannot be observed experimentally. Any observed level has meaning only for a particular sample size.

The observation of "no effect" for a group of animals may occur for one of two reasons: (1) The dosage level may indeed by below the theoretical no-effect level; or (2) the number of animals tested may have been inadequate to give a significantly high probability of detecting a biologically important change. For example, a test on 20 animals may show no deleterious effect, but a test on 100 animals, tested under the same conditions, may show one or more animals exhibiting deleterious effects. Similarly, for a graded response, a small sample may fail to provide enough statistical precision to detect a change from baseline, whereas a larger sample may. Thus, an observed "no-effect level" has no absolute meaning since it depends on sample size and poorly estimates the theoretical no-effect level; a better term would be the "no observed effect level."

However, data from experiments in which no effects are observed are useful in placing limits on the probable incidence of effects. For example, if no animals out of 100 animals displayed a deleterious effect, it can be stated with 99 percent confidence that fewer than 4.5 percent of animals tested under these conditions would exhibit deleterious effects. If this level of risk were too high, more animals could be tested. For example, observance of zero animals affected out of 1000 tested results in an upper 99 percent confidence limit of only 0.46 percent. To reach an extremely low acceptable risk level in this manner generally requires a prohibitively large number of animals.

With past practice of selecting some arbitrary fraction of no-effect level as a limit for exposure no estimate of risk is obtained. However, a fairly conservative estimate of the risk can be made by employing the one-hit (one-particle) theory (Food and Drug Administration Advisory Committee on Protocols for Safety Evaluation, 1971). This theory states that for low dosages, if an experimental dosage is divided by a factor f, then its upper confidence level of the risk is also divided by the factor f. Such an approach will often result in near-zero dosages for extremely small acceptable risks. For example, if zero deleterious responses were observed in 450 animals at a dose d, it can be stated with 99 percent confidence that the true response rate is less than 1 percent (one out of 100). The predicted dose for risk of one out of 1,000,000 would then be $10^{-4} d$.

An alternate means of estimating low risk exposure levels involves extrapolation from parametric dose–response curves. Many different empirical mathematical models may be fitted to a set of experimental data (Finney, 1964). The probit and logistic curves have been commonly used in biology, for example, and both curves may fit equally well in the region of experimental observations (2–98 percent response range) but give widely different estimates for extrapolated responses. For example, the probit curve will predict a dosage level approximately 140-times higher than the logistic curve for extrapolation to a dosage expected to elicit one response in 1,000,000 animals. In some instances (Doll, 1967) linear dose–response curves have been reported; often, however, these cover only a relatively limited response range.

There is no assurance that the dose–response curve observed in the experimental range of dosages will apply at extremely low response levels. Mantel and Bryan (1961) suggest the use of a presumably conservative slope of one probit for each factor of 10 in dosage level for extrapolating to low levels of carcinogenic risk.

A more recent approach to the extrapolation of laboratory findings to the establishment of standards or limits for human populations (Albert and Altshuler, 1973) has taken into account age at the time of the appearance of an adverse effect, as well as the frequency of its occurrence: For example, in the case of cancer from external sources, it has been shown, experimentally and in humans that, with lower doses, cancer appears later—that is, at increasing ages. Under this concept, and assuming the availability of reliable data, it should be possible to establish limits that would place the earliest occurrence of malignancy at an advanced age, or no more than 10 percent incremental likelihood of cancer at age 95.

SUMMARY

In the past, toxicologists have not only made the laboratory assessments of toxicity, but in many instances they have made the final judgment as to the social course to be taken on the basis of a particular set of findings. Instead, the technical experts should be charged with securing an objective independent determination of the extent, nature, and frequency of adverse effects. They should be asked to explain the relative gravity of these effects for the target system, be it humans or wildlife. Similarly, other qualified technical experts should be requested to make an objective assessment of the benefits of use and of alternative materials or processes. However, the final judgment as to a trade-off between an adverse health effect and a desired benefit is a social decision and should be made with the participation of those who are affected. This is not to say that technical experts using their technical expertise will not participate, but it does state that they should not be the sole judges of determining the balance between the benefit and the risk.

The dose–response curve is a valuable tool for assessing the safety of a chemical compound. Estimates of low effect levels are part of the information leading to the ultimate designation of safe and acceptable levels. The statistical problems of extrapolation from experimental dose levels to very low levels and the estimation of appropriate errors are particularly troublesome but can be handled if care is taken in the design and analysis of the experiments and the interpretation of results.

Without supporting experimental evidence, however, statistical analysis will never be capable of making the critical extrapolation from laboratory animals to man.

REFERENCES

Albert, R.E., and B. Altshuler. 1973. Considerations relating to the formulation of limits for unavoidable population exposures to environmental carcinogens. In C.L. Sanders, R.H. Busch, J.E. Ballou, and D.D. Mahlum, eds., *Radionuclide Carcinogenesis.* Proceedings of the Twelfth Annual Hanford Biology Symposium.

AEC Symp. Ser. No. 29 CONF-720505. National Technical Information Service, Springfield, Va. pp. 233–253.

Doll, R. 1967. *Prevention of Cancer: Pointers from Epidemiology.* Nuffield Provincial Hospitals Trust, London. 144 pp.

Finney, D.J. 1964. *Statistical Method in Biological Assay*, 2nd ed. Hafner Publ. Co., New York. 668 pp.

Food and Drug Administration Advisory Committee on Protocols for Safety Evaluation. 1971. Panel on Carcinogenesis report on cancer testing in the safety evaluation of food additives and pesticides. *Toxicol. Appl. Pharmacol.* 20:419–438.

Freireich, E.J., E.A. Gehan, D.P. Rall, L.H. Schmidt, and H.E. Skipper. 1966. Quantitative comparison of toxicity of anticancer agents in mouse, rat, hamster, dog, monkey, and man. *Cancer Chemother. Rep.* 50:219–244.

Mantel, N., and W.R. Bryan. 1961. "Safety" testing of carcinogenic agents. *J. Natl. Cancer Inst.* 27:455–470.

Part Three

HUMAN
HEALTH
EFFECTS

VI

Introduction

The major determinants of the effects of chemicals upon the health and well-being of the individual and society are (1) the nature of the chemical *per se*, (2) the duration of time over which the chemical interacts with the individual, and (3) the quantity of the chemical present. Thus, if a relatively large amount of a chemical acts over a short period of time, the effects are expressed acutely, i.e., promptly, in a readily noticeable fashion, and frequently in a self-limiting manner. If, however, relatively smaller quantities of a chemical act over a protracted length of time, the expression of the interaction occurs over a longer period as a chronic effect and the relation between cause and effect is less apparent.

As science has expanded its understanding of the effects of chemicals on human health, certain specific health effects produced by chemicals, for example, acute and chronic intoxication, have become more clearly perceived. Yet other effects are only now becoming apparent; the subtlety of such phenomena as chemical induction of cancer, or modification of nervous behavior, has escaped delineation until only recently. Studies of the mechanism of transferring genetic information through generations of cells have also revealed that these vital processes might be altered by chemicals resulting in mutagenesis or teratogenesis.

Primary among these determinants of the action of chemicals upon biological systems is that of the *quantity* of the chemical which con-

93

fronts biological matter. *Thus, a chemical—any chemical—is a poison only as a consequence of the quantity with which the host must deal.* Conversely, the same chemical which produces ill effects when present in relatively large quantities would not necessarily be expected to produce any untoward effect in lesser amounts. In many instances such smaller quantities of these same chemicals are necessary to life itself as is found with some trace elements (for example, Fe, Cu, Mg) and vitamins A and E.

From this consideration of quantity is derived another important factor: the time span over which the quantity of a chemical is presented for handling by living tissues. Thus, a large quantity of a chemical can produce an ill effect if biological systems are confronted with this quantity in a single exposure. However, deleterious consequences may not occur if the same large quantity is encountered over a protracted time span. This stems from the fact that a multitude of finely tuned defense mechanisms are available to cope with limited quantities of many chemicals. This also reflects the evolutionary reality that, over time, biological systems have been continually confronted with exogenous chemicals and compensatory mechanisms have evolved to enable survival. This perspective presents an external world, characterized by change, which has demanded that all biological matter develop the ability to deal with change.

Seen from this view, it is apparent that biological systems are characterized by the ability to change in response to change. Since there are limits to the capacity of organisms to respond and change generally, it is only when such response capacity is exceeded that untoward consequences ensue. It should be noted that, with some chemicals, there may be an accumulation of the chemical or its effect to the point where the injury is detectable. For the toxicologist, the integration of quantity and the time over which a chemical acts is subsumed within the term *dose*.

Another consideration must be noted as regards the properties of those chemicals which may be encountered by man. It is insufficient to refer to a toxic material in terms of an indefinite characterization of its atomic components: thus, the toxic potentials of mercury compounds cannot necessarily be defined by merely referring to the element itself. It is necessary to know the valence state of the mercury within a compound, and the specific physical and chemical properties, as these have a major role in determining toxicity. For example, while mercurous oxide is poorly, if at all, absorbed following ingestion (and thus has limited toxic potential), mercuric oxide, which is more soluble, presents altogether different possibilities. By contrast, the combination of mercury with other combinations of elements, as in the case of methylmercury, raises its toxicity to another order of magnitude greater than the element itself. Moreover, within the organomercury compounds, toxicity varies; thus, the aliphatic mercurials are much more toxic than the aromatic mercurials. Accordingly, it must be kept clearly in mind that toxicity is a property of the *specific* compounds that may be encountered.

When a biological system encounters a sufficiently large dose of a compound, which exceeds its defensive capacity, the expression of such failure is usually a change in function and/or structure. The relevance of an observed functional change to deleterious consequences is not always immediately clear. While a functional change may be the expression of a successful compensation, such change may also be the first expression of a train of events ultimately terminating in an undesirable consequence. Since the resultant may be apparent only with the passage of time, there is a risk of missing an important late effect. These problems of assessing functional change and its implications are dealt with by subsequent discussions in this section.

Understanding is usually less equivocal as regards the significance of structural change. Although structural and functional changes are the ultimate expression of effects induced by chemicals in biological systems, such expression cannot be automatically assumed to occur to the same extent, if at all, in every individual so involved. While the predictability of response to a specific chemical agent is reasonably high in purebred animal models, it is not absolute. That is, even in such pure strains, there is some genetically determined degree of variability, which may moderate or aggravate the degree of the response. In addition, most experimental testing studies are performed on healthy animals while, in any human population, there are wide variations of age and health. Thus, there may be a certain part of the population that will manifest severe responses to chemical doses that would cause little perceptible change in the majority of persons.

The human environment clearly contains a multitude of chemicals in various forms. The possibility of such agents acting together to cause effects that may be additive, synergistic, antagonistic, or independent is always present. While there are limits to our ability to describe or understand such interactions, the relatively small quantities of chemicals encountered in the general environment lessens the dangers. A reservation must be noted, however—the current inability to perceive an ill effect is no guarantee that one or more are not actually occurring.

The subsequent discussions in this section indicate that there is no one approach to evaluation of toxicity. Given the multiplicity of the possible responses of biological systems, an all inclusive standardized testing scheme, which considers all possible reactions, would be wasteful of limited resources if not impossible and such activities if carried out would still not guarantee complete safety. The extent and nature of tests should reflect (1) the possible level of exposure to be expected with intended usages, (2) the possible consequence that can reasonably be expected, and (3) a margin of safety between expected environmental levels and the dose that produces some adverse effect.

An inflexibly prescribed schedule of tests will *not* take advantage of new advances in our capabilities. At the same time, a thoughtless addition of new procedures will be wasteful of time and resources if not actually deceptive. From these considerations it is apparent that mature professional judgment must guide the design, development, and modification of test protocols. The aim of any reasonable testing program should be the development of sufficient, but not excessive, information necessary to make a decision that provides an appropriate degree of safety.

Although the testing process is extensively dealt with in this section, the foregoing considerations should serve to indicate that pretesting provides no *absolute* answers. While testing *can* provide some assurance, more complete assurance requires that the pretesting process cannot be considered the end step in hazard prevention. Accordingly, epidemiologic studies are essential. Such studies, by indicating changes in health status of populations, serve as late warning indicators, signalling for a re-investigation of the results of previously executed test processes.

Finally, it should be recognized by those concerned with human health that sources of information exist that have often been ignored in the past. Scientists engaged in studies of nonhuman, ecologic systems at the laboratory bench and in the field have gathered information regarding biological systems that has pertinence to humans. Ultimately, it is a truism that biological systems from the bacterium to man, operate in similar modes throughout one spectrum of life. Conversely, the data developed from study of mammalian and other genera by the toxicologist can serve some of the information needs of ecologic toxicologists. The much needed interchange of knowledge between these two interested groups is only now beginning.

VII

Acute and Subchronic Toxicity

Toxicity is the capacity of a chemical to produce injury; safety is the practical certainty that injury will not result from a specific use of that chemical. Thus, any safety judgement must take into account both the kind and severity of the toxicity and the use or, more specifically, the level and route of human exposure.

A "toxic substance" may be defined as an agent which can produce adverse effects on a biological system. However, this is a simplistic definition since it can be applied to almost any common and, sometimes, essential chemical, such as water, oxygen, table salt, vitamins, alcohol, carbon dioxide, etc.—as well as to industrial chemicals, pesticides, fertilizers, household chemicals, etc.—when such chemicals are administered at high enough levels by the appropriate route of administration. No chemical is absolutely—only relatively—safe. It is, therefore, more appropriate to define *toxic substances* as agents which have a potential for producing adverse effects on living systems only as a result of exposure under conditions of normal use or predictable misuse.

Any chemical can be shown to produce adverse effects if sufficiently high doses are used. The investigations of "potential hazard" as applied to a chemical include a demonstration of the toxicological properties of

97

an agent by appropriate test procedures and a determination of an exposure level that does not produce detectable adverse effects by the same procedure. For man, the margin of safety of an agent is evaluated by relating to the predicted human exposure the maximum exposure level in experimental animals that produces no detected adverse effects. An agent with a small margin of safety has a high potential for producing adverse effects, and, conversely, an agent with a large margin of safety has a low potential for producing adverse effects. The margin of safety of an agent may vary under different conditions of exposure and therefore each chemical may have several margin-of-safety ratings, depending upon different uses.

The potential hazard of any chemical is directly related to the dose. Degree of exposure (dose) may

1. be sufficiently massive to be lethal;
2. produce permanent changes;
3. produce temporary changes that may be serious;
4. produce temporary changes that are not injurious, but which may be discomforting; or
5. not cause detected changes by present procedures.

Acute toxicity can be defined as exposure to a test agent for 24 hours or less. This definition will provide for the 24-hour exposure period often used in dermal procedures and the 1 to 8-hour periods often used in the inhalation procedures.

The term "acute toxicity" has often been used to define the immediate (usually 24 hours or less) effects of an agent on the animal; it is more appropriate to use longer periods of observation after the single exposure in order to detect any delayed effects arising over an extended period of time. The 24-hour period of observation may detect primarily pharmacodynamic activity, although other biological mechanisms might be so altered as to cause death or other effects within a longer period of observation. A prolonged observation period would also permit detection of effects that might be related to anatomical, biochemical, or hematological changes that would not cause immediate death.

Acute toxicity studies are needed in safety evaluation for two distinctly different reasons: One is as a screening procedure to aid in identifying compounds of such low toxicity that, when considered in relation to a proposed use of low exposure, extensive investigations to make a judgement of safety are not justified. The other is as a type of acute toxicity procedure designed to delineate the specific toxic effect, and mechanism thereof, which might be associated with a massive exposure or a normal use associated with a high level of exposure to a compound. This latter type of study is designed to assist in the development of an appropriate clinical management program for individuals involved in a misuse or accident and to assist in appraisal of the safety of a particular use involving significant human exposure, even though that exposure might be chronic in nature. Such studies can aid in identifying target organ effects which may be valuable in the proper design of chronic studies.

In the screening type of acute toxicity procedure, the amount of material to which an animal is exposed is so massive that it generally bears no practical relationship to the expected human exposure. It is reasonable to establish maximum exposure levels (e.g., 5000 mg/kg orally, 3000 mg/kg dermally, etc.) for each acute procedure, which can be used to predict that the agent is essentially acutely nontoxic if no adverse effects are detected.

A decision process based on both parameters of experimentally derived toxic effects and estimated exposure levels should be developed through subchronic studies in an effort to identify those compounds and uses which merit chronic studies. In other words, as the knowledge of exposure level changes and toxicity information becomes available, further testing may not only be desirable but necessary. However, that there may be circumstances other than those which warrant chronic studies is recognized. Structural characteristics may indicate the need of a carcinogenic bioassay. No short-term or subchronic tests are known that can give assurance of the presence of possible carcinogenic activity.

When a new chemical is presented for evaluation of toxicologic hazard, the chemical and physical characteristics of the material must be considered so that appropriate steps can be taken to assure adequate exposure of the animal to the chemical in the various procedures. The chemical stability of the agent, vapor pressure, solubility, particle size, etc., can be of importance.

Before any judgment regarding health hazard can be made, it is necessary to know the intended use and the anticipated route, frequency, and level of exposure to man. The type of exposure being considered is generally that likely to result from the normal usage of chemicals rather than from an abnormal situation such as would result from a spill.

The commercial product being studied should contain a typical level of impurities. If the impurities contribute significantly to the human health hazard this will be reflected in the toxicity of the commercial product. Whether the toxicity of a commercial product is due to the principal ingredient or an impurity is immaterial from the point of view of health protection, as long as its toxicity is detected. Recognition that the toxicity is due to an impurity can be helpful to the producer since removal of this impurity could reduce the toxicity of the commercial product sufficiently to permit its use.

At the time a new chemical is submitted for evaluation, experience in man may be available to a limited extent because of exposure during manufacturing procedures. Adverse effects obtained from this experience would provide information useful in the toxicologic evaluations and would take precedence over negative animal data. Many chemical industries evaluate the safety of chemicals in animals as a routine procedure for protection of personnel.

It is recognized that present federal and state laws require knowledge of acute toxicity data for many chemicals manufactured today. These laws, in general, are designed to provide those data necessary for proper labeling and for obtaining proper industrial working environments and safe handling of bulk chemicals during transportation. A toxic substances law would expand the responsibility of EPA to include those chemicals that get into our environment either as end products or as degradation products and present potential hazards from relatively low level exposures for long periods of time. Acute data do not provide information directly applicable to these problems. However, to the experienced observer, information gathered from these acute and subchronic studies help determine the design of future studies and is the base from which all toxicological studies start.

ACUTE TOXICITY STUDIES

Acute Oral Toxicity

Acute oral toxicity studies, commonly the first step in investigations of toxicity, are designed to elicit the qualitative and quantitative nature of the toxic effects from a one time oral exposure to a large dose of a chemical. The dosages are selected to provide data for estimating the lethal dose for 50 percent of a group of animals (LD_{50}) and the slope of the dosage–mortality curve. Accordingly, the number of animals per dosage should be sufficient for such statistical evaluation. The chemical should be administered as a liquid or in an appropriate carrier, which facilitates absorption. It is essential to note the type, time of onset, severity and duration of all toxic signs. Observations of the animal should continue until signs of toxicity are absent in survivors, at which time gross pathologic examination should be made. A flat dosage–mortality curve or a delay in onset of and recovery from toxic signs are suggestive of potential for cumulative toxicity and thus the need for longer term testing.

Acute Dermal Toxicity

The ability of some chemicals to penetrate intact and abraded skin and produce systemic toxicity is well known, and steps should therefore be taken to evaluate this possibility. Skin permeability has been measured *in vivo* (Bartek *et al.*, 1971) in rat, rabbit, pig, and man with the use of radioactive labeled compounds (^{14}C and ^{35}S). The results generally indicate that rat and rabbit skins appear to be several fold more permeable than the skin of pig or man. The subject was reviewed by Barr (1962).

The albino rabbit is the animal most frequently used in assessing dermal toxicity. However, mouse, rat, guinea pig, and dog have also been used. After an appropriate exposure period, excess material is removed, and the local changes and any gross signs of toxicity are noted. Animals should be observed for a proper period of time and postmortem studies performed. A LD_{50} value estimated on the basis of several properly spaced dosage levels is useful but may not be obtained because of poor dermal absorption or low toxicity.

Acute Inhalation Toxicity

Man's contact with environmental chemicals in the community, home, or industrial environment is likely to include inhalation. Exposure by inhalation is probably the most time consuming and expensive of all toxicological dosing procedures. In the interest of utilizing effectively the limited personnel and facilities available for conducting inhalation studies, it is recommended that considerable flexibility be incorporated in planning inhalation studies in order that the required studies be toxicologically relevant and technically feasible. (This recommendation is particularly applicable to aerosol exposures.) It is expected that protocols designed for individual materials or classes of materials will have to be developed and that considerable judgment will have to be exercised in deciding which procedures are appropriate.

Inherent toxicity is defined as the ability of the chemical to exert an adverse effect on a biological system if it reaches the vulnerable point(s) in the biological system. An inhaled material can either exert a systemic effect or it can produce an effect on the respiratory tract itself. Systemic effects can usually be determined much more easily with dosage by other routes than by inhalation, assuming the same systemic dose by the two routes. If the material produces a systemic effect by another route it is usually proper to assume that inhalation at similar dosage would produce at least as great an effect; therefore, it is good operating procedure to postpone the inhalation experiments or to perform them last, although inhalation might be the most likely route of exposure. It is quite possible to base a "no-go" decision for a material likely to be inhaled on results of exposure by routes other than inhalation.

The effects on the respiratory tract itself can be measured only by inhalation. These may be transient or may be irreversible effects, including death. The most common direct effect is acute chemical irritation, which might affect any part or parts of the conducting airways or the gas-exchange surfaces. The acute effects are usually reversible, unless so severe that they produce pulmonary edema or such severe inflammation that the lung is no longer functional. These effects can be readily detected in animals. To enhance the sensitivity of this classical approach, pathological bacteria may be introduced into the animal lung following exposure to common pollutants as an adjunctive study.

An example of the kind of sensitive technique required to identify biologic activity at levels of nitrogen dioxide common to the Los Angeles basin will illustrate this point. Endothelial cell damage and death of pulmonary macrophages have been observed at moderate levels of nitrogen dioxide by standard methods. The technique necessary to demonstrate abnormalities of pulmonary function at 1 ppm or less has involved tests of the capacity of the mouse lung to clear bacteria. Although this system may be regarded by some as a test of the mechanism of action of a toxic chemical, the fact remains that animals exposed to chemicals that are injurious to macrophages in the above system are consequently more susceptible to infection.

This example supports the recommendation encouraging the development of methods that can measure animal effects from environmental chemicals at levels of exposure which exist or are expected to be attained in the environment. Such methods may not be useful as a routine screening technique. However, when a prospective environmental chemical is shown to have some effect at concentrations above those expected for human exposure, two decisions can be made. The chemical may be limited to concentrations that are lower than the minimum effective concentration in test animals by a large safety factor, or permissible concentrations can be determined more realistically by the use of more sensitive assay methods.

Another effect occasionally seen in the respiratory tract is an asthmatic type sensitization, which would not be manifest for some time after the first or possibly multiple exposures. This is apparently a rare phenomenon, but the effect produced can be extremely serious. Animal models have been of limited utility for predicting this type of inhalation sensitivity, although it has been adequately demonstrated in man as a result of industrial exposure, for example, to toluene diisocyanate and to cotton dust. There is therefore great risk of missing this toxic manifestation in examining new materials in animals.

Objectionable odors cannot be detected by animal experiments, although they can present serious problems for humans in the use of materials.

The three types of materials to be considered are gases, volatile liquids, and aerosols. In all three there should be concern with probable concentrations. For gases, this will depend almost entirely on the rate of usage under a given set of operating conditions. Since the gas is completely diffusible in any enclosed space, the concentration can be estimated from the quantity of gas released; however, it should be analytically determined during the experiment. Exposure to a volatile liquid is limited by the liquid's ability to evaporate at a given temperature so that a saturated vapor exposure gives an upper limit in concentration. For both gases and liquids, the solubility of the agent in water has a dominant influence on the access of the agent to the various parts of the respiratory tract. Highly soluble irritant gases will attack the upper respiratory tract, while those having limited aqueous solubility will penetrate deeply into the lung. The ability of the material to produce inflammation or, if absorbed, to produce systemic effects, will determine its toxicity. In the case of volatile liquids, the contribution of a simultaneous skin exposure that might result in percutaneous absorption and an increase in systemic toxicity must also be taken into account.

The group of materials most difficult to characterize and to obtain inhalation exposure data for are the aerosols. These are airborne particulates, which may be solid or liquid and which may remain airborne sufficiently long to be inhaled. There are significant engineering difficulties in producing an experimental aerosol for animal exposures. The system must resemble actual human exposure conditions, especially as far as particle size is concerned. This is important since the site of attack and deposition within the pulmonary tree is governed almost entirely by the physics of its air currents. In general, the smaller the particle, the deeper its penetration and the more serious its effects become.

SUBCHRONIC TOXICITY STUDIES

Subchronic toxicity procedures are designed to determine the adverse effects that may occur during repeated exposure over a period of a few days to usually three months (90 days). The subchronic procedures usually include the routes of exposure expected for man. The exposure levels used in these procedures are lower than in the acute toxicity procedures and lethal effects are not necessarily an end point. Instead, by the use of many types of observations (behavior, body weight, hematology, biochemistry, function and extensive postmortem studies) more subtle types of adverse effects can be detected. A high exposure level that is judged to be sufficiently large to produce adverse effects and at least one lower exposure level that is not expected to produce adverse effects are used. Intermediate exposure levels may be introduced if considered necessary. The number of animals (mice, rats, or any other mammalian species) should be sufficient for statistical confidence. Observations should include signs of toxicity, food consumption, growth rate, hematology, urine analysis, appropriate clinical studies, gross pathologic examination, organ weights, and microscopic pathology. Recovery studies can be included if the changes observed indicate that this type of procedure is necessary. The subchronic procedures provide a better baseline than acute studies for the design of chronic studies.

Systemic effects due to cumulative exposure may also be investigated by subchronic oral toxicity methods. Appropriate mammalian species may be selected and dosage should continue for at least 21 days. The dosage range should include several levels—from no observed effect up to and including maximum tolerated levels. Gross observations for toxic signs should be made during the exposure period. Upon completion of the study all animals are sacrificed and organ weights determined and histopathology of body organs performed. (*See also* Appendix B.)

If the calculated acute dermal LD_{50} is at or below 3 g/kg and/or produces significant toxicological effects and exposure is likely to be long term or at high concentration, dermal studies of 21–30 days or 90 days duration are in order. Abraded and unabraded test sites on a significant number of animals of both sexes should be used (the abraded skin should be freshly scarified once a week).

ACUTE IRRITANCY AND SPECIFIC EFFECTS STUDIES

A variety of test methods for detection of irritancy has been developed and used to evaluate the hazardous properties of chemicals. The problems and pitfalls associated with such predictive methods are, for the most part, well known and, certainly, a full discussion is well beyond the scope of this paper. Adequate references are available for general procedures as well as for the utility and shortcomings of some of these methods.

Eye Irritation

One of the most crucial screening tests for new chemicals or reformulated products is the eye irritation test in which the animal of choice is usually the albino rabbit; however, dogs, cats, and primates have also been used.

The problem of correlating animal data with human experience is a serious factor in the decision process. There is, at this point in time, no definitive study indicating that any animal model system is ideally suited for reliably predicting eye irritancy in man. The general procedure, in most instances, is to place a measured amount of the material in the albino rabbit eye and observe the reactions over a period of time, for example, 1 h to 21 days. The areas of the test eye which are evaluated are the cornea, iris, and conjunctiva. A sufficient number of animals should be tested and the effects of washing should be compared with unwashed eyes. The data should reveal the nature and extent of injury as well as recovery. In addition to the immediate and delayed reactions, the effects of washing, pain, and anesthesia are of particular importance in evaluating hazard.

It is absolutely essential that a clear distinction between those substances that produce only "transient irritation" and those that produce "substantial injury" be made. Substances that produce primarily conjunctivitis and clear within 2–3 days with no delayed type reactions generally require no further investigation. Materials that produce serious corneal injury or internal injury to the eye, with or without pain, are serious hazards and appropriate controls should be placed on their use.

Dermal Irritation

Primary Irritation   In evaluating the hazards of human skin contact with any chemical substance for primary irritation, one relies heavily on data obtained from laboratory animals. Generally, the albino rabbit is useful in conducting contact irritation studies. Probably the most widely used procedure is that developed by Draize *et al.* (1944). Alternate species, such as the guinea pig, have also been used to compare primary irritation scores obtained with rabbits on a limited number of compounds. The guinea pig skin has been shown to provide similar information to that obtained with rabbits (Roudabush *et al.*, 1965). In addition to rabbits and guinea pigs, primates and minipigs have also been used.

Chemicals or drugs can be applied to the clipped back or belly, on intact and abraded test sites, for periods of exposure that range up to 24 hours. A statistically significant number of test sites should be available for evaluating each chemical. The irritation—erythema and edema—should be graded after removing the patch and washing the treated area, and at regular intervals for two or three days.

Human patch testing is sometimes fraught with difficulty. There are a number of articles that describe predictive test methods (Rieger and

Battista, 1964; Brunner, 1967; Lanman *et al.*, 1968; Battista and Rieger, 1971).

A recent study (Phillips *et al.*, 1972) compared the irritancy of a dozen chemicals in man and rabbit using the standard Draize test. One of the conclusions drawn from this investigation was that the animal data accurately predicted the results observed on man for nonirritants and severe irritants. The animal test lacked the sensitivity to discriminate mild-to-moderate irritants, which were successfully separated in human tests.

Generally speaking, agents that cause primary irritation or corrosive effects are not selective in their action. They will affect animal and human skin alike after sufficient time and at appropriate concentrations. In addition, the system that is selected should have appropriate sensitivity, and should be capable of interpretation as a graded response.

Acneform Eruptions (Chloracne)   Certain chemicals and drugs are capable of producing skin lesions that resemble acne vulgaris. While this type of reaction is primarily associated with certain industrial exposures, as in the use of insoluble cutting oils in industrial manufacturing processes, it is not limited to industrial situations. Chlorinated hydrocarbons—chlornapthalenes, chlordiphenyls and chlorodiphenyl-oxides—are strongly acnegenic. The condition not only affects employees in manufacturing plants but also construction workers exposed to materials incorporated in wire insulator materials. It generally develops after a month or more exposure and can affect any exposed part of the body. The condition "chloracne" occurs after exposure to chlorinated organic compounds, and the resulting irritation to skin appears as an occlusion of the follicular orifice. The mechanism of the reaction is uncertain.

If there is any probability that technical grade chemicals may contain trace quantities of chloracnegens they should be screened by applying small amounts of material daily on a repeated basis to the inner surface of the rabbit ear. The phenomenon is manifested by production of comedones with subsequent hyperplasia of the entire ear.

Sensitization   Some chemicals are capable of producing allergic sensitization upon repeated contact with the skin. *Contact allergens* (eczematous allergens) can be defined as substances that, although not necessarily irritating on first contact, produce a skin response (*de novo* or enhanced) after a latent period. The latent or incubation period, is estimated to range from 4 to 30 days. The reaction time, time between contact of the allergen and the first sign of reaction in a sensitive subject, is generally not less than 12 hours and often reaches its peak in 48 hours. Contact allergens, for the most part, are simple chemical haptens combining with a macromolecule to form an antigen: Poison ivy (antigen) is a mixture of substituted catechols. Contact allergens can be demonstrated experimentally in both animal and man. Features of contact allergenic dermatitis are itching, erythema, edema, vesiculation, and—in severe cases—purpura and necrosis.

Cross sensitization may occur: Individuals that show a sensitivity to one substance may also show a sensitivity to other compounds which are structurally related, and to which they have had no previous exposure. Cross sensitization can also occur with products that have been changed from their original form via body metabolism.

The animal of choice in sensitivity testing is the albino guinea pig. Following the guinea pig studies, carefully conducted clinical studies *may be* carried out on humans. If the test material elicits strong positive reactions on guinea pigs, there is no valid reason for conducting similar studies in man. The material may be considered unsafe where significant human skin contact is anticipated. If the guinea pig tests are negative, further well-controlled investigations should be carried out in small groups of human volunteers if dermal exposure is expected. If these studies are also negative, it may be prudently assumed that the material involved is *not a strong sensitizer*. The judgment at this point may be to go next to a customized actual use test in a few test market areas— 30,000 to 50,000 people, for example, may be involved for a retail household product. It should be recognized, however, that the lack of controls and follow-up present serious drawbacks to this attempt. Alternate techniques, however, are just not available.

As is frequently the case, the gray area (borderline situations) in interpolation of sensitivity test data seems to be the greatest problem, and problems with false negatives or false positives are possible because of the small populations tested.

Photosensitization   Photosensitivity reactions can be demonstrated when predisposed individuals are exposed to light of wavelengths between 280 and 430 nm (2800–4300 Å). The introduction of a chemical substance into a biologic system by any route is capable of sensitizing that system to light so that a photodynamic chain of events is initiated in which molecular oxygen plays a vital role in the destructive reaction. Photosensitizers may also act as free radical initiators, which may cause damage to intracellular membranes. The mechanism of action is still poorly understood.

New environmental chemicals that resemble structures of well-known photosensitizers should be tested, as should chemicals where the biotransformation and metabolic pathways indicate similar structures to known photosensitizers. Up until the last decade or so photosensitivity testing with laboratory animals was not successful. Simultaneous advances in several areas of technology have improved test methods so that guinea pigs, rabbits, rats, and mice are routinely used. However, there is still a significantly high incidence of *false negatives* with these laboratory animals.

If the test results obtained on the basic chemical and finished formulations are *negative*, the panel would consider the material generally safe for its intended use. No further studies would be required. It is important that the procedures chosen be sensitive and that their limitations be recognized.

Oral Irritation and Corrosive Effects

Predicated on the experience that it is reasonable and foreseeable that a chemical substance can be ingested, especially by children under 5 years, studies for potential corrosive effects may be appropriate. Generally, the initial test data from preliminary exposures to skin or eye or both may be indicative of a potential hazard. Certainly with severe irritants the test is indicated. Varous species of animals have been used—rabbit, rat, dog, and cat. The material is administered on the posterior aspect of the animal's tongue and the animal is allowed to swallow normally. The animal is returned to its cage and allowed access to water but no food for the first 24 hours. After 24 hours two of the animals are sacrificed and complete gross necropsy performed. The examination includes the oral cavity, tongue, adjacent pharyngeal structure, trachea, esophagus extending to the cardiac incisure and stomach. The selected tissues may be preserved in neutral buffered formalin for subsequent microscopic examination as necessary, depending upon the gross observations. The surviving animals are allowed access to food and water after the first 24-hour period and sacrificed at 96 hours. These animals are likewise examined, and evaluation for corrosivity is based on *visible* effects on the anatomical structure as examined at necropsy. Each material can then be classified according to standard procedures.

Aspiration Toxicity   Chemicals that may not normally be classed as toxic by oral administration may produce more serious results when aspirated. Of particular importance are liquid hydrocarbon preparations, which may be readily aspirated and result in a fulminating chemical pneumonitis. This type of exposure is an acute problem which can occur in a few seconds with very severe consequences. A test procedure for the evaluation of aspiration hazard has been described (Gerarde, 1963).

Pharmacodynamics *Pharmacodynamics* is defined as the study of the biochemical and physiological effects of chemicals and their mechanisms of action on living systems. Although this is the broad definition, it is interpreted to encompass the area of metabolism of a chemical—including the absorption, distribution, biotransformation, storage, and excretion of chemicals. These factors, coupled with dosage, determine the concentration of a chemical at its target site and, accordingly, the magnitude and duration of its effects. Another area of pharmacodynamics is the correlation of action as a function of chemical structure. The results of the pharmacodynamic studies are used by the toxicologist in planning study protocols. Pharmacodynamic evaluations are an aid to the toxicologist in helping to explain or predict toxic action of a chemical but, alone, are not an end point in toxicologic study.

The experienced observer is capable of detecting and grading responses in experimental animals from an objective standpoint, while also obtaining valuable impressions of behavioral effects. The latter signs, reflecting effect on or subtle changes in mood, perception and general behavior, cannot be adequately described instrumentally. Gross observational techniques permit the rapid characterization of a wide continuum of signs, varying from minimal effects of questionable significance through fairly discrete toxicologic patterns of effect. Translation of these results into qualitative and quantitative terms can piece together general toxicologic and behavioral profiles. This type of information can, in experienced hands, lead to prognostications of what to expect in subchronic and chronic studies where known compounds provide the experience for such prediction. Not only do these signs themselves provide useful information, but equally important as pharmacodynamic formation are the time of onset and duration of signs with regard to absorption, biotransformation, distribution, storage, and excretion in relation to the target site.

These statements are based on observations and interpretations from acute studies in intact animals. In order to have a truly meaningful understanding of pharmacodynamic action of a chemical, the next step would be to undertake specific studies using classical pharmacologic preparations for blood pressure, respiration, gut motility, salivary flow, etc., and to determine the specificity of the test chemical on these systems as a function of dosage. Similarly, classical isolated organ, enzymatic and biochemical study can also be applied to further understand the chemical mechanism of action and fate. The selection of such studies should be left to the investigator and his innovation.

Environmental chemicals can be many and varied in structure and activity. Their use can result in multiple exposure levels and routes. These conditions make it necessary for the investigator to use his own judgment about what specific special studies available to him are to be applied. He should use his experience in structure activity relationships and the results of acute studies to plan and undertake such studies as may be needed to provide him a better understanding of the mechanism of action of environmental chemicals so that he may predict with reasonable certainty the consequences of man's exposure.

Short-Term Tests

The use of short-term tests with nonmammalian animals or with isolated mammalian organs or cells in toxicology, genetics, mutagenesis, teratogenesis, and carcinogenesis has been under investigation. However, it is felt that the state of knowledge has not reached the point at which such systems can be used to fully evaluate the toxic, or non-toxic, effects of environmental chemicals. At best they can be considered as screening tests with the recognition that they may not be useful in predicting the effects on the intact animal. Until these short-term tests are validated as being reliable for predicting effects in man, they cannot be accepted in lieu of the more standard and acceptable toxicologic procedures. However, the need and the promise is so great that an intensive search for and trial of them is urgently needed. Additionally, such tests are often critically useful in elucidating biological and/or chemical mechanisms. Some currently available short-term test systems are described in Appendix A.

Biological Interactions

Numerous cases of biological interactions have been reported. These have been observed principally with drugs and pesticides. Interactions can take the form of a less-than-additive biological response from simultaneous exposure to two or more chemicals, antagonism, or a more-than-additive response, potentiation. From the point of view of health protection, potentiation alone constitutes a problem.

Potentiation may be pharmacological or biochemical in nature. Chemicals affecting the same target system may exert more-than-additive effects when administered at pharmacologically active dosages. In the biochemical phenomenon, one chemical may inhibit an enzyme responsible for the detoxification of another chemical so that the latter chemical has a greater opportunity to exert its toxic effect on the target system. Conversely, some chemicals stimulate enzyme systems, which convert other chemicals to more toxic metabolic products.

All of the interactions are of concern in the evaluation of health hazard at levels of exposure that exert pharmacological or biochemical effects. This is the case with drug administration, accidental exposure, and, in some cases, occupational exposure. However, it is economically and physically impossible to test all possible combinations of potential pollutants for potentiation. Such studies should be limited to those (1) whose expected exposure pattern is simultaneous and at levels approaching those known to produce biological effects, (2) whose chemical structure closely resembles known potentiation combinations, and (3) whose target organs or mechanisms of action are the same and to which there will be simultaneous exposure. However, the goal in environmental management should be to restrict the level of all chemicals in the environment to a level that has no pharmacological or biochemical effect on man. If, in fact, this goal is achieved, we will concomitantly control the hazard of harmful interactions in the population from normal use of these chemicals.

PRIORITY JUDGMENTS

In summary, the following considerations must be reviewed with each chemical in our environment.

- nature of the final product which contains the chemical
- "quantity" (dose) of that product
- route of exposure
- duration of exposure—single, infrequent, constant (lifetime)
- population at risk
- human experience
- animal toxicity studies

Because of the tens of thousands of natural and synthetic substances present in the environment, it becomes necessary to establish a reasonable system of priorities for the further study of those substances not yet fully evaluated. To study every chemical to the same extent would represent an unjustifiable expenditure of effort that did not contribute significantly to protection of public health. It is neither practicable nor necessary to undertake experimental toxicological studies of every chemical to which man is exposed; to do so would be to assign equal importance to problems of unequal risk. This would deny the value of experience in assessing probable risk. All environmental exposures must be subjected to scientific evaluation, but not all exposures require experimental toxicological study. The economic and, indeed, the scientific merit of performing chronic, reproductive, carcinogenic, mutagenic, behavioral studies on all chemicals is questionable. The vast majority of man-introduced chemicals in our environment are in final products, which, because of their nature, markedly reduces exposure levels (dose).

The first step in this dilemma therefore, should be the preparation of guidelines for classifying chemicals into categories, such as (1) recognized as probably safe because of adequate and valid use experience, (2) of low priority of concern because the use level is at such an insignificant or trivial level, and (3) critical.

To provide optimum assurance of public safety within the existing limitations of capabilities available, toxicological facilities and skills for evaluating safety must be concentrated on environmental situations in which there is a reasonable expectation that exposure to chemicals may cause real hazards. It is clear that materials being widely distributed into the environment so as to place a large segment of the population at risk would be assigned a high priority for risk–benefit assessment, including toxicity tests. Conversely, those materials which are encountered in trace quantities by a limited population or even a large population would be given a lower priority. It is equally clear that, if the trace quantity is well below the known level of toxic effect, an even lower priority may be assigned.

It may be further argued that, if the trace level of a contaminant is well below the lowest known toxic levels, then it may reasonably be concluded that there is little probability of its presenting a significant risk to public health and therefore it may be designated toxicologically unimportant, requiring little or no actual testing. To insist that nothing can be assumed to be safe without direct experimental toxicological evidence implies that safety must be proved experimentally before the proof of safety can be considered unnecessary. This is contrary to the need for establishing priorities for using our limited resources for toxicity testing. Thus, there is urgent need to arrive at more specific guidelines for estimating levels that can be considered toxicologically unimportant.

The evaluation of toxicity data for judging the safety or hazard associated with the material can *only* be made in the light of the anticipated amount and circumstances of human exposure.

If the anticipated human exposure is very close to, or perhaps greater than, the maximum dose that produces no observable effect in an adequately sized group of experimental animals, then consideration (with adequate group size) should be given to the type and extent of controls to be applied in order to reduce human exposure to acceptable levels. The acceptable risk determination includes an evaluation of the benefits to the individual and to society of the proposed exposure and an evaluation of the nature and severity of the anticipated effects.

In practice, the knowledge of toxicity of a material should keep pace with the development of information about its proposed uses and the associated human exposure. A series of such studies of increasing complexity should be proposed, which are designed to minimize investment in unnecessary research. The following is a suggested guide to categorization.

1. *High Priority*—Those compounds not having a safety margin of 1000 or more in a 90-day subchronic test and which are either (1) produced in high volume, (2) are chemically related to some known carcinogens, (3) are chemically nonreactive so as to lead to persistence in the environment, or (4) have an intended use involving extensive public exposure require professional evaluation.

2. *Intermediate Priority*—Those compounds that produce acute toxic effects at doses less than 3000–5000 mg/kg and/or whose use can be expected to result in repetitive exposure levels of greater than 0.01 mg/kg/ day require subchronic toxicity studies in order to determine need for in-depth evaluation, i.e., chronic, reproductive, behavioral testing.

3. *Low Priority*—Those compounds that have low acute toxicity (i.e., produce acute toxic effects only at levels greater than 3000–5000 mg/kg) and/or whose use cannot be expected to produce human exposure rates in excess of 0.01 mg/kg/day may be considered low priority for testing.

SUMMARY

Definitions are presented of toxicity and safety, toxic substances, acute studies, margin of safety, and subchronic studies. With these in mind, a rationale has been developed for establishing priorities for additional studies. This takes into account the quantity of environmental chemicals to which man is likely to be exposed; the frequency, extent, and route of exposure; and certain basic values obtained in acute and subchronic toxicity studies.

Routes of probable exposure have been discussed, including oral, dermal, eye, and inhalation. Special problems of hypersensitization, photosensitization, and aspiration exposure have been considered. The roles of pharmacodynamic studies (including metabolism, storage, and excretion) and biological interaction have been defined and discussed.

REFERENCES

Barr, M. 1962. Percutaneous absorption. *J. Pharm. Sci.* 51:395–409.
Bartek, J., J.A. Labudde, and H.I. Maibach. 1971. Skin permeability *in vivo:* Rat, rabbit, pig, and man. *J. Invest. Dermatol.* 56:409.

Battista, G.W., and M.M. Rieger. 1971. Some problems of predictive testing. *J. Soc. Cosmet. Chem.* 22:349–359.

Brunner, M.J. 1967. Pitfalls and problems in predictive testing. *J. Soc. Cosmet. Chem.* 18:323–331.

Draize, J.H., G. Woodard, and H.O. Calvery. 1944. Methods for the study of irritation and toxicity of substances applied topically to the skin and mucous membranes. *J. Pharmacol. Exp. Ther.* 82:377–390.

Gerarde, H.W. 1963. Toxicological studies on hydrocarbons. IX. The aspiration hazard and toxicity of hydrocarbons and hydrocarbon mixtures. *Arch. Environ. Health* 6:329–341.

Lanman, B.M., W.B. Elvers, and C.S. Howard. 1968. The role of human patch testing in a product development program. *Proc. J. Conf. Cosmet. Sci.,* Washington, D.C. pp. 135–145.

Phillips, L., M. Steinberg, H.I. Maibach, and W.A. Akers. 1972. A comparison of rabbit and human skin response to certain irritants. *Toxicol. Appl. Pharmacol.* 21:369–382.

Rieger, M.M., and G.W. Battista. 1964. Some experiences in the safety testing of cosmetics. *J. Soc. Cosmet. Chem.* 15:161–172.

Roudabush, R.L., C.J. Terhaar, D.W. Fassett, and S.P. Dziuba. 1965. Comparative acute effects of some chemicals on the skin of rabbits and guinea pigs. *Toxicol. Appl. Pharmacol.* 7:559–565.

SUGGESTED READINGS

Barnes, J.M., and F.A. Denz. 1954. Experimental methods used in determining chronic toxicity. *Pharmacol. Rev.* 6:191–242.

Giovacchini, R.P. 1972. Old and new issues in the safety evaluation of cosmetics and toiletries. *Crit. Rev. Toxicol.* 1:361–378.

National Academy of Sciences–National Research Council. Food Protection Committee. 1970. *Evaluating the safety of food chemicals.* Washington, D.C. pp. 49–55.

U.S. Food and Drug Administration. 1968. *National Conference on Indirect Food Additives.* Abstracts of presentation, Feb. 13–14. Ace-Federal Reporters, Inc., Washington, D.C.

Zbinden, G. 1963. Experimental and clinical aspects of drug toxicity. *Adv. Pharmacol.* 2:1–112.

VIII

Chronic
Toxicity

There are many chemical agents in the environment that interact with biological systems to produce effects deleterious to the health and well-being of man only after prolonged and repeated exposure. These constitute chronic toxicity. The experimental study of chronic toxicity should be designed to reveal those exposure levels that are harmful or adverse and also those that appear to produce no adverse effects.

The need for chronic toxicity studies became apparent when it was realized that target organs found in acute experiments are not always the same as those following repeated exposure over long periods of time approaching a lifetime. Cause–effect relationships are not as apparent in chronic studies as they are in acute exposures. The observable toxic response may be the result of storage of the chemical, of action of its metabolites in body tissue with subsequent mobilization and redistribution, or just the repeated and additive insult on target organs, enzymes, hormones or other body systems, or a long delayed response to a single or time limited exposure.

Since industrialization led to widespread introduction of chemicals into the environment, techniques were needed to estimate the potential hazards of the consequent long-term exposure. In many instances man could be expected to be exposed for a lifetime; hence, chronic toxicity has come to be regarded as studies in animals for *their* lifetime or a very significant portion thereof.

In designing chronic toxicity studies consideration must be given to many factors among which are the known effects obtained from acute and subchronic studies, the estimated level and circumstances of human exposure, and any available human experience—for example, occupational exposure.

Repeated exposures result in continued chemical–biological interactions, which may produce continued changes in the status of the affected biological system. The interval between repetitions of exposures may be sufficient to permit total recovery, but, if not, the residual effects may accumulate to the point of producing overt injury. The chronic exposure experiments need to be patterned after such anticipated human exposures. The delayed consequences following a relatively few chemical exposures also necessitate extended follow-up.

The need for chronic testing may also be determined by knowledge of metabolic fate of the host–chemical interactions. However, present limitations in our knowledge are readily apparent, even where the action and metabolic fate of a compound are known. The predictability of metabolism and toxic consequences of chemical analogs is limited. Such limitations are further extended by a paucity of knowledge of the quantitative and qualitative details of all but a few metabolic pathways. Finally, even where some pathways have been tested in man, there is no certainty that these necessarily represent the course of biotransformation in the entire exposed human population. Accordingly, the need for mature professional judgment cannot be overemphasized.

Studies of this type are in the nature of a major research effort, require allocation of substantial sums of money, facilities and personnel, and will generally be in progress for many months or several years. Each study will have unique problems and objectives and will require the utmost in skilled planning and mature professional judgment. Although the objectives may vary considerably, they will generally be of the following sort:

- to follow, for long periods of exposure, the extent and progress of any changes that might have been seen in shorter studies, and to evaluate general factors in the health of animals such as growth, life span, mortality, nutrition, patterns of disease, appearances of organs and tissues, causes of death, tumors, reversibility or permanence of symptoms or changes, and other factors;
- to select species that will be most likely to give useful predictions for human effects, based on a knowledge of their known similarity to

man in response to this or similar chemicals, the ability to elicit in them certain classes of adverse response of interest, and other factors;

- to arrive at estimates of the safety margin between man's expected exposure level and the level in animals where significant adverse effects will be observed;
- to pick up delayed adverse effects not seen in the short-term studies and to establish dose levels for both their presence and absence; and
- to determine whether changes are present that might be suspected on the basis of experience with chemicals of similar structure or similar biological effects.

PRINCIPLES

The classical approach to the study of chronic toxicity of substances has been described in documents of the National Academy of Sciences (NAS), FDA, the World Health Organization (WHO), and others. This approach involves studies in two or more species of animals for periods of time ranging from many months to several years, during and after exposure to the agent in question with appropriate doses and routes of administration. A variety of specific tests, conducted at prescribed intervals during each study, allows assessment of anatomic and functional changes. These changes are measured by the use of biochemical, physiological, pathological and behavioral methods. These permit quantitation of adverse effects as opposed to changes that may occur spontaneously in concurrent control animals.

As a result of awareness of new and unforeseen effects of chemicals, new test procedures have been added to the armamentarium of chronic toxicology. In particular, teratogenic and mutagenic tests were stimulated by the experience of the thalidomide tragedy. [*See* Chapter X.]

The information from such highly structured animal studies and human experience has provided a basis for safety evaluation including definitions of no-effect levels, safety factors, acceptable daily intakes, and threshold limit values related to the pattern of use. Some of these terms have severe limitations. [*See* comments on terminology in Chapter V.]

A constructive approach, which minimizes the possibility of unforeseen chemically induced tragedies, should effectively utilize and build upon existing knowledge to formulate research programs that will provide a realistic assessment of the hazard that potentially might be associated with the use of a new chemical agent. *No set of routine animal investigations will be universally applicable for definition of the toxicologic properties of all substances.* All decisions regarding safety must be tentative and subject to subsequent reviews undertaken in the light of experience or with the development of more discriminating methodology for the study and interpretation of toxicologic hazard.

The urgent need is to recognize that chronic toxicity evaluations require a sophisticated multidisciplinary approach that applies expert professional judgment in utilizing advanced and newly developed scientific knowledge and techniques. This approach requires that no inflexible course be charted based upon regulations or past practices.

CONSIDERATIONS IN PLANNING THE CHRONIC TOXICITY STUDY

Although it is evident that these studies require individual planning, there are some general considerations, in addition to those described above, that pertain to all long-term studies. Some of these are described elsewhere in this document. [*See* Chapters IV–XI and XX.]

Chemical

Knowledge of the purity and nature and amount of impurities in the substance, provision of adequate supplies of the substance of a grade similar to that expected to be used, complete permanent records of analysis of all batches used, retention of samples for future reference, and appropriate analytical methods for use in documenting dosage (stability of the chemical under the conditions of storage, dilution, and incorporation in the diet) or for biochemical monitoring or metabolic studies—are considerations in obtaining chemical samples for testing. Such materials are usually a mixture of the desired product plus other process-derived contaminants, both or either of which may be biologically active. In addition, there is a further need for information regarding process changes which result in a modification of product composition. Furthermore, the potential hazards of the compounds produced by environmental transformation and the interactions with other environmental chemicals must be recognized and assessed by those responsible for toxicological testing.

Test Species

Knowledge of life history, diseases, nutritional requirements, and metabolic peculiarities, housing requirements, acclimation of animals, and the like—are considerations in obtaining experimental animals. Although opinions differ as to the merits of special versus optimum diets, the latter are generally more useful. Many studies fail because of lack of consideration of this factor.

Appropriate Numbers and Subgroups of Animals

Planning for serial sacrifices of animals in the course of the study, statistical considerations essential to planning, and documentation of the identification, history and fate of each animal—are considerations in obtaining a broad enough sample. Although the considerations above seem obvious, experience shows that matters of this sort are of vital importance in the success of such studies and are sometimes inadequately done.

Selection of Observations

This will depend on the specific needs of the study, but most studies will include the general health factors—body weight gain, food consumption, appearance, etc. Experience has shown that these general responses are of great importance, especially at lower dosage levels approaching those of anticipated human exposure.

Target organ or target system studies may provide an additional rational basis for the design of chronic studies. The results of a well-designed study will alert investigators to specific anatomical, physiological, and biochemical parameters requiring special attention. The effects of low levels of environmental substances have resulted in a search for more efficient and specific detection, methods which are now common components of chronic studies. Some samples follow.

Pathologic Change The most readily perceived change is manifested by modifications in biological structure as seen grossly and microscopically. The usefulness of this *criterion of alteration* derives from evidence that changes in structure reflect changes in function. However, structural alterations alone cannot be used to define functional changes. At best these relationships are only suggestive, and their significance must be pursued either by additional studies or by a correlative evaluation of the findings in other components of the chronic toxicity study. A knowledge of the reversibility of a morphologic change is of utmost importance in judging the significance of such alterations. This problem is well exemplified by the judgment required to assess such structural changes as adaptive hyperplasia or hypertrophy. These latter changes may be reversible or, indeed, the precursors of malignant alteration. The ultimate assessment of the significance of these modifications depends upon structural, biochemical, and physiological findings as well as professional judgment.

Although electron microscopy is not considered a routine procedure for detecting pathologic change, it may be useful in toxicity studies for the confirmation of suspected alteration or to define a pathological event or mechanism. Electron microscopy has its role in toxicity studies in confirming a suspected alteration or in defining a pathological event, but should not be used in "fishing" with the hope of uncovering a pathologic change (Grice, 1972).

Change in Organ Weights   Many long-term studies, especially by the oral route, have shown that enlargement of certain organs without histologic change (e.g., the liver and kidney) constitutes one of the most frequent and sometimes the only gross change. More recent biochemical studies show that this response of the liver is in the nature of a reversible hyperplasia, often indicating induction of microsomal enzymes. Regression of the enlargement can be demonstrated by withdrawal of the agent, and microsomal and electron-microscope studies help to confirm the nature of this change. Evaluation of this rather frequent type of response is extremely useful since it is important to differentiate it from other types of more serious and permanent liver enlargements.

The wide variety of liver function tests now available may help resolve the nature of changes. For example, biliary effects may be accompanied by elevated serum alkaline phosphatase, and characterization of the elevated enzyme by electrophoresis may pinpoint its source. The use of modern excretory studies of liver function (e.g., indocyanine green clearance) provide a powerful tool to detect early changes in this aspect of liver function.

Results of Renal Function Studies   The application of techniques of modern renal physiology in such studies is practical in some cases, especially in larger species. Clearance studies have been used successfully in evaluating toxic effects.

Results of Lung Function Studies   A variety of lung function studies have been used, *e.g.*, resistance and compliance studies. These are particularly valuable for inhalation exposures.

Changes in Central Nervous System Responses   Careful observations by a skilled scientist or well-trained technician may pick up changes in responses, performance, or behavior, especially in larger species. Certain species seem to be much more sensitive to central nervous system (CNS) effects: The response of the cat and chicken to demyelinating agents resembles that of man. Various neurophysiological techniques can be applied, especially in larger species and simians. Electroencephalogram (EEG) responses may be useful. Evaluation of CNS effects remains one of the greatest challenges for the toxicologist. [*See* Chapter XI, Effects on Behavior.]

Results of Hematologic Studies   In addition to routine study of peripheral blood, additional tests may be useful (e.g., the reticulocyte count as evidence of stress on the red cell system, search for Heinz bodies in the case of amines, platelet counts, and prothrombin time for clotting function). Biochemical studies may help evaluate red and white cell responses.

Change in Metabolic Response   A knowledge of biochemical pathways, rates and modes of excretion, storage, and nature of metabolites is of great importance in evaluating responses. The concept of a target organ and relation of levels in that organ is based on such knowledge. Such knowledge is necessary to understand the kinetics of absorption, excretion, and accumulation. The selection of appropriate species depends in part on metabolic data. Placental transfer of agents requires this information. [*See* below, Additional Considerations.]

Results of in vitro *Studies*   Although these have not as yet found wide acceptance and use, and extrapolation to the whole animal or to man is difficult, it can be anticipated that, with sufficient comparative study of *in vitro* and *in vivo* results, useful data will be developed. For example, human and animal pulmonary macrophages can be easily obtained and exposed to agents and biochemical or other tests applied. *In vitro* transformation of cells with carcinogens has been accomplished. Such studies require extensive comparison with *in vivo* approaches with positive and negative controls to give assurance as to their utility. [*See* Appendix A, Short-Term Tests.]

The above examples of some selective approaches to the search for adverse effects or their absence are only a few of the many that are available to the toxicologist, but it is clear that the decisions as to safety in chronic studies can best be made by an intelligent application of the principles described above.

ADDITIONAL CONSIDERATIONS IN THE ASSESSMENT OF CHRONIC TOXICITY

Protection of the public from the adverse health effects of chemicals in the environment requires special consideration of individuals having an abnormally high susceptibility to the action of these agents. This higher than normal susceptibility of an individual may be due to such normal characteristics of life as sex, age, race and genetic makeup or to unique idiosyncracies of metabolism, immunology, or allergy. These are discussed in the following paragraphs.

Sex and Age of Test Animal

Sex-linked variations in response are routinely studied by use of both sexes in chronic investigations.

Age dependent variation in response to toxic agents may also merit special consideration. In this event, animal models representative of age-susceptible organs can be put to toxic chemical stress. The immature status of the endocrine system in the young may dictate that pre-adolescent animals be tested by exposure to agents that target on this organ system. Similarly, the known high incidence of cardiovascular disease in the elderly might require use of animal models that mimic this human population. Such animals may then be tested by chemicals under investigation. Further development of relevant animal models that meet special needs is required.

Route of Administration

The important consideration which determines the route of administration in chronic studies derives from the prediction of the expected portal of entry. Where such potential exposures indicate that the gastrointestinal tract represents the route of entry into the body, principles of proper oral dosing are well established and applicable. Where the pulmonary tract represents the probable locus of action of a chemical, chronic inhalation exposure—though difficult—should be undertaken. However, even in such cases, other factors may make it necessary to consider other routes of administration. [See Chapter VII, Acute and Subchronic Effects.] If it is determined by subchronic studies that the reaction of an agent is exerted primarily upon lung tissue and poses no apparent risk of systemic distribution, it might still be necessary to consider oral dosing, as in the case of extrapulmonary effects of asbestos. A variable proportion of inhaled agents eventually find their way into the gastrointestinal tract via tracheobronchial clearance and swallowing.

Except in the case of carcinogenesis studies, dermal application usually is carried out for relatively short periods in subchronic studies; however, special circumstances may indicate the need for longer skin exposure studies.

It is apparent from the foregoing that choice of the appropriate route of administration cannot be made in a *pro forma* fashion.

Special Risks Due to Inborn Errors of Metabolism

The 92 presently known human genetic disorders identified by a variation in a specific enzyme can be grouped into five general categories [*see* Table 3 and Appendix C] (McKusick, 1970). In the design of research protocol it is important to note that, with few exceptions, genetic errors of metabolism give rise to exaggerated toxic responses, so-called hypersensitivity or hypersusceptibility reactions. A notable example is the glucose-6-phosphate dehydrogenase deficiency (other examples are present in Appendix C). This genetic defect is widespread (Beaconsfield *et al.*, 1965) and can explain the hyperactive response, hemolytic crises to a wide variety of chemicals (Table 4) in those individuals with a G-6-PD deficient red-cell enzyme system. It is of interest to note that not all of the consequences of this defective enzyme system are deleterious—such individuals may be resistant to malaria and cancer. In many cases structural relationships to known chemicals are adequate to alert the informed toxicologist; however, much work remains to be done in

TABLE 3   Categories of Genetic Variation in Man

Category	Example
1. Essential substance missing or deficient	α_1 Antitrypsin deficiency
2. Enzyme system missing or deficient	Glucose-6-phosphate dehydrogenase
3. Alteration in cellular transport of metabolite	CS_2 sensitivity
4. Abnormal antibody production	Reaginic antibodies to allergenic pollen antigens in "hayfever" cross-reacting to certain industrial chemicals
5. Presence of abnormal protein	Hemoglobin S in sickle-cell anemia

TABLE 4 Some Hemolytic Industrial Chemicals

Acetanilid	Cresol	o-Nitrochlorobenzenes
		Oxygen (Hyperbaric)
Amyl nitrite	Dinitrobenzenes	p-Phenylenediamine
Aniline	Dinitrotoluenes	Phenylhydrazine
Arsine	Guaiacol	Phosphorus
Benzene	Hydroxylamine	Selenium dioxide
Benzidine	Lead	Stibine
Carbon tetrachloride	Methylcellosolve	Tetrachloroethane
Chlorate	Naphthalene	Toluidine
Chloronitrobenzenes	Nitric oxide	Toluylenediamine
Chloroprene monomer	Nitrites	Trinitrotoluene
Antimalarial and numerous N-containing drugs	Nitrosamines	

SOURCE: Stokinger and Mountain (1963).

this area. Some interesting advancements using special inbred strains of mice—for example, in muscular dystrophy—are being made.

INTERPRETATION OF TOXICITY DATA

The toxicologist (with others) must be involved in judging the importance of observed effects, especially whether they are adverse or not adverse, as well as their significance if they are adverse.

Nonadverse Effects

Nonadverse effects were previously defined as the absence of changes in morphology, growth, development, and life span. The significance of functional alterations that result from chemical exposure, however, is more difficult to evaluate.

In terms of functional alterations, nonadverse effects can be considered as changes that

1. occur with continued exposure and do not result in impairment of functional capacity or the ability to compensate for additional stress;

2. are reversible following cessation of exposure, if such changes occur without detectable decrements in the ability of the organisms to maintain homeostasis; and

3. do not enhance the susceptibility of the organism to the deleterious effects of other environmental influences—chemical, physical, microbiological, or social.

The following examples derived from use of serum enzyme activity determinations have been given by Cornish (1971) and illustrate the problems involved in the assessment of functional change.

- Considerable changes may transpire as indicators of biochemical function without encroachment upon reserve capacity inherent in such systems.
- Significant changes in enzyme activity may reflect reversible functional change, which has no deleterious implications.
- Elevated serum enzyme activity may reflect a compensatory, feedback-directed, response to stress.
- Current methodology may not reflect the state of enzymatic activity at the critical receptor.
- Marked species variations of enzymatic alterations occur in response to insult.
- The effect of cellular enzymes may demonstrate marked time dependency.
- Choice of the proper enzymatic indicator of change is dependent upon knowledge of the specific organ or organs affected.

Similar consideration is necessary for the evaluation of other biochemical, physiological, hematological, and behavioral manifestations of change. The presence of change alone is not necessarily indicative of pathologic alteration.

In terms of morphologic criteria, nonadverse effects are somewhat less readily defined. Limitations on the ability of the investigator to make such judgments will be evident in subsequent discussions of the criteria that establish the existence of undesirable biological alterations (i.e., adverse effects).

Adverse Effects

With increasing dosage in the continuum of the dose–response relationship, the region is generally entered where the effects are clearly adverse. Thus, adverse effects may be defined as changes that

1. occur with intermittent or continued exposure and that result in impairment of functional capacity (as determined by anatomical, physiological, and biochemical, or behavioral parameters) or in a decrement of the ability to compensate for additional stress;
2. are irreversible during exposure or following cessation of exposure if such changes cause detectable decrements in the ability of the organism to maintain homeostasis; and

3. enhance the susceptibility of the organisms to the deleterious effects of other environmental influences.

The detection of adverse effects begins with gross observations of the intact animal in terms of growth, appearance, and activity. The next point of discrimination is at the organ-system level, wherein changes of a biochemical and physiological nature are assessed. These are followed by an examination of morphological changes at the gross and cellular levels in sacrificed animals or biopsy material.

HUMAN SURVEILLANCE

Appropriate human toxicologic information, where available, is more relevant than that obtained from animal exposure. In particular, human dose–response data are of great importance to sound regulatory action. Experimental exposures of man to toxic or possibly toxic substances are severely limited by ethical considerations. Therefore, we must depend on information obtained from the study of accidental or normally occurring exposures. Such data are obtained by clinical and/or epidemiological methods. Exposure situations available for study are most frequently found in association with occupation, but may occur in relation to hobbies, household activities, consumer use, etc. Most such exposures are at low-to-moderate levels, but accidents offer the possibility of obtaining some data on the effects of higher levels as well. Every effort should be made to maximize the amount of information obtained from these naturally occurring study opportunities, particularly in the case of new or inadequately studied substances.

In laboratory studies of toxic substances, certainty of cause–effect relationship is approached by means of control of variables; in epidemiologic observations, this is not possible. In some cases variables can be measured and adjusted for; others can be controlled by the use of suitable comparison groups, which do not have the exposure under study. Some degree of uncertainty frequently remains. Certainty of cause–effect relationship is further assessed in epidemiologic work through consistency of findings. This requires several studies of exposed and comparison groups. For these reasons, it is important to seek out and employ all available exposure study opportunities in man until a clear understanding of the effects of the substance under observation is obtained.

Early Response

Manufacturers should not be required to perform experimental studies on humans except where all ethical protection is supplied. If such data are available, they should, of course, be furnished. Producers should be required to make full use of the human exposure situations that occur in the development and production of substances requiring evaluation. Where any such exposures occur routinely or accidentally, monitoring for exposure level and for effects should be maintained and recorded. Desirably, exposure records should exhibit not only average levels but also degree of variability and range. Personal monitoring and *in vivo* measurements of exposure (e.g., carboxyhemoglobin, blood lead) are desirable where possible. Detailed study of exposed and unexposed comparison groups is desirable with appropriate questions, examinations, and tests. Minor effects, which are not apparent in individual observations, can sometimes be detected by such group comparisons.

When accidental exposures occur in an industrial setting, the law requires that records be made and kept on the accident, that it be reported to the Occupational Safety and Health Administration (OSHA), and that the episode be open to investigation by them. Such exposure information will also be available if any such accidents have occurred with the substance under study.

Information obtained as described above will perhaps be meager or nonexistent for most new substances. If products already in use are being evaluated, such data may already exist and need not be generated anew if adequate. Even where no effects are found at ordinary or accidental exposure levels, information on well-documented harmless levels of human exposure will be of considerable value and use. In all cases in which EPA plans to require information of an occupational health nature from producers, this should be planned, and possibly carried out in cooperation with the National Institute of Occupational Safety and Health (NIOSH) and OSHA.

In the case of new substances where the preproduction toxicologic data are equivocal, and a strong suspicion remains that human exposure might result in deleterious effects, it would seem reasonable that EPA require that exposed workers be placed under surveillance, as described above, in order to learn whether or not significant effects or undesirable body burdens are apt to occur.

Chronic Toxicity

Chronic toxicity data on humans will, of course, not be available and cannot be required with new substances, except where it might be predicted upon the basis of acute exposure as discussed above. For substances already in production, such information may already be available or, in some cases, can be obtained. In cases where chronic injury is known or suspected to appear in a period of less than 5 or possibly 10 years, prospective investigation leading to accurate dose–response data, while difficult to obtain, is desirable. Chronic effects may appear only after 10 or 20 years; in such cases, prospective studies are of limited immediate value due to the long waiting period for results, and uncertainties as to completion. Retrospective studies based on the experience of previously exposed groups, where applicable, are useful; however, accuracy and dose data are usually less adequate in such studies than in prospective ones. Epidemiologic studies are now required of industry by occupational health legislation and several are under way; therefore, a requirement for such studies is appropriate.

Retrospective investigation of this kind is best carried out in a reconstructed work population beginning as far back as practical, preferably 20–30 years minimum. All employees who were exposed, even though only for a short period, should be included. Comparison groups of unexposed persons should be selected with great care: More than one is frequently desirable; both morbidity and mortality effects should be studied. Some long delayed effects are the result of continued overexposure; others are probably due to briefer exposure followed by a long incubation period. Data should be obtained and analyzed in such a way that both these hypotheses can be examined. The inclusion of individuals who worked for only a few months or years many years ago in the study population will be useful in such analyses. Although reconstruction and follow-up of such populations is difficult and time consuming, it has repeatedly been carried out successfully and yielded valuable information of both a negative and positive nature.

Reproductive Performance

In any case where a teratogenic and/or mutagenic potential has been identified in mammalian test systems for a new chemical, it is useful to examine the reproductive history of both sexes of occupationally exposed persons. Teratogenic effects may be manifested in the immediate pregnancies and offspring of these individuals and may be inferentially suggested in terms of increased frequency of spontaneous abortion, especially during the first trimester. The effect may be only a missed menses. In addition, the usual observations should be made or be available on fetal deaths, perinatal deaths and the morbidity and mortality among the live births surviving beyond 24 hours.

Reproductive effects may be transient and related only to the time period of occupational exposure; thus, performance before and after exposure may sometimes serve as control observations.

Genetic damage may be transmitted through both sexes and would have short and long-term components. The short-term effects would be similar to those described above and represent essentially the dominant lethals. These are more transient and largely eliminated via successive germ cell cycles of replenishment. Long-term mutation rate changes are extremely difficult to detect except under rigorous conditions of genetic ascertainment and are, therefore, not expected to be quickly or easily derived.

These rather straightforward observations on reproductive performance all involve measures routinely made on hospital deliveries. They include— in addition to the prenatal and perinatal losses—birth-weight, congenital malformation or defect (single and multiple), and diseases or difficulties involving the respiratory, gastro-intestinal, genito-urinary, and hemato-poietic systems. Although there is a prospective epidemiologic aspect to this surveillance, it can be of short duration and involve routine observation and, therefore, need not be economically demanding. There is considerable normal variation in these measures of reproductive performance, so any set of observations should involve adequate samples; many hundreds to thousands of events may need study if significant deviations are to be detected. Therefore, reproductive history examinations are not recommended for those cases of occupational exposure where no reasonable teratogenic or mutagenic threat is conceivable. However, for the case of a new use for an old compound, the retrospective analysis of such reproductive records may be appropriate.

Carcinogenesis

The demonstration of the relationship between cigarette smoking and lung cancer is a striking example of the importance of human surveillance for the study of cancer in man. Other less publicized clinical and epidemiological studies of human populations have led to the identification of a variety of carcinogenic substances in man's environment, and full utilization of already existing data sources should be most productive in the future. Two major efforts should be made in this regard. First, study of well-defined occupational groups should be undertaken on a large scale to identify previously unsuspected carcinogenic hazards. Second, special surveys should be made of occupational groups employed in the production and use of agents identified as potential carcinogens through chemical and biological screening.

Other Toxicologic Studies of Humans

The Environmental Protection Agency has broad responsibilities for evaluation and control, which extend beyond the limits required by legislation on toxic substances: Here, also, information on toxicity to man may be obtained by epidemiologic methods. Study opportunities similar to those available in the occupational health field and others of a different nature are available for use. Some such studies have been carried out by or for government agencies, and the experience gained forms a valuable base for further work. It is particularly important to make use of existing situations in which the effects of low and moderate exposure levels over long periods may be evaluated. A program of such studies to supplement the work generated by toxic substances legislation should be undertaken. Since other agencies—for example, NIOSH, the National Institutes of Health (NIH), FDA, and the Atomic Energy Commission (AEC)—are also interested in such studies, coordination would be required. Some possibly useful opportunities are considered below.

Accidental exposures to toxic substances frequently occur outside industry. They are usually not studied carefully, or, if studied, the useful toxicologic information obtained is not made accessible or optimally used. Follow-up for study of residual injury is rarely done either at the time, or later by reconstructing a previously exposed group for evaluation. Methods of making better use of these opportunities should be explored.

Many situations exist in which groups outside of industry are exposed to hazardous or possibly hazardous substances over long periods due to location of residence, differences in mode of living, pursuit of hobbies, unusual food or water sources, etc. Some of these have, of course, been studied, but many others still await exploitation. They are particularly useful for the evaluation of prolonged exposures above the usual level. Such information is needed for regulatory action. An important resource for such investigations is the Committee on Epidemiology and Veterans Follow-Up Studies of the National Research Council.

Toxicologic screens cannot be considered infallible, nor do we have screening systems in all hazardous areas. Therefore, watchfulness and alertness for trouble are constantly needed. A generation ago and earlier, much effort was expended to increase and improve health record systems for various uses. One of these uses was to analyze health records for indications of excessive unexpected illness in time, place or group. Vital record units are currently so preoccupied with maintenance and routine reports that special studies are rarely done. It is currently fashionable to discourage systematic exploration of existing records for discrepant occurrences by terming such work "fishing expeditions." Nevertheless we need a program that exploits morbidity and mortality data systems for useful clues to the existence of unrecognized important hazards. All localized phenomena found will not be of environmental origin, of course, but many will be.

In recent decades a number of unexpected epidemics of disease from toxic chemicals have been found, for example, thalidomide and tri-orthocresyl phosphate. All, or nearly all, of these have been found in-itially by alert medical practitioners. A modest center for reporting sus-pect observations, investigating these, and stimulating such reporting would be desirable. At present this is our most clearly functinal warning source. Previously, there were organized activities which acted as a focus for the collection of such episodic data—for example, the Epidemic In-telligence Service of the Public Health Service (PHS). However, such activities have essentially lapsed. It would be worthwhile attempting to reactivate these programs with this particular end in mind.

Another aspect of the problem is that the environmental effects phenomena searched for may occur but may be extremely difficult to isolate. Analytic studies of data that can be assembled from existing records are very difficult because the population is very mobile in a country such as the United States and vital records are kept by multiple jurisdictions. Analytic studies would be greatly facilitated if appropriate record linkages were established. For example, if Social Security Ad-ministration files were to be used as a ready means of follow-up for par-ticular cohorts of interest and death were the outcome under investiga-tion, the fact of death could be determined only if the state in which it occurred is known to the investigator. While alphabetical indices of death are maintained by the various health departments, there is no national centralization of these indices. A central national index that provided the identifying information necessary to locate the death certificate filed in the states and other registration areas would greatly facilitate those studies where the outcome of concern involved a high probability of death. This matter was somewhat more comprehensively discussed in the 1970 Report of the Task Force on Research Planning in Environ-mental Health Science, *Man's Health and the Environment—Some Re-search Needs* (Nelson, 1970).

UTILIZATION OF CHRONIC TOXICITY DATA

The toxicologist's task is a deliberate professional assessment of those fac-tors that define the chemical–biological interaction and their considered utilization in chronic studies. Using these data, public policy makers will determine whether this margin of safety is acceptable. This determination utimately will revolve about the need or importance of a chemical in the promotion and maintenance of society's well-being.

When the toxicity or epidemiological studies are completed, the data derived are used in defining the margin of safety between the highest level for which no adverse effect was observed in groups of suitable size and the anticipated level of public exposure. Such values must also take into account possible excursions above these anticipated levels, which arise from misuse or poorly controlled applications, as well as a judgment as to the range of susceptibility in exposed populations.

SUMMARY

Generally speaking, the classical chronic toxicity test is supported as the only available technique for assessment of long-term human health hazards. This approach involves studies in two or more species of animals for long periods of time at several dosage levels. A detailed list of the principal considerations used in planning the chronic study are presented. A variety of specific tests, especially histopathology, conducted at various time intervals throughout the study allow assessment of anatomical and functional changes. The species used should be those which will provide the most reliable data for predicting human effects. Dosage level selection should permit the development of a dose–response curve. With this information, a professional should be then able to arrive at estimates of human health hazards and anticipated exposure levels.

Emphasis is placed on appropriate human data where available. The value and limitations of clinical and/or epidemiological data are discussed.

REFERENCES

Beaconsfield, P., R. Rainsbury, and G. Kalton. 1965. Glucose-6-phosphate dehydrogenase deficiency and the incidence of cancer. *Oncologia (Basel)* 19:11–19.

Cornish, H.H. 1971. Problems posed by observations of serum enzyme changes in toxicology. *Crit. Rev. Toxicol.* 1:1–32.

Grice, H.C. 1972. The changing role of pathology in modern safety evaluation. *Crit. Rev. Toxicol.* 1:119–152.

McKusick, V.A. 1970. Human genetics. *Ann. Rev. Genet.* 4:1–46.

Nelson, N., *Chairman.* 1970. *Man's Health and the Environment—Some Research Needs.* Report of the Task Force on Research Planning in Environmental Health Science. National Institute of Environmental Health Sciences, U.S. Department of Health, Education, and Welfare. U.S. Government Printing Office, Washington, D.C.

Stokinger, H.E., and J.T. Mountain. 1963. Test for hypersusceptibility to hemolytic chemicals. *Arch. Environ. Health* 6:495–502.

SUGGESTED READINGS

Barnes, J.M., and F.A. Denz. 1954. Experimental methods used in determining chronic toxicity. A critical review. *Pharmacol. Rev.* 6:191–242.

Beyer, K.H., Jr. 1966. Perspectives in toxicology. *Toxicol. Appl. Pharmacol.* 8:1–5.

Boyd, E.M. 1968. Predictive drug toxicity: Assessment of drug safety before human use. *Can. Med. Assoc. J.* 98:278–293.

Brodie, B.B. 1964. Kinetics of absorption, distribution, excretion, and metabolism of drugs. In Nodine, J.H., and P.E. Siegler, eds., *Animal and Clinical Pharmacologic Techniques in Drug Evaluation.* Year Book Medical Publishers, Chicago. pp. 69–88.

Detweiler, D.K., and D.F. Patterson. 1965. The prevalence and types of cardiovascular disease in dogs. *Ann. N.Y. Acad. Sci.* 127:481–516.

Dixon, R.L., R.W. Shultice, and J.R. Fouts. 1960. Factors affecting drug metabolism by liver microsomes. IV. Starvation. *Proc. Soc. Exp. Biol. Med.* 103:333–335.

Fitzhugh, O.G. 1955. Procedures for the appraisal of the toxicity of chemicals in foods, drugs and cosmetics—chronic oral toxicity. *Food, Drug Cosmet. Law J.* 16:712–719.

Goldenthal, E.I. 1968. Current views on safety evaluation of drugs. *FDA Pap.* 2(4):13–18.

Gay, W.I., ed. 1965. *Methods of Animal Experimentation.* Vols. 1, 2. Academic Press, New York.

Herrick, A.D., and M. Cattell, eds. 1965. *Clinical Testing of New Drugs.* Revere Publishing, New York.

Laurence, D.R., and A.L. Bacharach, eds. 1964. *Evaluation of Drug Activities: Pharmacometrics.* Vols. 1, 2. Academic Press, New York.

Mantegazza, P., and F. Piccinini, eds. 1966. *Methods in drug evaluation.* Proceedings of the International Symposium held in Milano, 20–23 Sept. 1965. North-Holland Publishing Co., Amsterdam.

National Academy of Sciences–National Research Council. Food Protection Committee. 1960. *Principles and Procedures for Evaluating the Safety of Food Additives.* NAS–NRC Publ. No. 750. National Academy of Sciences, Washington, D.C.

Paget, G.E., ed. 1970. *Methods in Toxicology.* F.A. Davis Co., Philadelphia.

Peck, H.M. 1966. Evaluating the safety of drugs. *BioScience* 16:696–701.

Rašková, H., ed. 1968. *Mechanism of Drug Toxicity.* Proceedings of the Third International Pharmacological Meeting, São Paulo, 24–30 July 1966. Pergamon Press, Oxford.

Ribelin, W.E., and J.R. McCoy, eds. 1965. *The Pathology of Laboratory Animals.* Charles C Thomas, Springfield, Ill.

World Health Organization. 1966. *Principles for Pre-Clinical Testing of Drug Safety.* ITS Tech. Rep. Ser. No. 341. Geneva.

IX

Chemical
Carcinogenesis

A variety of agents, including ultraviolet light and ionizing radiation, certain viruses, and many different chemical moieties, are known to cause cancer in experimental animals. There is strong reason to believe that a high proportion of cancer in humans is due to environmental factors (Searle, 1970). Whether these act alone or in concert with viruses has not been established. Nevertheless, while most human cancers are of unknown etiology, we have come to regard cancer as a disease with definite environmental causes and one that can largely be prevented by suitable action. The first line of defense against cancer is to identify carcinogens in the environment and, by appropriate measures, to eliminate or reduce their presence to minimum levels.

The procedures for evaluating the carcinogenic potential of chemicals have been reviewed several times during the past decade by national and international advisory groups (Consultative Panel on Carcinogenesis on Environmental Carcinogenic Risks, 1968; NAS–NRC, 1969; WHO, 1969; Berenblum, 1969; FDA, 1971; *Ad Hoc* Committee on the Evaluation of Low Levels of Environmental Chemical Carcinogens, 1971). As indicated in the introduction to this section of the report, the induction of tumors is a chronic response; that is, observations on animals exposed to single or repeated dosing must usually continue for long periods of time because of the long latency period in the development of tumors. Thus, carcinogenesis bioassay is, in a sense, a chronic toxicity study. However, the special nature of these observations and the gravity of this disease are such that special emphasis must be placed upon this extremely important topic. Progress in the field of cancer research and the experience from programs of carcinogen bioassay make it necessary to frequently reconsider the principles and details of procedures of this problem.

LONG-TERM BIOASSAYS

Choice of Species

It has generally been accepted that rodents represent the only feasible test system for large-scale screening. This is based not so much on the established similarities of rodents to man, or on a biochemical, physiological or anatomical basis, but rather on the feasibility of testing large numbers of compounds in a comparatively short time. Experience has shown that the rat, mouse, and Syrian hamster are the genera of choice. Experience has also shown that carcinogenic screening in rodents gives reliable identification of carcinogenic materials, although the tumors observed in rodents are not necessarily found in the same tissues or organs in other species. The dog is of limited utility as a test animal, since a positive test may take 7 years or more. The susceptibility of simians to chemical carcinogenesis has been established for several species and for several groups of chemicals, but again the long latency period, particularly before negative results can be evaluated, argues against their routine use for carcinogenesis screening.

Choice of Strain

In screening bioassays the randomly bred animal is preferred over the inbred animal. However, inbreds are recommended for specific bioassay of compounds belonging to chemical groups previously tested in specific inbred strains. There is reliable information on these special strains for several tissues including the mammary, respiratory, and lymphatic systems.

Mode of Administration

The route of administration generally should be the same as the route by which man receives the compound. The mouse skin is suitable for testing compounds for skin carcinogenesis. The oral route is preferred for chemicals that man will receive in his food. Administration in the diet is preferred to oral intubation, which is, however, very useful in certain circumstances. It is important to recognize that dietary factors, such as lipids, can result in different rates of absorption in animals and man and, in other ways, modify the carcinogenic response to a given agent.

For the bioassay of material in which the normal route of entry is through inhalation, administration to the respiratory tract should be included in the screening system. This is essential because a given agent may be peculiarly capable of eliciting tumors in the respiratory organs, or, conversely, the respiratory tract—by virtue of its defense mechanisms— may be refractory to tumors induced by a particular agent. Three methods of exposure are applicable:

1. exposure by inhalation;
2. instillation of the material by means of intratracheal injection; and
3. introduction of the material by implantation (e.g., impregnated pellet).

Inhalation exposure is the most natural method of exposure of the respiratory tract. However, physiological and anatomical differences between test species and man preclude direct extrapolation to man of data on inhalation of particulates by animals. This method has been relatively unproductive in demonstrating the carcinogenic effect of even the most potent hydrocarbon carcinogens administered alone in high concentrations over long periods. Thus, its applicability as a routine bioassay method for environmental carcinogens appears limited. Its routine use should probably be reserved for more definitive evaluation of substances that have been shown by other means to have carcinogenic potential for the pulmonary tract.

Intratracheal injections permit repeated application of controlled doses of test material for long periods of time. Evaluation of the influence of cocarcinogenic factors can be carried out by introduction of material with the suspected carcinogen or, in the case of volatile or gaseous agents, concomitant inhalation exposure. Objections have been made to this method on the grounds of dose variability from site to site within the lung and production of foci of chronic inflammation due to the presence of sequestered particles.

Incorporation of the test material into a substance such as beeswax, with subsequent implantation into the lung tissue, assures continuous application as the agent is eluted gradually from the pellet. This method is, of course, inapplicable for gases and volatile liquids. It has been widely used for lung tumor induction by benzo[a]pyrene and 7,12-dimethylbenz[a]anthracene when introduced with large amounts of particulate matter (e.g., iron oxide (Fe_2O_3) or carbon particles). The introduction of the particles with the tumorigenic agent appears to increase the likelihood of a positive outcome. Squamous tumors of the larynx, trachea, and bronchi, together with tumors of other cell types, have been induced by these techniques.

In contrast to the above dosing methods, the subcutaneous route of administration has certain advantages and should not be ignored. Although it is less readily extrapolated to conditions of exposure encountered by man, it allows the testing of chemicals available only in small amounts and requires minimal handling of the animals. Sarcoma production at the injection site leaves little ambiguity regarding its relation to the injected chemical. The question of whether or not the carcinogenic effect may be the result of introduction of a solid material that, by its physical properties, may cause the neoplastic response can be answered by study of appropriate controls, the nature of the injected material, and the histopathology of tissue at the site of injection.

Characterization of the Animal

It is essential to maintain animals in a good state of health and to monitor this by observations on weight gain and food utilization. The viral profile of the test animal may be of value when comparing results in different laboratories.

The hormonal status of the test animal is important since the induction of many experimental tumors is hormone dependent. Depression of immunological tolerance by cortisol and other immunosuppressants frequently enhances carcinogenesis.

Consideration should be given to the comparability of absorption, retention, distribution, metabolism and elimination of the chemical in the test species and in man in order to develop confidence in extrapolation of animal data to man.

The exposure of the test animal should encompass most of the total life span. However, termination of the test and control animals is recommended when the cumulative mortality reaches 75 percent. Care must be exercised to avoid autolysis; moribund animals should be killed, rather than allowed to die.

It is of interest that some experiments started on 1-, 1½-, and 2-year-old rats indicated a comparable lung tumor incidence in all groups, even though the life expectancy of the older group was much shorter. This observation must be kept in mind when considerations of latency period are being made. In other experiments, the older animals were equally or more resistant.

Histopathology

Regardless of the bioassay method, the decision as to whether the lesion produced is cancerous or noncancerous is dependent upon morphologic criteria. Such decisions are not always clear-cut, and a large element of individual judgment based on experience in tumor diagnosis is required. However, familiarity with a particular experimental model is very helpful in arriving at the diagnosis of malignancy in experimentally induced tumors.

The decision of whether a lesion is benign, precancerous, or malignant is based on (1) the morphologic character of the tumor mass in question, i.e., variation in size and cell appearance, increase in number of mitoses, presence of abnormal mitoses and degree of variation from normal in the organizational pattern of the cells; and (2) invasion of the capsule or surrounding tissue or metastases to distant points. Distinguishing squamous metaplasia from squamous cancers and unraveling the many hyperplastic states induced by chronic inflammatory effects due to toxic substances must be accomplished, not only by careful attention to histologic criteria, but also by following the biological event to its eventual termination in any particular model. Pulmonary and hepatic adenomas are particularly difficult, and the investigator must not only distinguish between benign adenoma and carcinoma, but he must also pinpoint the progression from adenoma to carcinoma. The weight to be given to multiple pulmonary adenomas as contrasted to solitary adenomas in the lung should be stated in the experimental protocol and systematic criteria worked out in advance.

Considerable differences exist between various species of rodents and specific inbred strains regarding the incidence of spontaneous benign neoplasms: For instance, A-strain mice commonly develop pulmonary adenomas, whereas C57B1 mice do not. Hamsters are singularly free of such lesions. In tumor bioassays in rats involving the lung, characterization of malignant lesions is complicated by the presence of chronic pneumonitis; thus, it is important, where possible, to obtain animals of known source, free of complicating disease, and virus-defined for cancer bioassays and to become familiar with the biological peculiarities of the particular species and strain being used.

Data Collection

It is impossible to have too much data. The minimum requirements for data collection as outlined in the UICC technical report (Berenblum, 1969) are recommended. When tumors can be observed by inspection or palpation, thrice weekly examination provides the most careful check.

This, together with weekly weighings, provides a reasonable and careful evaluation of the general health of the animal and its response to the test material locally and systemically; it also forewarns the investigator that death may be impending, thereby permitting a careful autopsy without autolysis.

TRANSPLACENTAL CARCINOGENESIS

Prenatal determinants of cancer in man have long been suspected. This suspicion has been based upon (1) the occurrence of congenital cancer—tumors that grow to large size *in utero*, (2) peaks in mortality soon after birth, primarily for cancers of the same cell type as occur congenitally (e.g., teratoma, neuroblastoma, primary liver cancers, Wilms' tumor and leukemia), (3) the concurrence of certain cancers and congenital malformations, and (4) an increase in childhood leukemia related to high maternal age or low birth order. Whether specific chemicals pass the placental barrier to produce these effects in man is unknown. However, a most dramatic development was recently reported by Herbst *et al.* (1971a). In retrospective epidemiological studies, stilbestrol therapy during pregnancy was shown to induce clear-cell adenocarcinoma of the vagina of the daughter 14–22 years later (Greenwald *et al.*, 1971; Herbst *et al.*, 1971b).

Transplacental carcinogenesis is a well-recognized phenomenon in experimental animals exposed to appropriate agents *in utero*, especially direct-acting alkylating agents such as alkylnitrosoureas. Dunn and Green (1963) observed cancer of the vagina and other sites in mice after a single dose of diethylstilbestrol given at birth. The class of organic nitroso compounds has been found to include many potent carcinogens (Druckrey *et al.*, 1967; Magee and Barnes, 1967). This class of compounds is of particular significance to man since it has been shown in rodents that these compounds may be formed *in vivo* by reaction of nitrite ion and secondary (or tertiary) amines and amides in the gastrointestinal tract in amounts sufficient for carcinogenesis in distant organs (Sander and Buerkle, 1969; Sander, 1970) or for transplacental passage to the fetus, with subsequent development of tumors after birth (Ivankovic and Preussmann, 1970).

Many substances that are potent carcinogens in adult animals are weakly active transplacentally because they require enzyme-mediated metabolic conversion into reactive intermediates, and these may not be formed in fetal tissues due to lack of the necessary enzymes.

Genetics plays a crucial role in determining what tumors will result from exposure to a carcinogen. In most of the transplacental experiments performed in rodent species, the major types of induced tumors have been essentially the same as those found in the same species of animals treated during adult life. These constitute a spectrum of organ specificities and histological patterns characteristic of each species. Thus, transplacental ethylnitrosourea in the rat causes neurogenic tumors, especially gliomas and schwannomas (Ivankovic and Druckrey, 1968), while in the mouse the same compound yields principally lung tumors, hepatomas and lymphomas (Rice, 1969), but very few neurogenic tumors (Searle and Jones, 1972). It is not established that the human tumors most characteristic of infancy and childhood—neuroblastoma, retinoblastoma, Wilms' tumor—can result from prenatal exposure to chemicals. However, Wilms' tumor is associated with a spectrum of non-inherited developmental anomalies (Miller *et al.*, 1964), and statistical studies have suggested that both retinoblastoma and Wilms' tumor may result from two successive mutations possibly caused by exogenous agents, the first of which can involve either germinal or somatic cells (Knudson, 1971; Knudson and Strong, 1972).

A representative list of transplacental carcinogens is provided in Table 5. A substantial proportion of these compounds, especially methylmethanesulfonate and the alkylnitrosoureas, are also potent mutagens. Chemicals whose structures do not suggest carcinogenic activity *a priori* have been found to be transplacental carcinogens, presumably as a result of metabolic transformation to reactive compounds.

Relatively few substances have been tested adequately for transplacental carcinogenic activity, and no studies have been reported in simians or carnivores. In the rodents, however, a frequent finding has been that latency periods for many types of tumors are not greatly reduced from those expected in animals exposed to carcinogens in adult life, and often comprise more than half the normal life spans of rats and mice. Obviously, then, transplacentally treated offspring must be kept for their lifetime, or at least 18–24 months, in order to evaluate their responses properly.

Animal testing for transplacental carcinogenesis is not yet at a reliable state of predictability for human risk. Surveillance of human cancer occurrence should reveal exceptional clustering such as the above mentioned cases of vaginal cancer. A tumor registry data bank is the only present hope of identifying compounds not now under suspicion in human oncogenesis. These observations in man then lend themselves to hypotheses that can be tested in the laboratory so that ultimately a testing procedure may be available.

CHEMICAL AND PHYSICAL PROPERTIES

In testing any material for possible carcinogenic effect, it is most desirable to know the actual chemical composition of the material in ques-

TABLE 5   Transplacental Carcinogens and Target Organs

Compound	Species	Target Organ	Reference
Ethyl carbamate (urethan)	Mouse	Ovary	Vesselinovitch *et al.* (1967)
	Mouse	Lung	Larsen (1947); Smith and Rous (1948)
Propylnitrosourea	Rat	Nervous system	Ivankovic and Zeller (1972)
Ethylnitrosourea	Rat	Nervous system	Ivankovic and Druckrey (1968)
	Mouse	Lung, liver	Rice (1969)
	Mouse	Nervous system	Searle and Jones (1972)
Methylnitrosourea	Rat	Nervous system	Jänisch *et al.* (1972)
Methylnitrosourethan	Rat	Multiple	Tanaka (1973)
Diethylnitrosamine	Rat	Kidney	Wrba *et al.* (1967)
	Mouse	Lung	Likhachev (1971)
Dimethylnitrosamine	Rat	Kidney	Alexandrov (1968)
Cycasin (methylazoxy-methyl-β-D-glucoside)	Rat	Jejunum; multiple	Spatz and Laqueur (1967)
1,2-Diethyl-hydrazine azoethane azoxyethane	Rat	Nervous system	Druckrey et al. (1968)
Benzo[*a*]pyrene	Mouse	Lung, skin	Bulay and Wattenberg (1970)
Methyl methanesulfonate	Rat	Nervous system	Kleihues *et al.* (1972)
Diethylstilbestrol	Human	Vagina	Herbst *et al.* (1971a,b)

tion. Such knowledge will not only increase the reliability of the conclusions, but also will help furnish leads concerning compounds of similar structure. Many commercial compounds of environmental importance are diluted with stabilizers, extenders or fillers, or contain impurities from the manufacturing process. It is desirable to test the compounds as they are used commercially.

Vehicles

Controls receiving vehicle alone are always necessary. If the materials being tested for carcinogenicity are not water soluble, a uniform suspension in steroid suspending vehicle (SSV) or Klucel may be indicated.

However, it must be kept in mind that suspending vehicles usually contain a hydroxycellulose and/or a polysorbate (Tween) of some type and these can enhance the effect of some carcinogens (Niskanen, 1962).

Food oils are useful for less-soluble materials. The oils should be fresh, obtained in sufficient quantity for the entire study if possible, and stored in a freezer to prevent deterioration. Some food oils contain antifreeze materials and antioxidants, which may affect the action of the test compounds. Cottonseed oil, unless refined by superheated steam processing, may contain cyclopropenoid fatty acids, which can enhance the activity of some carcinogens (Lee *et al.*, 1968). Sesame oil that contains methylenedioxybenzene compounds may also act as a promoter of carcinogenesis (Morton and Mider, 1939). Therefore, controls receiving vehicle alone may not always be adequate for proper comparison.

Some of these variables may be overcome by using a properly purified synthetic oil like trioctanoin. However, some commercial lots of this material are toxic and samples should be checked before use in animal studies. Certain oily vehicles are digested slowly, thus releasing the material dissolved in them to the test animal's system at a slow rate.

Acetone and dimethyl sulfoxide are often used for skin painting experiments since they promote skin absorption and are of low toxicity. Dimethyl sulfoxide is not metabolically inert; animals so treated excrete some of it in the form of dimethyl sulfide.

Stability of Chemicals

The type of decomposition product obviously differs for each chemical: Aromatic amines oxidize to quinone imines; hydrocarbons to keto compounds; in the presence of light, dialkylnitrosamines undergo photolysis, producing oximes. Some of the alkylating or acylating agents, in the presence of moisture, will hydrolyze to inactive compounds. For example, β-propiolactone hydrolyzes to inactive 3-hydroxypropionic acid; N-mustards give hydroxylalkylamines. Certain environmental chemicals, specifically the bis-ethylenedithiocarbamates (agricultural fungicides), spontaneously decompose forming ethylene thiourea, which is a thyroid carcinogen. Aromatic amines are more stable as their salts.

Proper storage of carcinogens—generally in a dry, cold, dark place in an inert atmosphere (argon or nitrogen)—will retard decomposition.

Stability in Vehicle for Administration

Any compound likely to undergo hydrolysis should be administered in a nonaqueous medium. Preferably, solutions should be made up fresh for each administration unless the stability of the compound in the vehicle has been demonstrated. The stability of compounds that are mixed in the diet should also be monitored. In many cases, determining stability in the diet may involve a new set of analytical problems.

Evaluation of Priorities in Bioassay

Overall priorities in bioassay should be given to those substances which are most likely to make contact with the greatest number of people most frequently, i.e., to those which are widely used and appear in many products to which people are exposed. Persistence in the environment, especially if the compound finds its way to man through the food chain, must also be considered.

The chemical structure of the material and its similarity to known chemical carcinogens should be taken into account. Structure–activity correlations and a knowledge of what functional groups are associated with carcinogenicity of the molecule can furnish some leads concerning suspect compounds. However, total reliance on structure–activity relationships as an index of carcinogenic risk is a hazardous venture. If the only reason for testing a material of little environmental importance is that its structure is closely akin to that of a known carcinogen, it is not necessary to give it high priority for testing.

As more information on new structures becomes available, the old guidelines must often be discarded: For instance, it was once assumed that to be carcinogenic, an aromatic amine needed at least two aromatic rings. Now, more thorough tests of the simpler aromatic amines have shown that such a premise does not hold. Similarly, tests of fairly simple aliphatic substances have shown that they can be very active carcinogens in certain cases, for example, bis(chloromethyl)ether (Van Duuren *et al.*, 1972).

The subject of molecular geometry and carcinogenic activity of various aromatic and heterocyclic compounds has been extensively reviewed (Arcos and Argus, 1968). The comprehensive paper on 65 *N*-nitroso compounds (Druckrey *et al.*, 1967) affords some leads as to which structures are more likely to be active. Despite the deficiencies, a few simple leads can be summarized for classes of compounds:

1. Aromatic amines—If the amino group is in the most reactive or more readily substituted position of the aromatic nucleus, the compound is more likely to be carcinogenic than if the amino group is in another position. Amino groups adjacent to a ring annulation are less likely to be associated with carcinogenic activity. Blocking a position usually involved

in metabolic hydroxylation of an aromatic amine by a methoxy, fluoro, or methyl group can yield a more carcinogenic substance.

2. Amino azo dyes—Blocking certain positions of the rings can also enhance hepatocarcinogenic potency.

3. Polycyclic aromatic hydrocarbons—Linear condensed hydrocarbons are noncarcinogenic; those with a small number of rings (3 or less) and those with too large a molecular size (approximately 120 Å^2) are not active.

4. N-Nitroso compounds—Symmetrical and unsymmetrical dialkyl-nitrosamines are active; activity decreases as the length of alkyl chain increases. Diarylnitrosamines are inactive. Nitroso-alkyl or aryl ureas and amides are active, except for p-tolylsulfonyl-N-methyl-N-nitrosamide.

Aziridines, especially those with simple structures, are often carcinogens. Alkyl diepoxides and strained lactones or sultones—such as β-propiolactone or propane sultone—are active carcinogens. Thio compounds are suspect, as in the case of alkylthioureas and thioacetamide (but not diphenylthiourea).

Many compounds that have pronounced alkylating activity, for example, nitrogen or sulfur mustards, chloromethyl ether, and activated halo-compounds, are carcinogenic.

Only actual testing of a substance will establish its carcinogenicity. Experience can only yield an educated guess.

SHORT-TERM BIOASSAYS

In vivo *Testing: Sebaceous Gland Suppression and Hyperplasia*

Although the reaction of sebaceous glands to carcinogens was examined (Suntzeff *et al.*, 1955) and then abandoned, Chouroulinkov *et al.* (1969) have refined and standardized it for the study of potential carcinogens in tobacco smoke condensate and were able to show excellent dose–response relationships. This test may be useful also for the study of potential carcinogens for the skin. At present it can only be considered as a possible screening test for topically applied chemicals with carcinogenic potential.

In vitro *Testing: Cell Transformation and Mutagenesis*

Cell Transformation   At this stage of cancer research, it should be feasible to use cell transformation *in vitro* as one type of screening procedure to detect compounds and classes of compounds with potential carcinogenic activity. The assays can provide preliminary evidence of the need for further testing *in vivo*, if one is aware of the drawbacks as well as the advantages.

It is almost 10 years since the original demonstration (Berwald and Sachs, 1965) of a quantitative *in vitro* assay for chemical carcinogens. Since that time the conditions of the assay have been more precisely defined and expanded (DiPaolo *et al.*, 1971; 1972a) and several other quantitative assays have been developed (Chen and Heidelberger, 1969; DiPaolo *et al.*, 1972b). The use of such assays for studying the mechanisms of chemical as well as viral carcinogenesis is now generally accepted. Scoring of transformation is based on morphologic criteria with confirmation by transplantation into homologous hosts or immuno-depressed heterologous hosts.

Unlike oncogenic viruses, which induce virus-specific functions that can be followed biochemically and immunologically as adjuncts to morphologic screening of virus-cell interaction, chemical carcinogens do not yet offer such aids in quantitating their effects. The use of strictly morphologic changes for scoring transformation has been criticized in the past because it did not always correlate with transplantability; however, within a single assay system, these instances are probably rare.

There are essentially two types of tissue culture—organ culture in which fragments of whole tissue, generally from a single organ, are maintained, and cultures of single dispersed cells, which adhere to a glass or plastic surface and grow as monolayers. Organ cultures have been useful for studying the histologic effects of carcinogens on different cells in a whole tissue. Although hyperplasia frequently has been observed, there have been only a few reports of the induction in organ culture of cell transformation in which target cells produced carcinomas when transplanted into homologous hosts (Flaks and Laws, 1968; Dao and Sinha, 1972).

Although monolayer cultures involve the loss of the integrity of whole tissue, they would seem to be preferable for screening procedures because they are less time-consuming to set up and easier to score, and there is still only scant evidence that transformation can be readily achieved in differentiated cells in an organ culture.

Since various chemical carcinogens have different target cells *in vivo*, different cell types may have to be included in a screening system using monolayer cultures. However, if cell specificity *in vivo* is due to the physiologic function of the organ rather than the cell, the requirement for a specific cell type will be of less concern.

Primary cultures of whole embryos or single organs will have the greatest variety of cell types to serve as target cells, although assays based on their use are more difficult to reproduce consistently and to score by morphologic criteria. The use of established cell lines avoids these pit-falls but introduces the disadvantages of providing a single type of target cell, the possible loss of differentiated properties that may be involved in activation of the carcinogen, and the occurrence of spontaneous trans-formation in the untreated cell population.

Whether primary cultures or established cell lines have been used, the target cells in the quantitative assays currently being employed have been fibroblasts that, when inoculated into animals after transformation, produce sarcomas. This is apparently independent of whether or not the carcinogen is organ-specific *in vivo*. Whether this will be true of all car-cinogens cannot be stated at this time.

Recently it has been possible to establish primary and continuous cul-tures of differentiated mammary and liver epithelium (Lasfargues and Moore, 1971; Buehring, 1972; Potter, 1972). While many organ-specific functions may be lost in such cultures, the liver cells, for example, do produce carcinomas *in vivo* when inoculated after spontaneous or car-cinogen-induced transformation (Oshiro *et al.*, 1972; Williams *et al.*, 1973). These developments hold promise that, in the near future, cul-tures will be available for quantitative transformation assays in specific differentiated target cells.

The probable presence of latent viruses, especially of the RNA-contain-ing C-type group, in most, if not all tissues should not in itself be a de-terrent to the use of *in vitro* assay procedures any more than it is a deter-rent in *in vivo* assays. There are now available highly sensitive tests for assaying various virus-specific functions so that the indicator cells used in screening can be monitored, if desired.

As assay procedure developed for screening purposes is not necessarily dependent on understanding the mechanisms involved. There are several reports that cells infected with exogenous leukemia virus or shedding endogenous virus are more susceptible to chemically induced transforma-tion than cells which are not synthesizing virus (Freeman *et al.*, 1971). This may or may not be a direct effect of the virus, but it does indicate that the more sensitive infected cells may be preferable for screening purposes.

Furthermore, it has recently been shown that the synthesis of virus antigens and complete infectious virus can be induced in noninfectious normal cells by treatment with mutagens or carcinogens (Weiss, *et al.*, 1971; Teich, *et al.*, 1973). Again the mechanism is not known, but this property of carcinogens might also be exploited in a screening system.

Since many carcinogens require metabolic activation to the ultimate carcinogen, transformation assays done in cells lacking the required en-zymatic activity may give false negative results. This may be overcome by (1) including enzyme inducers in the cultures, (2) cocultivating the indicator cells with irradiated cells possessing enzymatic activity, or (3) exposing the test cells to the carcinogen during fetal life *in utero* (Marquardt and Heidelberger, 1972; DiPaolo *et al.*, 1972a). One should be aware, however, that both *in vitro* and *in vivo* there is undoubtedly a very delicate balance between metabolic activation and inactivation of a carcinogen, and that whether or not enzyme induction will inhibit or en- hance transformation will depend on the interaction of many factors— the carcinogen, the cells, the inducer, the time schedule, etc.

Mutagenesis   The question of whether or not a mutagenic event is a req- uisite for carcinogenesis is a long-standing one. Although many mutagens had been shown to be carcinogenic, other known carcinogens were shown *not* to be mutagenic. Recent experiments in which the activated forms of carcinogens were used have indicated a greater correlation between mutagenesis and carcinogenesis than was indicated previously (Corbett *et al.*, 1970; Ames *et al.*, 1972a, b). Consequently, interest has been re- vived in the possibility that all carcinogens are mutagens and that assays for mutagenicity can be used for preliminary screening of potential car- cinogens. At this time, however, the demonstration that a particular com- pound has mutagenic activity can be considered, in terms of carcino- genicity, as merely indicative of potential reactivity with host cell DNA. The compound should thus be given priority status for testing for car- cinogenic activity.

MODIFYING FACTORS

This topic is of importance in extrapolating carcinogenesis data regarding the hazard to man's health; unfortunately, it depends on varied mecha- nisms and defies analysis. Yet, this problem will frequently prevent the consideration of a no-effect threshold. In animal experiments, most studies have been focused on mouse skin, where the carcinogenic effect of a polycylcic hydrocarbon can be significantly enhanced by application of plant products such as croton oil (Mottram, 1944). The same effect, however, can also be produced by painting the skin with a simple hydro- carbon, like dodecane, a common constituent of petroleum (Horton *et al.*, 1957).

Other noncarcinogenic chemicals have been identified that can potenti- ate the carcinogenic response as much as 1000-fold (Bingham and Falk, 1969). This enhancing effect is not limited to a specific type of carcinogen or a unique tissue, but has been observed for tissues other than the skin.

So far, no acceptable short-term test for cocarcinogenesis has been developed; however, the long-term tests can be modified since the effect is noted when the latency period is shortened. Thus, an end point, at less than a year or so, is attainable.

It is known that precancerous changes associated with cocarcinogenesis are reversible. Therefore, their early recognition and attempts at their control in the environmental situation are of utmost concern.

Carcinogenesis is dependent, in part, on overcoming normal protective mechanisms that rid the organism of foreign materials. The physiologic importance of removal of foreign matter from the lungs by mucus secretion and ciliary action or by phagocytosis is familiar. That these mechanisms can be impaired on exposure to various environmental toxicants has been well documented.

The process of enzyme induction of nonspecific oxidases and conjugases, a mechanism which allows for ready elimination of foreign chemicals, is not always to the advantage of the organism. This is particularly true when the metabolic product is a carcinogen. Conversely, chemicals that will inhibit enzyme induction include the economically useful pesticide synergists (Falk and Kotin, 1969). Other inhibitors, such as carbon monoxide, exert their effect on cytochrome P_{450}, an essential cofactor for certain induced enzymes (Estabrook et al., 1963).

The process of DNA repair, which normally is quite efficient in excising altered nucleotide sequences, can be inhibited by certain chemicals. These have, so far, not been studied in detail, and it is likely that some environmental chemicals will be found to block repair enzymes (Gaudin et al., 1971).

The use of immunosuppressive drugs concomitant with organ transplantation has frequently led to the appearance of cancer, suggesting that the normal immunologic surveillance and control of nests of incipient tumors have been interrupted (Fahey, 1971). Therefore, chemicals that overcome these essential host defenses must be given due consideration as cofactors in carcinogenesis.

Nutritional factors are important in carcinogenesis since they affect the outcome of tumor development in many ways. Considerable attention has been paid to the process of enzyme induction, which depends on adequate intake of protein, essential lipid components, members of the vitamin B family and vitamin E. However, when the requirements for enzyme induction are met, it cannot be predicted if a carcinogen requiring metabolic activation will be more or less potent since multiple enzymes may be involved. For certain precarcinogens requiring N-hydroxylation, evidence exists that the detoxicification mechanism may take priority over the pathway leading to the proximate carcinogen (Lange, 1967).

Chemicals that cause enzyme induction may be dietary contaminants, for example, the frequently discussed chlorinated hydrocarbons (DDT) or prescription drugs (barbiturates). They are usually not present in high enough concentrations to make a significant contribution to enzyme induction.

When requirements for enzyme induction are not met, the results of exposure to a carcinogen may be unpredictable; the usual target tissue may not be affected but a different organ may respond by developing cancer (Swann and McLean, 1968). In general, however, under conditions of protein depletion or semistarvation, the cancer incidence due to a carcinogen is decreased significantly or completely absent. Conversely, overeating may produce an increased risk for cancer.

The dietary lipid components may also contribute minute amounts of toxic compounds such as the tetrachlorodibenzo(p)dioxins or closely related compounds introduced into the environment as impurities of pesticides. In contrast to the pesticides with which they are associated, the "dioxins" are not degraded rapidly and, therefore, may accumulate in lipids. Plant fats may also contain components which act as cocarcinogens. Some have been identified in cottonseed oil (Lee *et al.*, 1968) and sesame oil (Morton and Mider, 1939). Far less well understood, however, is the effect of high fat diets on the carcinogenesis that has been observed with a variety of fats of plant or animal origin and carcinogens affecting different target tissues (Gammal *et al.*, 1967; Carroll and Khor, 1970).

The importance of vitamin A in protecting the lung from carcinogenesis by polycyclic hydrocarbons has been documented (Saffiotti *et al.*, 1967).

From these few observations it becomes clear that diet plays an important role, and variation in diet may yield variable and sometimes contradictory results. Standardization of diets would be most desirable. Although not necessarily best for the health of the animal, the diet may have to be shifted to a higher fat content to be more comparable to the human diet and allow the expression of some cocarcinogenicity of fats.

It is difficult, at present, to determine if commercial diets can be obtained that are free of, and adequately monitored for, contaminants like DDT and PCB's; that contain fats from identified sources; and that have no seasonal variation in protein quality and tryptophan or vitamin content. Semisynthetic diets will be a good choice if agreement can be reached about which ingredients should be present at what levels, keeping in mind that some ingredients may be protective and others cocarcinogenic. It is likely that too much protocol may lead to the choice of a diet that is not the most suitable for all carcinogenesis programs. The highest dose of carcinogen to be used in tests should not interfere with adequate food intake or body weight gain.

SUMMARY

1. Rodents are the animals of choice for carcinogenesis tests because of their convenience, comparatively short life span and proven susceptibility to a broad range of carcinogenic agents. For most purposes two rodent species will suffice and it would not normally be practical to use larger, longer-lived animals because of the time required.

2. Inbred strains have special advantages in specific instances, but may lack susceptibility to certain classes of compounds. Therefore, randomly bred animals, despite greater variability in response, are preferred for routine testing.

3. Concurrent positive controls with known carcinogens of analogous structure are most desirable. Concurrent negative controls of adequate size are essential.

4. Ideally a semisynthetic basal diet of demonstrated nutritional adequacy is preferred for carcinogenesis studies. At the very least, a diet which meets established specifications regarding the absence of additives, pesticides, mycotoxins, and other specified components should be used.

5. Carcinogenesis tests should include several dose levels to allow the demonstration of a dose–response relationship. The highest dose administered should not cause more than a minimal depression of weight gain or any gross pathology in any tissue or organ in subchronic toxicity tests.

6. Adequate numbers of animals—for example, 40–50 of each sex at high dosage levels—should survive more than 18 months in order to establish absence of carcinogenic activity. Also, the study should preferably not be terminated until cumulative mortality has reached close to 75 percent in a group showing apparently negative results. Larger sample sizes are required for testing weaker carcinogens.

7. The viral profile of test animals should be ascertained.

8. Strains with a high incidence of spontaneous tumors are not suitable for *routine* carcinogenicity studies.

9. If transplacental exposure is a possibility, carcinogenesis studies should begin ideally prior to conception and the offspring should continue to be exposed for life.

10. Neonatal animals should be used to test substances to which human infants may be uniquely exposed.

11. When technically feasible, the route of administration should include the likely route of exposure of man.

12. Every effort should be made to identify environmental cocarcinogens or promoters, and to develop adequate test systems for them.

REFERENCES

Ad hoc Committee on the Evaluation of Low Levels of Environmental Chemical Carcinogens. 1971. *Evaluation of Environmental Carcinogens, Report to the Surgeon General USPHS April 22, 1970.* U.S. Senate Subcommittee on Agricultural Research and General Legislation of the Committee on Agriculture and Forestry, 92nd Congress, March 23–26.

Alexandrov, V.A. 1968. Blastomogenic effect of dimethylnitrosamine on pregnant rats and their offspring. *Nature* 218:280–281.

Ames, B.N., E.G. Gurney, J.A. Miller, and H. Bartsch. 1972. Carcinogens as frameshift mutagens: Metabolites and derivatives of 2-acetylaminofluorene and other aromatic amine carcinogens. *Proc. Natl. Acad. Sci.* (USA) 69:3128–3132.

Ames, B.N., P. Sims, and P.L. Grover. 1972. Epoxides of carcinogenic polycyclic hydrocarbons are frameshift mutagens. *Science* 176:47–49.

Arcos, J.C., and M.F. Argus. 1968. Molecular geometry and carcinogenic activity of aromatic compounds. New perspectives. *Adv. Cancer Res.* 11:305–471.

Berenblum, I., ed. 1969. *Carcinogenicity testing.* A report of the Panel on Carcinogenicity of the Cancer Research Commission of UICC. International Union Against Cancer. Tech. Rep. Ser., Vol. 2. Geneva.

Berwald, Y., and L. Sachs. 1965. *In vitro* transformation of normal cells to tumor cells by carcinogenic hydrocarbons. *J. Natl. Cancer Inst.* 35:641–661.

Bingham, E., and H.L. Falk. 1969. Environmental carcinogens: The modifying effect of cocarcinogens on the threshold response. *Arch. Environ. Health* 19:779–783.

Buehring, G.C. 1972. Culture of human mammary epithelial cells: Keeping abreast with a new method. *J. Natl. Cancer Inst.* 49:1433–1434.

Bulay, O.M., and L.W. Wattenberg. 1970. Carcinogenic effects of subcutaneous administration of benzo[a]pyrene during pregnancy on the progeny. *Proc. Soc. Exp. Biol. Med.* 135:84–86.

Carroll, K.K., and H.T. Khor. 1970. Effects of dietary fat and dose level of 7,12-dimethylbenz[a]anthracene on mammary tumor incidence in rats. *Cancer Res.* 30:2260–2264.

Chen, T.T., and C. Heidelberger. 1969. *In vitro* malignant transformation of cells derived from mouse prostate in the presence of 3-methylcholanthrene. *J. Natl. Cancer Inst.* 42:915–925.

Chouroulinkov, I., P. Lazar, C. Izard, C. Libermann, and M. Guérin. 1969. "Sebaceous glands" and "hyperplasia" tests as screening methods for tobacco tar carcinogenesis. *J. Natl. Cancer Inst.* 42:981–985.

Corbett, T.H., C. Heidelberger, and W.F. Dove. 1970. Determination of the mutagenic activity to bacteriophage T4 of carcinogenic and non-carcinogenic compounds. *Mol. Pharmacol.* 6:667–679.

Consultative Panel on Carcinogenesis on Environmental Carcinogenic Risks. 1968. Report. Ministry of Health, London.

Dao, T.L., and D. Sinha. 1972. Mammary adenocarcinoma induced in organ culture by 7,12-dimethylbenz[a]anthracene. *J. Natl. Cancer Inst.* 49:591:593.

DiPaolo, J.A., P.J. Donovan, and R.L. Nelson. 1971. *In vitro* transformation of hamster cells by polycyclic hydrocarbons: Factors influencing the number of cells transformed. *Nature: New Biol.* 230:240–242.

DiPaolo, J.A., R.L. Nelson, and P.J. Donovan. 1972a. *In vitro* transformation of Syrian hamster embryo cells by diverse chemical carcinogens. *Nature* 235:278–280.

DiPaolo, J.A., K. Takano, and N.C. Popescu. 1972b. Quantitation of chemically induced neoplastic transformation of BALB/3T3 cloned cell lines. *Cancer Res.* 32:2686–2695.

Druckrey, H., R. Preussmann, S. Ivankovic, and D. Schmaehl. 1967. Organotrope carcinogene Wirkungen bei 65 verschiedenen N-Nitroso-Verbindungen an BD-Ratten. *Z. Krebsforsch.* 69:103–201.

Druckrey, H., A. Ivankovic, R. Preussmann, C. Landschütz, J. Stekar, U. Brunner, and B. Schagen. 1968. Transplacental induction of neurogenic malignomas by 1,2-diethyl-hydrazine, azo-, and azoxyethane in rats. *Experientia* 24:561–562.

Dunn, T.B., and A.W. Green. 1963. Cysts of the epididymus, cancer of the cervix, granular cell myoblastoma, and other lesions after estrogen injection in newborn mice. *J. Natl. Cancer Inst.* 31:425–455.

Estabrook, R.W., D.Y. Cooper, and O. Rosenthal. 1963. The light reversible carbon monoxide inhibition of the steroid C21-hydroxylase system of the adrenal cortex. *Biochem. Z.* 338:741–755.

Fahey, J.L. 1971. Cancer in the immunosuppressed patient. *Ann. Intern. Med.* 75:310–312.

Falk, H.L., and P. Kotin. 1969. Pesticide synergists and their metabolites: Potential hazards. *Ann. N.Y. Acad. Sci.* 160:299–313.

Flaks, A., and J.O. Laws. 1968. Pulmonary adenomata induced by carcinogen treatment in organ culture. Influence of duration of treatment. *Br. J. Cancer* 22:839–842.

Food and Drug Administration. Advisory Committee on Protocols for Safety Evaluation. 1971. Cancer testing in the safety evaluation of food additives and pesticides. Report of the Panel on Carcinogenesis. *Toxicol. Appl. Pharmacol.* 20:419–438.

Freeman, A.E., P.J. Price, R.J. Bryan, R.J. Gordon, R.V. Gilden, G.J. Kelloff, and R.J. Huebner. 1971. Transformation of rat and hamster embryo cells by extracts of city smog. *Proc. Natl. Acad. Sci.* (USA) 68:445–449.

Gammal, E.B., K.K. Carroll, and E.R. Plunkett. 1967. Effects of dietary fat on mammary carcinogenesis by 7,12-dimethylbenz[a]anthracene in rats. *Cancer Res.* 27:1737–1742.

Gaudin, D., R.S. Gregg, and K.L. Yielding. 1971. DNA repair inhibition: A possible mechanism of action of co-carcinogens. *Biochem. Biophys. Res. Commun.* 45:630–636.

Greenwald, P., J.J. Barlow, P.C. Nasca, and W.S. Burnett. 1971. Vaginal cancer after maternal treatment with synthetic estrogens. *New Eng. J. Med.* 285:390–392.

Herbst, A.L., H. Ulfelder, and D.C. Poskanzer. 1971a. Adenocarcinoma of the vagina: Association of maternal stilbestrol therapy with tumor appearance in young women. *New Eng. J. Med.* 284:878–881.

Herbst, A.L., H. Ulfelder, and D.C. Poskanzer. 1971b. Registry of clear-cell carcinoma of genital tract in young women. *New Eng. J. Med.* 285:407.

Horton, A.W., D.T. Denman, and R.P. Trosset. 1957. Carcinogenesis of the skin. II. The accelerating properties of aliphatic and related hydrocarbons. *Cancer Res.* 17:758–766.

Ivankovic, S., and H. Druckrey. 1968. Transplazentare Erzeugung maligner Tumoren des Nervensystems. I. Äthyl-nitroso-harnstoff (ÄNH) an BD IX-Ratten. *Z. Krebsforsch.* 71:320–360.

Ivankovic, S., and R. Preussmann. 1970. Transplazentare Erzeugung maligner Tumoren nach oraler Gabe von Äthylharnstoff und Nitrit an Ratten. *Naturwissenschaften* 57:460.

Ivankovic, S., and W.J. Zeller. 1972. Transplacental blastomogenic action of propyl-nitrosourea in BD rats. *Arch. Geschwulstforsch.* 40:99–102.

Jänisch, W., D. Schreiber, R. Warzok, and J. Schneider. 1972. Die transplazentar Induktion von Gaeschwülsten des Nervensystems. Vergleichende Untersuchung der Wirksamkeit von Methyl- und Äthylnitrosoharnstoff. *Arch. Geschwulstforsch.* 39:99–106.

Kleihues, P., Chr. Mende, and W. Reucher. 1972. Tumours of the peripheral and central nervous system induced in BD-rats by prenatal application of methyl methane-sulfonate. *Eur. J. Cancer* 8:641–645.

Knudson, A.G., Jr. 1971. Mutation and cancer: Statistical study of retinoblastoma. *Proc. Natl. Acad. Sci.* (USA) 68:820–823.

Knudson, A.G., Jr., and L.C. Strong. 1972. Mutation and cancer: A model for Wilms' tumor of the kidney. *J. Natl. Cancer Inst.* 48:313–324.

Lange, G. 1967. Ablauf der Induktion von Mikrosomen-Enzymen in der Kanin-chenleber. *Naunyn-Schmiedebergs Arch. Exp. Pathol. Pharmakol.* 257:37–38.

Larsen, C.D. 1947. Pulmonary-tumor induction by transplacental exposure to urethane. *J. Natl. Cancer Inst.* 8:63–70.

Lasfargues, E.Y., and D.H. Moore. 1971. A method for the continuous cultivation of mammary epithelium. *In Vitro* 7:21–25.

Lee, D.J., J.H. Wales, J.L. Ayres, and R.O. Sinnhuber. 1968. Synergism between cyclopropenoid fatty acids and chemical carcinogens in rainbow trout (*Salmo gairdneri*). *Cancer Res.* 28:2312–2318.

Likhachev, A. 1971. Transplacental blastomogenic action of *N*-nitrosodimethylamine in mice (in Russian). *Vopr. Onkol.* 17:45–50.

Magee, P.N., and J.M. Barnes. 1967. Carcinogenic nitroso compounds. *Adv. Cancer Res.* 10:163–246.

Marquardt, H., and C. Heidelberger. 1972. Influence of "feeder cells" and inducers and inhibitors of microsomal mixed-function oxidases on hydrocarbon-induced malignant transformation of cells derived from C3H mouse prostate. *Cancer Res.* 32:721–725.

Miller, R.W., J.F. Fraumeni, Jr., and M.D. Manning. 1964. Association of Wilms's tumor with aniridia, hemihypertrophy, and other congenital malformations. *New Eng. J. Med.* 270:922–927.

Morton, J.J., and G.B. Mider. 1939. Effect of petroleum ether extract of mouse car-casses as solvent in production of sarcoma. *Proc. Soc. Exp. Biol. Med.* 41:357–360.

Mottram, J.C. 1944. A sensitising factor in experimental blastogenesis. *J. Pathol. Bact.* 56:391–402.

National Academy of Sciences–National Research Council. Food Protection Com-mittee. 1969. *Guidelines for Estimating Toxicologically Insignificant Levels of Chemicals in Food.* National Academy of Sciences, Washington, D.C.

Niskanen, E.E. 1962. Mechanism of skin tumorigenesis in mouse. *Acta Pathol. Microbiol. Scand.* (Supplement) 159:4–77.

Oshiro, Y., L.E. Gerschenson, and J.A. DiPaolo. 1972. Carcinomas from rat liver cells transformed spontaneously in culture. *Cancer Res.* 32:877–879.

Potter, V.R. 1972. Workshop on liver cell culture. *Cancer Res.* 32:1998–2000.

Rice, J.M. 1969. Transplacental carcinogenesis in mice by 1-ethyl-1-nitrosourea. *Ann. N.Y. Acad. Sci.* 163:813–827.

Saffiotti, U., R. Montesano, A.R. Sellakumar, and S.A. Borg. 1967. Experimental cancer of the lung: Inhibition by vitamin A of the induction of tracheobronchial aquamous metaplasia and squamous cell tumors. *Cancer* 20:857–864.

Sander, J. 1970. Induktion maligner Tumoren bei Ratten durch orale Gabe von N,N'-Dimethylharnstoff und Nitrit. *Arzneimittelforsch.* 20:418–419.

Sander, J., and G. Buerkle. 1969. Induktion maligner Tumoren bei Ratten durch gleichzeitige Verfütterung von Nitrit und sekundären Aminen. *Z. Krebsforsch.* 73:54–66.

Searle, C.E. 1970. Chemical carcinogens and their significance for chemists. *Chem. Br.* 6:5–10.

Searle, C.E., and E.L. Jones. 1972. Tumours of the nervous system in mice treated neonatally with *N*-ethyl-*N*-nitrosourea. *Nature* 240:559–560.

Smith, W.E., and P. Rous. 1948. The neoplastic potentialities of mouse embryo tissues. IV. Lung adenomas in baby mice as result of prenatal exposure to urethane. *J. Exp. Med.* 88:529–554.

Spatz, M., and G.L. Laqueur. 1967. Transplacental induction of tumors in Sprague-Dawley rats with crude cycad material. *J. Natl. Cancer Inst.* 38:233–245.

Suntzeff, V., E.V. Cowdry, and A. Croninger. 1955. Microscopic visualization of the degeneration of sebaceous glands caused by carcinogens. *Cancer Res.* 15:637–640.

Swann, P.F., and A.E.M. McLean. 1968. The effect of diet on the toxic and carcinogenic action of dimethylnitrosamine. *Biochem. J.* 107:14P–15P.

Tanaka, T. 1973. Transplacental induction of tumors and malformations in rats treated with some chemical carcinogens. *In* L. Tomatis and U. Mohr, eds., *Transplacental Carcinogenesis*. IARC Sci. Publ. No. 4, p. 100-111. International Agency for Research on Cancer, Lyon.

Teich, N., D.R. Lowy, J.W. Hartley, and W.P. Rowe. 1973. Studies of the mechanism of induction of infectious murine leukemia virus from AKR mouse embryo cell lines by 5-iododeoxyuridine and 5-bromo-deoxyuridine. *Virology* 51:163–173.

VanDuuren, B.L., C. Katz, B.M. Goldschmidt, K. Frenkel, and A. Sivak. 1972. Carcinogenicity of halo-ethers. II. Structure–activity relationships of analogs of bis(chloromethyl)ether. *J. Natl. Cancer Inst.* 48:1431–1439.

Vesselinovitch, S.D., N. Milhailovich, and G. Pietra. 1967. The prenatal exposure of mice to urethan and the consequent development of tumors in various tissues. *Cancer Res.* 27:2333–2337.

Weiss, R.A., R.R. Friis, E. Katz, and P.K. Vogt. 1971. Induction of avian tumor viruses in normal cells by physical and chemical carcinogens. *Virology* 46:920–938.

Williams, G.M., J.M. Elliott, and J.H. Weisburger. 1973. Carcinoma after malignant conversion *in vitro* of epithelial-like cells from rat liver following exposure to chemical carcinogens. *Cancer Res.* 33:606–612.

World Health Organization. 1969. *Principles for the testing and evaluation of drugs for carcinogenicity.* ITS Tech. Rep. Ser. No. 426. Geneva.

Wrba, H., K. Pielsticker, and U. Mohr. 1967. Die diaplazentar-carcinogene Wirkung von Diäthylnitrosamin bei Ratten. *Naturwissenschaften* 54:47.

SUGGESTED READINGS

Arcos, J.C., M.F. Argus, and G. Wolf. 1968. *Chemical Induction of Cancer.* Vol. 1. Part II. The nature of tumors. Concepts and techniques of testing chemical agents for carcinogenic activity. Academic Press, New York. pp. 303–465.

Benitz, K.-F. 1970. Measurement of chronic toxicity. In Paget, G.E., ed., *Methods in Toxicology.* F.A. Davis Co., Philadelphia. pp. 82–131.

Clayson, D.B. 1962. *Chemical Carcinogenesis.* Little, Brown & Co., Boston.

Falk, H.L. 1971. Anticarcinogenesis—an alternative. *Prog. Exp. Tumor Res.* 14:105–137.

Macpherson, I. 1970. The characteristics of animal cells transformed *in vitro. Adv. Cancer Res.* 13:169–215.

Magee, P.N. 1970. Tests for carcinogenic potential. In Paget, G.E., ed., *Methods in Toxicology.* F.A. Davis Co., Philadelphia. pp. 158–196.

Paul, J. 1970. *Cell and Tissue Culture,* 4th ed. Williams and Wilkins Co., Baltimore.

Tomatis, L., and U. Mohr, eds. 1973. *Transplacental Carcinogenesis.* IARC Sci. Publ. No. 4. International Agency for Research on Cancer, Lyon.

Weisburger, J.H., and E.K. Weisburger. 1967. Tests for chemical carcinogens. In Busch, H., ed., *Methods in Cancer Research.* Vol. I. Academic Press, New York pp. 307–398.

World Health Organization. International Agency for Research on Cancer. 1972. *IARC Monographs on the Evaluation of Carcinogenic Risk of Chemicals to Man.* Vol. 1. Lyon.

X

Environmental Chemicals as Potential Hazards to Reproduction

Reproduction encompasses the biological functions that are directly involved in the perpetuation of the species. Although the endocrinological and psychosexual backgrounds of reproduction are important in the overall process, they are not exclusively within the domain of reproduction and are consequently not dealt with in depth. Derangements in these broader aspects are likely to entail other toxicological manifestations than simply those relating to the quantity and quality of offspring. Attention is focused primarily on the events and processes that are directly involved in producing healthy offspring. For this presentation these events and processes are identified as follows.

Preservation of the germ line
Gametogenesis
Release and transport of gametes
Fertilization
Cleavage and blastocyst (preimplantation) stages
Implantation
Metabolic changes in the pregnant mother
Embryonic period—tissue differentiation and organogenesis
Fetal period—prenatal growth and functional maturation
Placental functions and maternal—conceptual relationships
Birth and adjustment to postnatal existence

Lactation and maternal care of offspring
Postnatal growth and maturation of offspring

SUSCEPTIBILITY OF REPRODUCTIVE PROCESSES TO ENVIRONMENTAL INFLUENCES

Areas of Vulnerability

It can be argued that, although some aspects of reproduction may be susceptible to some kinds of adverse environmental influences, protection against such influences would ordinarily be assured by earlier toxic manifestations in other systems. In fact, however, relatively little information is available on the comparative sensitivity of reproduction and of other functional parameters. In 1970 the Panel on Reproduction of the FDA Advisory Committee on Protocols for Safety Evaluation undertook to review the subject as it pertained to food additives and pesticide residues and concluded the following (FDA, 1970):

... It is illusory to place complete reliance on the thesis that a well-defined and well-conducted subacute toxicity study will detect changes in reproductive organs as well as changes in other biological systems.

Several of the reproductive processes cited above can undoubtedly be adversely affected by exposure to toxic substances in the environment. The following comments include some known examples and some situations wherein adverse effects might be suspected.

Mechanisms for Preservation of the Germ Line   In theoretical terms it can be assumed that nonlethal mutations within the germinal cell line will be retained and will tend to accumulate within such cells with time and succeeding cell generations (or mitoses). Therefore, the continuing presence of a mutagen at an effective level in the environment is likely to offer a more serious threat to future generations than a single acute exposure. In addition, recent observations suggest the existence of "supermutagens," which produce high frequencies of mutations at essentially nonlethal levels of exposure in submammalian test systems. All exogenous mutagens might be assumed to produce additive genetic effects that ultimately contribute to and enhance the genetic load in human populations, although the possibility of repair or selective elimination of defective germinal cells cannot be fully evaluated at this time. The transmissibility of toxicologic manifestations to future generations is the characteristic feature of mutagenesis, and occupies a unique place in toxicology.

Gametogenesis   Interference here would be manifested by slowed or arrested germ cell production, production of defective cells with reduced fertility, production of cells bearing heritable changes, or by interference with the normal development of the fertilized ovum. Lowered fertility would result from a reduced rate of production or a reduced fertilizing capacity of the gametes; however, this would have to be distinguished from reduced fertility that might be secondary to structural or functional abnormalities elsewhere in the reproductive system. Effects of ingested chemicals on gametogenesis may be revealed in gross quantitative terms by semen analysis, by histologic examination of the testes, or by measurement of overall fecundity.

Germ Cell Transport   Little is known of the factors affecting this parameter in man, and most of the available information concerns factors (e.g., infections) not applicable to this survey. However, animal studies indicate germ cell transport can be interfered with by a variety of agents including those that affect smooth muscle motility and reproductive secretions. Transport of the fertilized zygote depends on normal muscular, ciliary, and secretory activity in the upper part of the female genital tract, and interference with such activities might well be responsible for reproductive failure. The extent to which fertilization and implantation are likely to be adversely affected by extrinsic factors is not well known and deserves more study. Little attention has been given to the possible entry of foreign substances into secretions elaborated by male and female accessory sex organs, and the effects of such foreign substances in the glandular secretions of the reproductive tract of either sex on spermatozoa, ova, or zygotes is much in need of systematic research.

Fertilization, Blastocyst Formation, Implantation   Termination of pregnancy at this critical period could result from insult directly to the zygote, or indirectly by altering the uterine environment in some manner that would prevent implantation. Unless there were long-term exposure resulting in persistent infertility, such effects might be extremely difficult to recognize. Many of the same concerns apply here as were expressed above regarding transport of germ cells.

Metabolic Changes in the Pregnant Female   The maternal organism is, in some ways, more vulnerable during pregnancy: For example, detoxification mechanisms are altered. In addition, the maternal organism experiences alterations in pathways of metabolism: Protein, carbohydrate, and lipid metabolism are all altered in pregnancy. It is well known that pregnant women may have unusual appetites, either diminished during periods of nausea or increased in respect to certain items of diet. Under these conditions of limited hepatic reserve, abnormal metabolic patterns, or unusual dietary habits, the pregnant woman may become more susceptible to exogenous agents. Certain substances may specifically interfere with the maintenance of the pregnancy, such as substances which inhibit enzymes related to steroid biosynthesis or which are diabetogenic.

It is not known what initiates spontaneous labor, but it is known that a group of substances can either stimulate (oxytocin or ergot derivatives) or retard (epinephrine) the progress of labor. It is conceivable that substances with similar actions might exist among the large number of chemicals in the environment.

Embryo   The high and variable susceptibility of the conceptus to environmental influences during the period of embryonic organogenesis has been fully reviewed elsewhere (Wilson, 1973a). This is the time when a great majority of teratological effects are induced, and the conditions of exposure and types of agents that represent particular concerns are summarized later in this chapter.

Fetus   Although the fetus is generally considered less vulnerable to exogenous chemicals than the embryo, this generalization is valid mainly in quantitative terms and as regards the type of developmental defects likely to be induced. Because the fetal period is characterized by physical growth and functional maturation, it is to be expected that adverse influences at this time are more likely to lead to growth retardation and postnatal functional abnormality than to the structural defects produced by stressing the embryo.

In experimental rodent species, transplacental carcinogens (Chapter IX) are most active during the latter half of gestation. Furthermore, the stages in the formation of primary oocytes by mitosis from oogonia—and early, vulnerable stages of meiosis as well—occur before or shortly after birth in many species, including mice, rats, and man. Thus, genetic damage that causes mutants to appear in a F_1 generation may well have been inflicted while the female parent was *in utero* or in early infancy.

Postpartum Infant   The infant may be unusually susceptible to chemicals in a variety of ways, for example, its immature metabolic systems may be unable to cope with foreign substances or even an excess of endogenous substances.

Lactation   Several different types of effects on lactation may occur. First, certain substances (e.g., steroid hormones) can decrease the quantity of milk and alter its quality. Second, there may be no primary effect on lactation but the substance may be excreted in the milk and render it unpalatable to the infant. Finally, some substances may be excreted in the milk that can have direct toxic effects on the infant. Of opposite concern would be the presence of substances, such as tranquilizing agents, that might enhance lactation so that persistent galactorrhea would occur.

Postnatal Function of the Offspring　Since certain developmental processes are not completed until after birth—for example, physical growth and structural and physiologic maturation of the central nervous system and some endocrine glands—it is to be expected that environmental chemicals may exert detrimental influences on these postnatal aspects of development. Aside from observations on postnatal survival and growth rates, little has been done in the way of experimental studies on postnatal functional alterations induced by environmental chemicals. An exception is the increasing concern about behavioral changes that may be induced either by prenatal exposure to substances that are mediated by the pregnant mother, or direct exposure of the immature postnatal animal. [*See* Chapter XI, Effects on Behavior.]

Factors To Be Considered in Testing for Toxic Effects

Toxic Effects on Reproduction vis-à-vis Other Systems　It may be argued that despite the unusual nature of hazards attending reproduction, protection against such adverse effects might be assured by other toxicity studies. If this were the case, it would not be necessary to emphasize careful testing of the processes of reproduction. The unique effects of mutagens and especially teratogens (e.g., thalidomide) confirm the dichotomous nature of toxicity in the healthy adult as compared to the maternal–fetal biological unit. Rodent fetuses can be at least an order of magnitude more sensitive to carcinogenic stimuli than adults, but this is not always the case with respect to either carcinogenesis or acute toxicity (FDA, 1970). Parental LD_{50}'s for certain substances may be as much as 300-times greater than embryonic LD's (Wilson, 1973a).

Areas of Greater Vulnerability　It is clear that toxic effects on reproduction selectively affect certain stages. There are many examples of this. Certain substances are known to interfere preferentially with spermatogenesis (Fox and Fox, 1967; Lee and Dixon, 1972). Hormonally active substances are known to affect ovulation, implantation, and lactation in the adult female or induce vaginal malignancy in offspring.

All reproductive processes referred to in the introduction have been demonstrated in experimental animals to be altered by exposure to certain environmental agents, but there is a large range in susceptibility to different exposure levels. Some reproductive processes do not manifest abnormalities until levels of exposure that severely affect the adult are attained, while other reproductive processes manifest abnormalities at exposures considerably below those affecting the adult. It is this potential susceptibility of certain reproductive phenomena that is of major concern since it can put the human species at risk because of this possible vulnerability at low environmental exposures. The most vulnerable aspects of the reproductive process are mutagenesis and teratogenesis. The following definitions of mutagenesis and teratogenesis have been agreed upon.

Mutagenesis is the induction of heritable changes in the genome of germinal and somatic cells. With respect to the germinal cells, these changes could be produced from the time of formation of the zygote through germinal cell development and maturation in the embryo, infant, and adult. In the adult male, the cell stage of greatest sensitivity in gametogenesis is essentially a function of the specific agent to which the individual is exposed. For instance, certain chemical compounds are known to be most active in the late postmeiotic stages of gametogenesis, other agents have been shown to exert their greatest action premeiotically, and still others show a bimodal or polymodal sensitivity distribution within gametogenesis. "Heritable changes" could be manifested in the F_1 generation as infertility, reduced fertility, pre- and postimplantation deaths, visible structural and functional anomalies, normal heterozygotes, or normal carriers of balanced translocations. Mutations in embryonic germinal or somatic cells are dependent on the mutagen reaching the embryo via the uterine fluid or by placental transport, rather than indirectly through the gonadal tissue of the infant and adult organism.

Teratogenesis is the induction of structural and/or functional development abnormalities by exogenous factors acting during gestation. During development it is conceivable that changes in the genome of embryonic somatic cells could contribute to abnormal development. Natural or induced mutations in embryonic somatic cells have been shown to contribute to abnormal embryonic structure and function, although the extent of this contribution is not known.

It is recognized that developmental abnormalities can be produced after parturition, so the gestational period is included in the working definition for teratogenesis. This was done in order to simplify the formulation of a protocol since the most readily monitored developmental abnormalities occur during the early stages of gestation. The phrase "functional developmental abnormalities" also needs some explanation. Broad usage of the word *teratogenesis* may be confusing since such classical teratogenic agents as radiation or some cytotoxic agents produce a triad of (1) structural and functional abnormalities, (2) embryonic death or resorption, and (3) intrauterine growth retardation. It is obvious that a proportion of embryonic death is due to the occurrence of a nonviable structural or functional abnormality; similarly, induced intrauterine growth retardation that is not recuperable during postnatal life is, in a sense, a form of teratogenesis. However, the value of recording separately the extent of embryonic death and growth retardation cannot be overemphasized; such a separation provides qualitative variations of the results, which facilitate the interpretation of the data. Some agents predominantly induce embryonic death while others result in a high percentage of viable malformations. Furthermore, the same agent can result in different effects at different stages of gestation. Therefore, it is essential that data on growth and embryonic death be separated from those on structural and functional abnormalities.

The question has been raised as to whether the mechanisms involved in teratogenesis and mutagenesis are sufficiently similar that testing might be combined in a single protocol for determination of safety in both areas. This concept may have arisen from the fact that a small percentage of known mutagens are teratogenic and, vice versa, a small percentage of known teratogens affect the genome. In other words, some developmental abnormalities result from mutation, and some somatic mutations may play a role in deviations from normal embryonic development. On the other hand, there are numerous compounds that are teratogenic and have no mutagenic potential. Furthermore, carcinogenesis overlaps teratogenesis and mutagenesis in that some, but not all, carcinogens may also be either teratogenic or mutagenic or both. Finally, in view of present incomplete understanding of the mechanisms of teratogenesis and mutagenesis, it would be foolhardy to infer that results from one area could be applied to the other. Since both teratogenesis and mutagenesis appear to be different processes—each involving highly sensitive aspects of reproduction—it is sensible to continue to study them as separate phenomena, either of which may prove to be the more sensitive under particular environmental conditions.

Substances Uniquely Toxic to Reproductive Processes   In this section the agents mentioned will not be restricted to those that are recognized as environmental pollutants because it is considered possible that all chemicals in the environment, regardless of the original intent of their use, may under certain conditions persist and accumulate in air, water, or soil and thus become pollutants.

Known and Possible Mutagens Chemical mutagens can be divided into three major categories. The first, and presumably of least concern as environmental pollutants, are the purine and pyrimidine analogs—mainly drugs—which cause mutation by incorporation into the primary structure of DNA. The second group consists of substances that chemically interact with DNA to produce new chemical bonds. This is the category of most obvious interest and concern in the area of environmental pollutants, and it contains many alkylating agents—including aziridines, nitrogen and sulfur mustards, nitrosamides, alkyl sulfates, alkyl alkane sulfonates, lactones, epoxides, aldehydes and alkyl halides. In addition, it contains certain oxidizing agents and agents that act catalytically to alter the structure of DNA. The last category of mutagens is comprised of those substances that become bound to DNA by their insertion between DNA bases (intercalation). This category of mutagenic agents includes some drugs. Since these substances are almost invariably of a polycyclic aromatic structure, they might be of significance as environmental pollutants.

Research over the past decade has provided considerable information on the essential chemical features of genetically active compounds. Indeed, to an appreciable extent, structural considerations alone have some predictive value in pinpointing potential mutagenicity. The problem, however, is more complex in that many of the substances that are genetically inert may be activated by metabolic reactions to active mutagens. This situation is similar to carcinogenesis in which it is known that many potentially active compounds require metabolic activation to attain carcinogenicity. On this basis, it is permissible to think in terms of promutagens and proximate mutagens, with obvious analogy to carcinogenesis. It is this former class, promutagens, that are the most cryptic and would accordingly present the greatest problem.

Known and Possible Teratogens Most known experimental teratogenic agents are chemicals, including some drugs, pesticides, solvents, and industrial effluents. Table 6 lists several classes of chemicals with representative examples of each that have been shown to be embryotoxic in one or more species of laboratory mammal. Certain of these classes, such as antibiotic, antineoplastic, and antimalarial drugs and all types of pesticides, might be suspect of having teratogenic potential because they were originally prepared for the express purpose of suppressing metabolism and growth. Until proven otherwise, it should be assumed that all of these substances in sufficient dosage are capable of impairing the high metabolic activity and growth of mammalian embryos and fetuses in spite of maternal homeostatic mechanisms and placental transport rates that tend to protect the fetus.

It is impossible to generalize about the teratogenic mechanisms, except to say that there is great diversity in the ways different chemicals

TABLE 6   Some Types of Drugs and Other Chemicals That Have Been Shown To Be Teratogenic in One or More Species of Laboratory Mammal

Chemical Group	Example
Salicylates	Aspirin, oil of wintergreen
Certain alkaloids	Caffeine, nicotine, colchicine
Tranquilizers	Meprobamate, chlorpromazine, reserpine
Antihistamines	Buclizine, meclizine, cyclizine
Antibiotics	Chloramphenacol, streptonigrin, penicillin
Hypoglycemics	Carbutamide, tolbutamide, hypoglycins
Steroid hormones	Triamcinolone, cortisone, testosterone
Alkylating agents	Busulfan, chlorambucil, cyclophosphamide, TEM
Antimalarials	Chloroquine, quinacrine, pyrimethamine
Anesthetics	Halothane, urethan, nitrous oxide, pentobarbital
Antimetabolites	Folic acid, purine and pyrimidine antagonist
Solvents	Benzene, dimethylsulfoxide, propylene glycol
Pesticides	2,4,5-T, carbaryl, captan, folpet
Industrial effluents	Some compounds of Hg, Pb, As, Li, Cd
Miscellaneous	Trypan blue, tryparanol, acetazolamide, etc.

NOTE: Teratogenic effects were usually seen only at doses well above therapeutic levels for the drugs, or above likely exposure levels for the environmental chemicals (from Wilson, 1973a).

act on living systems. Some are capable of causing mutations and chromosomal aberrations (Fishbein *et al.*, 1970; Kalter, 1971) as well as the more usual teratogenic manifestations. Others interfere with various aspects of the mitotic cycle (Malawista *et al.*, 1968) or interfere with nucleic acid synthesis or function (Schumacher *et al.*, 1969). In other words, virtually all of the teratogenic mechanisms that have been proposed (Wilson, 1973a) can be activated by one or more types of chemical agents.

Once access is gained to the parental bloodstream, it must be assumed that some fraction of all foreign chemicals may reach the germ cells and probably also the embryo or fetus *in utero*. Thus the critical question is, at what level and for what duration does exposure occur? In other words, are the parental homeostatic system and the embryonic and fetal placentae able to reduce the concentration sufficiently to avoid mutagenic and teratogenic effects in developing tissues?

The great majority of safety evaluation testing for both teratogenic and mutagenic potential is now and will doubtless continue to be directed toward chemical agents. This is not necessarily because these agents inherently involve greater risk than other agents but that, among the various types of potential causative agents, new chemicals are probably being introduced into the environment faster than all of the other factors combined. Numerous lists of chemicals and drugs known adversely to affect mammalian development are available in the literature (Kalter and

Warkany, 1959; Nishimura, 1964; Tuchmann-Duplessis et Mercier-Parot, 1964; Cahen, 1966; and others) and the subject as regards the teratogenic potential of drugs in man has been reviewed in detail elsewhere (Wilson, 1973b).

The problem of detrimental effects on development from environmental chemicals is by no means a new one (Warkany, 1971), although recent recognition of some previously unsuspected types of exposure emphasize the need for close scrutiny of other seemingly unlikely situations involving pregnant women. For example, neuromuscular abnormalities and failure to grow in a child have been attributed to lead poisoning as a result of consumption by the pregnant mother of moonshine whiskey (Palmisano, *et al.*, 1969), and a high abortion rate and the birth of a child with clubfeet among women working in a culture media preparation laboratory has been related to exposure to high selenium levels (Robertson, 1970).

Mercury, as well as lead, has been regarded with some suspicion for a number of years (Butt and Simonsen, 1950). However, the demonstration that industrial effluents into Minamata Bay and other coastal waters of Japan were responsible for a congenital form of *Minamata disease* was the first proven instance of organic mercury (i.e., methylmercury) having accumulated as a teratogenic pollutant. Several newborn babies exhibited multiple neurological symptoms resembling cerebral palsy. The mothers of these infants had eaten diets containing a large proportion of fish which, as a result of biological magnification through the food chain, had accumulated high concentrations of methylmercury (Matsumoto *et al.,* 1965; Harada, 1968). The fact that many of the mothers of affected babies did not themselves show symptoms of the adult form of the disease was another illustration of the greater sensitivity of the fetus than of the mother to many chemical agents. The same type of congenital mercury poisoning occurred in the United States (Snyder, 1971) when a mercury containing fungicide was applied to seed corn; the corn was fed to hogs, and meat from one of these was subsequently eaten by a pregnant woman. The teratogenicity of organic mercury has now been confirmed in mice (Spyker and Smithberg, 1972) and in hamsters (Harris *et al.*, 1972).

Several types of solvents have been shown to be teratogenic or otherwise embryotoxic in mammals: for example, acetamides and some formamides in rats (Thiersch, 1962), dimethylsulfoxide in hamsters (Ferm, 1966), benzene in mice (Watanabe *et al.*, 1968), and several alkane sulfonates in rats (Hemsworth, 1968). Similar incidents in man are largely unknown, but the possibilities of industrial or household exposure to such substances during early pregnancy should be thoroughly examined.

At least one report relates industrial exposure of pregnant women to solvents—such as xylene, trichloroethylene, methylchloroethylene, and acetone—and the subsequent birth of children with sacral agenesis (Kučera, 1968). The same author points out that a similar malformation can be induced in chicks by exposure of incubating eggs to xylene.

Among the great variety of pesticides, the defoliant 2,4,5-T has undoubtedly been most often linked with teratogenesis. This compound has recently been the subject of exhaustive review of all of its effects on mammalian reproduction (2,4,5-T Advisory Committee, 1971) with particular attention to possible teratogenic effects in man and laboratory animals. Claims have come from three areas of the world of embryotoxicity following alleged exposure during human pregnancy, namely, Vietnam (Cutting et al., 1970; Meselson et al., 1970), Globe, Arizona (Binns et al., 1970), and Swedish Lappland (Rapport, etc., 1971). When all available animal data and evidence from these localities was examined by qualified scientists, however, no basis could be found for regarding this herbicide as teratogenic in man.

Positive embryotoxicity is known to occur in laboratory animals after application of some other pesticides during pregnancy: Organophosphorus cholinesterase inhibitors—such as DFP, parathion, and methyl parathion—caused intrauterine death and growth retardation but no teratogenicity in rats (Fish, 1966); captan caused malformations in rabbits (McLaughlin et al., 1969); carbaryl produced terata in very high doses in guinea pigs but not in hamsters and rats, and thiram was teratogenic in hamsters (Robens, 1969). Courtney et al. (1970) reported on a large scale screening study in mice in which a number of pesticides were found to produce a statistically significant increase in the proportion of litters containing abnormal young. It was necessary to use large doses during the period of organogenesis to obtain the adverse effects mentioned.

It is noteworthy that DDT, the insecticide most often accused of adverse biological effects, has not been reported to be teratogenic in any mammalian species (Khera and Clegg, 1969). It appears that relatively few of the numerous pesticides now in use have been found to be teratogenic, a somewhat surprising observation in view of the fact that these compounds were developed for the specific purpose of arresting growth in or killing living organisms. However, it must be emphasized that many pesticides now in use have not been rigorously tested for teratogenicity at high dosage levels.

Possible Hazards to Other Reproductive Functions　Known environmental effects on human reproductive processes other than mutagenesis, teratogenesis, or transplacental carcinogenesis (Chapter IX) are usually detected by increased incidences of infertility, spontaneous abortion, prematurity or retarded postnatal growth or development. Thus, even though an environmental toxin (e.g., heavy metals, propylenechlorohydrin) might specifically act upon spermatogenesis, its activity might be detected only if men became infertile and appropriate correlative information were available. Nevertheless, about 10 percent of couples in the United States are infertile. Many cases have no other demonstrable abnormality; whether spontaneous abortion, failure of implantation, or failure of corpus luteum function is responsible cannot be ascertained.

Another recognized abnormality of reproduction in humans is a high incidence of premature birth. At present, the only etiologic correlations are socioeconomic. By implication, this includes deficient nutrition and inadequate medical care, but exposure to toxic substances may be increased in this segment of the population. Cigarette smoking has been implicated as a causal agent in prematurity. Thus, while it is difficult to cite specific examples of substances present in sufficient quantities to cause reproductive failures, the frequency of such failure and the existence of some substances in the environment already known adversely to affect reproduction in man or animals allows the possibility that other unrecognized effects may occur.

CRITIQUE OF EXISTING EVALUATIVE METHODS

The purpose of this section is to examine critically the existing methods for using animals to estimate risks to human reproduction from environmental chemicals. The intent is to discuss the methods as they are currently used and to highlight areas in need of better information and/or methodology. For the most part, concrete suggestions for improving currently used procedures will be reserved for later in the discussion.

Methods for Mutagenicity Testing

General Consideration   There is little basis in fact for the often made assumption that teratogenic test systems are more closely relevant to the health of man than are mutagenic tests. Both are important in the immediate and long-term welfare of man. Recent advances in genetics and biochemistry have established the fundamental molecular mechanisms of mutation (Fishbein *et al.*, 1970; Vogel and Röhrborn, 1970; Drake, 1970; Hollaender, 1971). Many similarities and differences between species on a broad phylogenetic scale are known: For instance, some of the mutations induced in the lower organisms have their counterpart in human populations. Furthermore, in specified instances, observed differences in sensitivity to mutagenic agents is attributable to well-delineated molecular processes that govern mutation rates. For example, the marked quantitative and qualitative differences in mutation induction at specific loci can be attributed to known differences in the ability to repair pre-mutational lesions.

Recent work with mammalian tissue culture systems, including human cells, shows an excellent quantitative correlation between induction rates of somatic cells *in vitro* and the germinal stem line of the intact mouse. However, such a correlation pertains only to proximate mutagens and, as was emphasized in an earlier section, the most difficult and demanding challenge concerns identification of those agents which are not mutagenic, *per se*, but depend upon metabolic conversion for the expression of mutagenic activity. Thus, pharmacokinetic considerations and the known variations among animal species are thought to constitute a serious problem and a vital issue in terms of the safety evaluation of specific agents. A variety of approaches to account for metabolic activation has been proposed, and a few of the approaches have been investigated in some detail. Among the original proposals was the well-known host-mediated assay, which initially utilized bacterial mutants as an indicator organism for recording genetic events arising from the metabolic activation of promutagens *in vivo*. It has been shown, for instance, that simple nitrosamines were genetically inactive when bacteria were exposed *in vitro*. However, when coupled to the host-mediated assay, metabolic activation of the nitrosamine—presumably by the liver—led to products which were powerful mutagens to the bacteria within the host-animal peritoneum. In recent years, attempts have been made to utilize other body cavities and tissues in the host-mediated assay to assess organ-specific activation. In addition, a variety of other indicator organisms have been employed, including yeast, *Neurospora*, and a variety of mammalian cells in culture. Still other approaches to metabolic activation have utilized drug-metabolizing systems *in vitro*, such as liver microsomal preparations from various mammalian species including man. The latter approach provides the obvious advantage of yielding information as regards species differences in metabolic activation. These are but a few of the ways in which the essentiality of metabolic activation can be ascertained.

In recent years, there has been a growing awareness of the genetic basis of human disease. Relaxation in the pressures of natural selection inherent in modern society increases the importance and impact of mutational drift. Mutations are thus able to enter the population, affect the gene pools, and contribute more significantly to man's genetic load than ever before. Modern society's burden to sustain genetically unfit individuals is dependent, in large part, on present and future use of chemicals that are mutagenic and as a result would serve to enhance the rate of mutational drift. The last two decades of research in laboratory animals and lower organisms have provided some understanding of the kinds of genetic damage that may be of importance for man (McKusick, 1968).

The two main categories of concern are gene mutations and chromosomal aberrations. Observations in man and other mammals demonstrate the types of gene mutation that occur and require consideration in the context of mutagenicity. The so-called "point" mutation, which may involve as little as a single purine or pyrimidine base in a gene containing a thousand or more such bases, has been demonstrated by the application of biochemical techniques to human population genetics. Two well-known examples are Lesch-Nyhan syndrome and sickle-cell anemia.

It is also evident that point mutations in mammals and man occur by a variety of mechanisms—for instance, by either base substitution or base addition or deletion. In addition, interstitial and small chromosomal deletions are known to occur in mammals and contribute to the spectrum of gene mutations. The second category consists of chromosomal aberrations and constitutes a small but well-defined disease burden in man as exemplified by Down's, Klinefelter's and Turner's syndromes. While these particular mutant genotypes normally arise as a result of nondisjunction producing an abnormality in chromosome number, translocations and other chromosomal rearrangements are also known in man. Certain of these aberrations, but by no means all, are heritable. Of lesser concern is a third category of genetic events with the potential of contributing mutant phenotypes. This refers to mitotic recombination and gene conversion which, while not demonstrated to occur in mammals owing to current inability to assess the event, has been shown to be of great significance in other eucaryotic systems. This problem, however, may be of greater relevance to carcinogenicity than as a threat to future generations. Nevertheless, this mechanism could well be of real significance to the developing germ stem line during embryogenesis. It should be emphasized that induced and natural gene mutations constitute the greatest concern as regards the genetic load in man and that, as an important generalization, gene mutations are expected to be retained within the population through a greater number of generations than chromosomal aberrations. This is not to imply that gene mutations impact only on gene pools, for it is evident that they also have potential for immediate F_1 generation effects.

There are two basic mechanisms by which mutation occurs. The first is obvious and has been recognized for some time: the direct interaction of a chemical agent with DNA to produce a premutational lesion. The second process of potential concern is the inhibition of normal repair processes by chemical substances acting either at the level of DNA, or conceivably at some lower level.

Gene Mutation   The primary purpose of assays for gene mutations is to assess changes that result in an alteration or complete loss of gene function at loci anywhere within the genome. To avoid biasing evaluation of the results, it is preferable to measure the genetic effect over the entire genome. Where a single gene is used to the exclusion of the rest of the genome, there is always the concern that the effects measured may be highly atypical and misleading. Unfortunately, assays applicable to the whole genome are not currently available in mammalian cells or intact mammals. It is, therefore presently necessary to rely on submammalian test systems for this kind of information. The parasitic wasp habrobracon (Smith and vonBorstel, 1971) and the two-component heterokaryon of the fungus *Neurospora* (de Serres and Malling, 1971) are ideally suited for this task. Because the relationship of specific locus analysis to events occurring elsewhere in the genome is ambiguous, it is deemed advisable that more than just a single locus be utilized in gene mutational assay systems.

Forward gene mutations are much preferred over reversions for assay purposes since, in most instances, they are less restrictive and will respond to a greater variety of genetic events than reverse mutations. Forward mutational assays that concern man should be preferentially selected over the corresponding reverse mutation assays. This particular approach is necessary to obtain the quantitative and qualitative information needed for making informed risk–benefit evaluations regarding environmental mutagens. In this regard, assays measuring reversions at specific loci, though highly specific indicators of genetic activity, fail to provide the information required for risk–benefit evaluation. It should be emphasized that mammalian cell lines heterozygous at specific loci are currently available, which are believed to register the full array of genetic damage that is important to man (Clive *et al.*, 1972). These systems are currently in use and would seem to provide important experimental material for safety evaluation as regards mutagenicity.

Such assays provide an adequate test of proximate mutagens but do not consider essential pharmacokinetic factors as they might apply to man. Thus, certain substances which cause mutations in the intact animal would appear genetically inert by *in vitro* analysis. Attempts to consider pharmacokinetic factors have essentially focused on the question of metabolic activation, and little consideration has been given to absorption, tissue distribution, rates of elimination, and clearance. While this has been true of the host-mediated assay, these are not necessarily unavoidable limitations. For instance, if mammalian cells were used as the indicator organism, it is possible to inject them intravenously and, theoretically possible with certain cell lines, to recover them from various sites to evaluate the problem of organ-specific activation. Thus, the indicator organism might serve as a bioassay for providing information regarding tissue distribution of the compound and/or its metabolites. One alternative to the host-mediated assay utilizes microsomal preparations from various organs to provide for metabolic activation *in vitro*. This approach, however, will only measure the potential of a compound and its metabolites to cause mutations but will not provide the quantitative (dosage level) data essential for risk evaluation.

Another especially promising approach for the detection of gene mutations is to screen for protein variants in blood serum or other body tissues or fluids. Protein variants can be detected either with starch gel electrophoresis or by cytochemical methods that can detect rare variants by differential staining. By using two mouse strains that have differences in the electrophoretic mobility of several serum proteins, it is not only possible to look for electrophoretic variants with alterations in activity, but also amorphs which have no enzyme activity.

Chromosomal Aberrations   The objective of assays for chromosomal aberrations is to determine whether exposure to the environmental agent will produce cells with abnormal numbers of chromosomes or chromosome rearrangements. Abnormal numbers of chromosomes usually arise by nondisjunction, giving rise to cells with either higher or lower chromosome numbers than exist in the standard diploid chromosome complement. Many types of abnormalities in structure can be produced, including gaps, breaks, and terminal deletions—as well as such rearrangements as dicentrics, rings, and reciprocal translocations. The latter three classes of chromosomal aberrations require both breakage and reunion, and these structural rearrangements can persist for many cell generations.

Cells with both abnormal numbers of certain autosomes and sex chromosomes, as well as cells with chromosomal translocations, are transmissible and these classes of chromosomal aberrations constitute a known hazard for the human population. Cells with other types of chromosomal aberrations, such as breaks, gaps and autosomal monosomy, usually die as the result of chromosomal imbalance. Gametes containing such structural abnormalities, if capable of fertilization, produce embryos which usually die during organogenesis.

Germ Cells   Assay systems for chromosomal aberrations in germ cells include the dominant lethal test, the translocation test, and direct cytological analysis of germ cells. In the dominant lethal test (Bateman and Epstein, 1971), a positive result is generally interpreted as presumptive evidence for the production of chromosomal aberrations. Because of the high spontaneous background of dominant lethality in most strains of rats and mice, the assay is relatively insensitive and does not supply the type of information required for evaluation of long-term genetic effects on the population. Nevertheless, it is one of the few tests that simulate the physiological and reproductive factors that are applicable to man. It is important to remember in interpreting the dominant lethal test that negative results can not be regarded as proof that the agent is nonmutagenic; it is possible that the converse is true. Recent studies with the F_1 progeny produced in the dominant lethal test (Generoso, 1973) have shown that this assay can be expanded and tests can be made on the viable F_1 progeny for the presence of reciprocal translocations. Since the spontaneous frequency of translocations is low, induced frequencies can be detected with much lower levels of exposure than induced frequencies of dominant lethality. In the translocation test, a particular type of chromosomal aberration that is transmissible within the human population can be identified.

An alternate method for obtaining cytogenetic information directly on the production of chromosomal aberrations in germ cells (Yerganian and Lavappa, 1971) is provided by recently developed techniques. These techniques can be used for direct spermatogenic analysis, as well as examination of the early states of embryogenesis. In fact, the differences in the morphology and staining reaction of the male and female chromosome complements in the early stages of embryogenesis makes it possible to identify the parent that has contributed an abnormal chromosome complement. The high level of technical sophistication required for this type of analysis currently limits the extent of large-scale implementation of these techniques.

Somatic Cells *In vitro* assays for chromosomal aberrations can be made directly on cells of various mammalian tissues (Cohen and Hirschhorn, 1971). Interphase cells from the bone marrow can be screened rapidly for micronucleii that are produced by various types of structural changes; anaphase cells can be examined for bridges that are produced by disjunction of dicentric and ring chromosomes; and metaphase cells can be examined for all of these aberrations, as well as additional types of chromosomal rearrangements.

The main problem with testing somatic cells for mutagenicity is uncertainty about how to relate the frequencies of genetic damage observed to the frequencies that might be expected in germ cells. An additional problem in somatic cell assays is that these cells are usually scored only for chromosomal breaks and gaps, and these aberrations are of questionable relevance with regard to heritable events of importance for man. Certain classes of reciprocal translocations can also be scored in such analysis. Thus, collection of data in somatic cells on the chromosomal aberrations of interest with regard to genetic hazards is largely without substantiation.

Mitotic Recombination and Gene Conversion Assays for mitotic recombination and gene conversion have generally been ignored as an important category of genetic damage for man. Both of these effects should be given greater consideration, however, since they provide a mechanism for making recessive genes homozygous in an initially heterozygous diploid cell. This category of effect is of greater importance for the individual than for the population. Somatic recombination can be of major consequence to the developing mammalian embryo, by permitting expression of deleterious recessive genes. It may also have an effect in the somatic cells of the mature adult: For example, it could represent a mechanism for the expression of recessive genes that might be associated with the development of certain neoplasms, although such association has been demonstrated only for dominant genes.

The only practical assay for somatic recombination and gene conversion uses diploid yeast (*Saccharomyces cerevisiae*) (Mortimer and Manney, 1971), but treatment can be made *in vivo* by using yeast as the indicator organism in the host-mediated assay. Thus, this test can be made not only on the original compound but also on the important products of mammalian metabolism. The test for somatic recombination and gene conversion is rapid and sensitive and is generally a good indicator of genetic activity. Furthermore, the frequencies of this class of genetic effect are often orders of magnitude higher than the frequencies observed for gene mutations and chromosomal aberrations.

Methods for Teratogenicity Testing

Since the thalidomide incident, progress has been made in devising test procedures that identify some potentially embryotoxic substances, but presently used procedures still do not provide all of the predictive value that is possible in view of present knowledge. Over the past 10 years a great many refinements of concept and procedure have been proposed by numerous investigators (Lorke, 1963; Fraser, 1963; Brent, 1964, 1969; VanLoosli and Theiss, 1964; Zimmermann, 1964; Ferm, 1965; Gottschewski, 1965; Frohberg and Oettel, 1966; Gibson *et al.*, 1966; WHO, 1967; Nomura, 1969; Palmer, 1969; Dyban *et al.*, 1970; Robson, 1970; Clegg, 1971; Fave, 1971; Tuchmann-Duplessis, 1972).

It is agreed that no single test or battery of animal tests will provide complete assurance that exposure to an environmental agent at a particular level in animals will quantitatively predict a teratogenic risk in humans. Some potential human teratogens will be uncovered by animal testing, but some agents will also be indicated as teratogenic when, in fact, the risk following human exposure may be negligible. There are many reasons why teratogenicity testing in animals is not entirely reliable; even if teratogens were tested in several hundred human pregnancies, there is the possibility that some chemicals with teratogenic potential for certain individuals would not be recognized. Until all of the mechanisms of teratogenesis in animals and humans are known, and all the differences between human beings and animal models are understood, teratogenicity testing in animals can only be regarded as a statement of probability that the test substance will or will not act similarly in man. The predictive value of animal tests, however, can be improved by attention to the factors discussed in the following paragraphs.

Duration of Exposure   The earlier practice of treatment throughout gestation has now been largely abandoned. Most protocols now specify treatment throughout the span of organogenesis of the species in use. This has the advantage that treatment covers the early formative and maximally sensitive stages of organ development; it also affords the convenience of an uncomplicated procedure. Nevertheless, continuous dosage throughout organogenesis may produce misleading results, a possibility less likely if the duration of treatment, in at least some test animals, is limited to no more than 3 or 4 days.

Changing Plasma Concentrations versus Changing Embryonic Sensitivities   The main objection to treatment throughout organogenesis is that it may activate maternal adaptative mechanisms (Burns, 1970), which could alter maternal plasma concentration and hence cause fluctuations in embryo dosage during a test period. Conversely, if the compound happens to be one that slows its own metabolism (e.g., by inhibiting metabolic enzymes or destroying liver tissue) an exaggerated effect might be expected after repeated treatment (Wilson, 1966). In either case maternal plasma level and accordingly, embryo dose as well, would change during the course of protracted dosage.

Masking of Later Teratogenicity by Early Embryolethality   Embryos in early stages of organogenesis are sometimes more subject to embryolethal than to teratogenic effects (Wilson, 1973b). This was pointedly illustrated in recent rat experiments: A single dose of cytosine arabinoside at 20 mg/kg of maternal weight on day 9 was sufficient to kill most of the embryos, whereas a single injection of this compound on day 12 at 100 mg/kg was found to cause 67 percent malformations, but no increase in lethality above control level (Ritter *et al.*, 1971). Continuous treatment with 20 mg/kg or more begun early in organogenesis would have led to the conclusion that this drug was only embryolethal.

Single versus Multiple Exposures Experimental demonstration that repeated treatment with a chemical agent may produce different embryotoxic results than a single treatment with the same compound was made by Robens (1969) using a number of pesticides. Groups of pregnant hamsters were treated on days 6 through 10 with the test compounds, while other groups were treated with smaller total amounts of the same compounds as a single dose on day 7 or 8 of gestation. Multiple treatments caused few developmental defects, even at high doses, but did cause some resorption and maternal death. The single treatments produced numerous defects in live-born young. A similar phenomenon was observed by King *et al.* (1965).

Misleading Results from Repeated Doses The ways in which long-duration dosage with chemical agents may interfere with teratogenicity testing are summarized in Table 7. That implantation can be prevented by prior treatment with thalidomide has been shown or presumed to occur in a number of instances (Lucey and Behrman, 1963; Wilson, 1970). Thus, a treatment regimen begun at a time prior to or coinciding with implantation could preclude the birth of offspring. The presence of many malformations in an embryo probably predisposes to intrauterine death, whereas the more limited pattern of defects expected from short-term dosage would more likely permit survival to term.

TABLE 7 Misleading Effects of Repeated Dosage Early in Pregnancy in Teratological Testing

Treatment Begun	Primary Effect	Secondary Effect, Capable of Altering Test Results
Before implantation	Interference with implantation	No issue
Early postimplantation	Embryonic death in early stages	No issue
Before, or in early, organogenesis	Induction of catabolizing enzymes	Reduced blood level during organogenesis
Before, or in early, organogenesis	Inhibition of catabolizing enzymes	Elevated blood level during organogenesis
Before, or in early, organogenesis	Liver pathology or reduced function	Elevated blood level during organogenesis
Before, or in early, organogenesis	Kidney pathology or reduced function[a]	Elevated blood level during organogenesis
Before, or in early, organogenesis	Saturation of protein binding sites[a]	Elevated blood level during organogenesis

[a] These effects have been demonstrated in experimental teratology but they exist in other toxicological situations.

Alternative Measures   The obvious alternative to treatment throughout organogenesis is treatment of different groups of animals for shorter
periods that consecutively cover the span of organogenesis. Treatment
on successive single days is both impractical and unnecessary. A reasonable compromise is to divide the period of organogenesis of the test
species into several short time spans (3–4 days for rats), with separate
groups of animals tested at each of these shorter spans. However, the
highest dose that causes no embryotoxicity during the short-term treatment should be tested continuously throughout the period of organogenesis in one group of test animals to observe cumulative effects that
may result from long-term treatment. Thus, by using both short-term
and long-term treatment groups, the predictive value of teratogenicity
tests could be appreciably increased.

Exposure Level and Range   A teratogenicity test should not be regarded
as complete until a dose is found that produces some embryotoxicity,
that is, intrauterine death, teratogenicity, or growth retardation.

   The Threshold for Embryotoxic Effects   Most, if not all, chemicals
can be shown to produce some type of embryotoxicity if applied in
sufficient dosage during an appropriate time in embryogenesis in one
or more species of animal (Karnofsky, 1965). The establishment of an
embryotoxic level of dosage is important because this is the logical starting point from which to extrapolate downward in setting a safe tolerance
level for chemicals that may be consumed by or brought in contact with
pregnant women. Technically the threshold of embryotoxicity could be
defined as either the highest no-observed-effect or the lowest effect level,
but absolute precision in this regard cannot be established experimentally.
A reasonable approximation would usually be sufficient in practice because the acceptable tolerance level for most environmental chemicals
would be set at a very small fraction of any known effect level. In any
event, if teratogenicity testing is to be put on a rational basis, the practice
of extrapolating downward from a minimal effect level to a safe tolerance
level must be accepted.

   Safe Tolerance Levels   A *safe* tolerance level is an empirically derived
dosage set somewhere below the minimal effect level, depending on the
nature of the compound, and presumed to be the permissible daily intake or exposure that causes no toxic effects in a great majority of individuals exposed. It will vary widely for different categories of chemicals, such as drugs, pesticides, and food additives, and will vary within
those groups according to the type of benefit expected from their use.

   Usage levels for chemicals that are less directly involved with man's
health and welfare than are drugs should be given much lower acceptable

exposure levels in reference to the embryotoxicity threshold in animals. Environmental pollutants should be tested for embryotoxicity when there is any reason to suspect appreciable exposure of pregnant women. A ratio of 1000:1 of the embryotoxic threshold level in test animals to average daily human exposure might be taken as an upper limit of tolerance for most types of chemicals, while a 10:1 ratio may be appropriate for agents of very high benefit or limited distribution.

Therefore, test doses should be chosen with the intention of identifying an embryotoxic threshold, which will then be used as a basis for extrapolating downward to an acceptable tolerance level. The setting of acceptable tolerance levels requires a value judgment of risk–benefit: Benefit will vary widely, and teratological testing in animals provides only a rough estimate of the risk under the best of conditions. Because of probable differences in the embryotoxic sensitivity of test animals and man, and the possibility of overexposure, human tolerance levels must be set as far as possible below embryotoxic levels in consideration of the circumstances relating to the presence of the chemical in the environment.

Choice of Test Animals   The first of many problems arising from the use of animals to assess teratological risks in man is the choice of the most appropriate species for the tests. Rats, mice, and rabbits have been the most widely used species for the practical reasons that they are readily available, inexpensive, easy to maintain and can be bred with relative ease in the laboratory. Unfortunately, none of these reasons has much scientific bearing on the central problem of the predictive value of tests with these species for environmental risks to human reproduction.

Disregarding economic considerations, the ideal animal for teratological testing would have the following characteristics: (1) the ability to absorb, metabolize, and eliminate the test substance in a manner similar to that of man, (2) the ability to transmit the substance and its metabolite across the placenta as does man, and (3) embryos and fetuses that have developmental schedules and metabolic pathways similar to those in the human conceptus. Existing comparative data are too limited for a judgment as to which animal is most like man in any of these regards; but it is already apparent that no presently used species, including simians, resembles man in all of these respects. Furthermore, it is evident that the degree of similarity to man exhibited by a given species varies from one test substance to another.

Number of Species and Which Species   The current practice of performing teratogenicity tests in at least two species would seem laudable in view of the foregoing comments. Unfortunately, however, much of the benefit that might be expected from a diversity of test animals is lost because of the widespread tendency to select all test species from the closely related rodents (rat, mouse, and occasionally hamster or guinea pig) and lagomorphs (rabbits and hares). Although these animals have several dietary, reproductive, and metabolic similarities, probably the most significant for this type of research is the fact that they all possess a highly specialized placental structure not present in higher mammals during the critical period of organogenesis—the inverted yolk sac placenta. The embryos of these species may be dependent on this atypical structure for all interchange of essential materials with maternal blood during the critical first few days of organogenesis, the time when embryos generally are most susceptible to embryotoxic influences. Evidence has accumulated that the yolk sac placenta is not only structurally, but very likely also functionally, different from the typical chorioallantoic placenta that serves other mammals (Everett, 1935; Padykula *et al.*, 1966; Beck *et al.*, 1967; Brent, 1971). Furthermore, Brambell (1957) showed that molecules the size of immunoproteins were much more readily transported across the yolk sac placenta than the chorioallantoic placenta.

Direct comparisons of the teratogenic susceptibility of rodents and rabbits, on the one hand, and of higher mammalian species, on the other, have seldom been attempted. In one study, comparison of the susceptibility of rats and rhesus monkeys to several drugs known to be teratogenic in one or the other species was made (Wilson, 1971). Particular care was taken to administer the drugs at comparable stages in development. Rats were found to show embryotoxic effects after lower doses of most of the compounds tested than did monkeys. Thalidomide was a striking exception to this rule, however, and serves to deter a hasty generalization that rats are always teratologically more sensitive than monkeys. Nevertheless, when the literature on experimental teratological studies was reviewed (Wilson, 1972), it became apparent that little or no teratogenicity was observed in simians to many chemical agents that are highly teratogenic in rats, mice, and rabbits. When dosage was increased sufficiently to elicit some embryotoxic response in simians, it was more often manifested as intrauterine death (abortion) or growth retardation than malformation. Further comparative studies of this type are needed, not so much to determine which of various test species has greater or lesser sensitivity to teratogenesis, but which reacts to given types of agents in ways most nearly comparable to those in man. As emphasized above, the choice of animals should ideally be based on similarities to man in plasma concentrations, in placental transfer, and in reactions within the conceptus for the compound being tested. Such data are not available for any compound today and a tremendous amount of research remains to be done if the choice of test animals, and thus the translation of experimental results to man, is to be made on a less empirical and more truly scientific basis.

Number of Animals per Test Group It has become customary to use 20 female rats or mice and 10 or more female rabbits at each dosage level when treatment is given throughout organogenesis. In general these numbers seem to have yielded sufficient numbers of offspring for statistical purposes in screening studies, but larger numbers are needed to establish precisely the lower end of dose–response curves. As suggested earlier, however, a shorter duration of treatment (3 instead of 10 days) with smaller groups of animals (10 rats or mice instead of 20) treated at several consecutive time spans in organogenesis, would probably yield more meaningful results, and would not greatly increase the total number of test animals. The tendency to use fewer rabbits than rats or mice reflects such factors as availability, cost and ease of breeding. These considerations become even more compelling when simians or other large species are used.

Genetic Background of Test Animals A question is sometimes raised as to the desirability of using inbred or other highly homogenous strains of animals in teratological testing. Accumulated experience over many years of experimental teratology has shown that intrastrain variability, in general, and spontaneous malformations, in particular, are reduced when stocks of animals with some heterogeneity in genetic makeup are maintained by closed-colony but not brother–sister mating (Palmer, 1969). Highly inbred animals, as would result from brother–sister matings, often show developmental defects unique to that strain, but they also may be particularly resistant to teratogenesis by certain agents. The best safeguard against being misled is to use a stock for which extensive cumulative control data are available, in addition to the concurrent controls run with each experiment. For example, when an unusual malformation occurs during a teratogenicity test, such background data can greatly facilitate interpretation by allowing the investigator to state that the defect has or has not occurred in a stated frequency among a large number of controls of the same stock examined in the same way over several years.

Health and Parity of Test Animals One must stress the need for cleanliness, adequate nutrition, constant temperature, and regular light–dark cycles to obtain reproducible results. The use of specific-pathogen-free animals adds little of value to teratogenicity testing. Such extraneous chemicals as pesticides should not be used in the vicinity of test animals either during, or for several weeks preceding, a test to avoid the possibility of the induction or inhibition of drug metabolizing enzymes.

Such enzymes can also be induced by aromatic bedding materials, especially conifer wood shavings, which should also be avoided. The use of specific disease control measures—such as daily dosing of simians with isoniazid as prophylaxis against tuberculosis—is preferable to the alternative, but its use during or immediately preceding the period of organogenesis in which a teratogenicity test is conducted is not advised.

The only reason for using parous dams is that some females, particularly rodents, are more likely to destroy or neglect the newborn of first litters than of subsequent ones, thus reducing the numbers of offspring available for postnatal study. For general reproduction studies in which possible effects on fertility are under scrutiny for the test substance, it would be desirable for all subjects to be proven fertile before the substance is administered.

Appropriate and Inappropriate Test Subjects   It has already been noted that no one animal species or group of related species is ideally suited for the evaluation of human teratological risks. Accumulated experience, however, has shown that certain groups of animals may offer advantages for particular types of use, whereas others have been found generally inappropriate. In the inappropriate category must be placed all species or test systems that lack the parental adaptive mechanisms by which mammals are usually able to reduce the dosage of most physical and chemical agents before they reach the conceptus.

The mammalian embryo and fetus benefit from a further and unique line of defense against chemical agents—the selective transport functions of the placenta. Most chemicals in the environment, inlcuding those in the maternal bloodstream, are subject to concentration gradients across the placenta, usually with the gradient favoring lower concentration in the conceptus than in maternal plasma. Although far from infallible, the placenta is so important as a dose-regulating device that its presence cannot be disregarded in realistic testing of the embryotoxic effects of environmental agents. Thus, nonmammalian forms are not appropriate for use in the safety evaluation of human embryotoxic risks. Avian and other nonmammalian embryos have contributed and doubtless will continue to contribute, greatly to studies on embryologic and teratogenic mechanisms; but the relatively static nutritional and excretory functions in the incubating egg are in sharp contrast to the fluctuating interchange that occurs in both directions across the placenta. Foreign substances introduced into incubating eggs may remain in a slowly diminishing pool for a relatively long time, whereas most compounds as well as their metabolites have a short half-life in maternal and presumably also in embryonic bloodstreams of mammals.

In vitro systems—whether involving whole embryo, organ, tissue, or cell cultures—are all inappropriate for use in embryotoxicity evaluation. Among the many other obstacles to achieving and maintaining conditions that would even approximate the *in vivo* state, the problem of circulation of nutrients and metabolites surely ranks as a major one. These variables superimposed on and possibly interacting with whatever stress is introduced by the test substance, would render results from *in vitro* cultures almost meaningless as compared with an embryo in dynamic balance with maternal homeostasis through the placenta.

As mentioned earlier, rodents and lagomorphs have one major disadvantage as test animals: Their embryos are dependent on the highly atypical yolk sac placenta during early organogenesis. Although this unique placental structure may not be wholly at fault, there is accumulating evidence that animals whose early embryos are dependent upon it for essential transport show embryotoxicity to lower doses of more chemical agents than do other mammals. On the other hand, the small size, short gestation period, large litter size, lack of seasonal breeding patterns, and ready availability of these animals add up to a strong inducement to continue their use in initial screening procedures. Not the least of the advantages is their modest cost, which permits the use of ample numbers for statistical evaluation of results.

Carnivores have not been widely used in teratological testing, but, in view of the urgent need for diversity in the choice of test animals (particularly for animals that do not possess the specialized placentation of the preceding group), it is hoped that investigators will be encouraged to explore further the use of these animals. All of the three species that can be maintained in the laboratory—ferret, cat, and dog—have the disadvantage of being seasonal breeders, usually having only one or two litters per year. On the other hand, they are polytocous and the gestation period is relatively short so that test results are available within 2 months or less after treatment.

Ungulates, such as the pig, sheep, and possibly the goat, seem to be promising subjects for use in the evaluation of human teratic risk. The agricultural background of these animals assures a wealth of information on the breeding performance of various stocks. Although they have not been used as extensively in pharmacological and toxicological investigations as some of the preceding species, a significant amount of information probably could be found. The larger size of these animals would require large samples of the test compound.

The advantages and disadvantages of simians have recently been reviewed (Wilson, 1972). To date only two genera, *Papio* (baboons) and *Macaca* (several species), have been demonstrated to be promising for use in the evaluation of human teratic risk. It is taken for granted that simians will not be used in mutagenicity testing or for preliminary teratogenicity screens, both of which uses require larger numbers than are practicable. In fact there is growing concensus that simians used in reproduction studies should be reserved for the teratogenicity testing of certain types of drugs in relation to possible use during human pregnancy. Even in these special situations, simians would be used only as the last step before clinical trial, after the test compound had been shown in nonprimate animals to have acceptably low levels of general embryo-toxicity. In view of the negative value, as regards human welfare, of most environmental chemicals, it is unlikely that the precision hopefully provided by simian tests would be needed to establish tolerance levels of such materials. Therefore, in general, simians would not be used to evaluate the hazards to human development of environmental chemicals except under unusual circumstances.

Current Methods for Testing Other Aspects of Reproduction

In a previous document (FDA, 1970), the suitability of the multigeneration test currently in use by the Food and Drug Administration was considered, in comparison with a battery of single tests. That review committee wrote

It would be desirable and intellectually more satisfying to have information about specific effects during various stages of the reproductive cycle. For example, answers to the following questions would be useful. Is the toxicity in terms of LD_{50} of the mother and fetus the same? Are there differences in effects in immature and mature animals? Does the substance concentrate in the placenta, gonads, or elsewhere in the reproductive system? Are there specific histopathologic or gross effects in the pituitary in the male and female gonads, or in the secondary sex organs? Has libido been influenced? Are there effects on formation and maturation of the gonads and gametes, transport of the gametes, on combination of the gametes, on implantation, and on continued function of corpus luteum and the placenta? Is there a normal onset and completion of parturition? Is lactation normal? Is the quality of the milk favorable? Do the offspring have congenital malformations or abnormalities? Do the offspring carry altered genetic potentials? Exhaustive studies of each of the questions asked above would be expensive and time-consuming. A distinct advantage of the three-generation test is that it gives an overall view of reproductive function which is not achieved by single specific tests. For example, a "standard" reproduction study gives us information on fertility and pregnancy in the case of the F(0) or parent generation. Observations of the F(1) generation would determine the effects of a substance upon the uterine environment and upon lactation as well as on post-weaning growth and development. The F(1) animals which have been exposed continuously to this substance from the time of conception would reveal changes in reproduction characteristics acquired during the periods of embryogenesis, infancy, puberty, and reproductive maturity. The accumulation of a potentially toxic substance would be determined by the reproductive performance of the F(1) generation and observation of the growth and development of the F(2) generation. It is debatable whether or not enough new information is derived from the F(3) generation of reproduction studies as presently performed to justify the effort. There is an occasional report of an effect showing up in a later generation which did not appear earlier. In each case, the investigator must determine the value of additional generations on the basis of data accrued to that point. However, as a minimum a reproduction protocol should include a study of the progeny of parents who themselves have been exposed to the test substance from the time of conception to reproductive maturity.

The panel concurs that the three-generation test is probably the best measure available for assessing overall reproductive efficiency. It could be expanded by observing the animals for their lifetime for normal rate of growth and maturation, as well as for the appearance of tumors or chronic disease.

SUGGESTIONS FOR ENHANCING THE PREDICTIVE VALUE OF ANIMAL TESTS

Monitoring Human Populations

Because of marked species differences, animal data cannot be confidently extrapolated to man. In the opinion of the panel, there is no substitute for data collected on human beings. The advent of very sensitive techniques now makes it possible to examine adsorption, metabolism, storage, accumulation, excretion, and metabolic conversions in man with relative ease and with little danger. However, it is difficult to see how information regarding deleterious effects from environmental substances can be obtained in human beings except by long-range monitoring and by close scrutiny of accidents and situations involving occupational exposure where the levels are much higher than would be expected in the general population. Prospective clinical studies should be taken advantage of when possible.

Several approaches to the collection of data directly applicable to man are possible. Tracer studies can demonstrate absorption through various routes and provide some information on metabolic pathways and potentially toxic metabolites. Another form of human testing might involve metabolic studies with fragmented tissue systems or even tissue culture. A third approach to human testing would be ongoing monitoring. At the present time the best experimental data, even if from several animal species, may not be closely relevant to man. Once a compound is made generally available on the basis of safety evaluation studies in animals, the final answer regarding safety will come from human experience. Therefore, a program of continued monitoring is very important. Such monitoring, rather than being a casual alertness for reports of adverse effects, should be a planned, deliberate effort to obtain useful data. Although the results of animal studies may provide suggestions regarding feasible designs for monitoring, the possibility of major qualitative differences existing between man and experimental animals would indicate a need for alertness concerning possible unexpected human effects.

A monitoring program should include (1) accumulation of data on levels of intake of different substances similar to that of FDA "market basket" surveys for radioactivity and pesticides; (2) routine random examinations of postmortem and surgical specimens to determine accumulations of the compounds in human tissues, and a correlation of such "body load" data with clinical and pathological data from the same patients; (3) development of techniques for eliciting information from the medical profession regarding unusual manifestations or disorders that might result from environmental factors, such as expanded disease registries and improved uniform death certificates; (4) establishment of epidemiologic studies utilizing the working populations in chemical manufacturing plants; and (5) epidemiologic studies in a selected population during market surveys, prior to release of new substances for general use.

Multilevel Teratogenicity Testing

It has been emphasized that there is no one animal species that can be considered ideal for evaluating human teratological risk. There is also uncertainty as to which of the criteria (i.e., phylogenetic proximity, metabolic relatedness, similarity of placental transfer, or similarity of embryonic reaction) relative to man should receive major emphasis in designing protocols. A great deal of research remains to be done before all of the information needed for making the wisest choice will be available. In the meantime, testing and research on mechanisms must not only be continued but, in view of the rate of environmental change, it should be intensified.

Unfortunately, experience with any one agent cannot always be used in designing protocols for testing other agents, not even agents of the same class. For example, thalidomide would be particularly unsuitable as a model of the embryotoxic properties of other drugs because (1) the disparity between maternal and embryonic toxicity is greater than for any other teratogen, (2) it produces an atypically flat dose–response curve in simians, the most sensitive species, and (3) the range of effective doses varies widely among susceptible species. It should be noted that any or all of these observations are instant clues to the need for more thorough study of chronic toxicity. Nevertheless, some standardization of testing procedures is necessary and the following suggestions are thought to represent an acceptable amalgam of the numerous procedures and objectives that have been proposed (Brent, 1972; Wilson, 1973a).

Table 8 lists the many factors that one should consider when establishing guidelines for animal testing protocols to screen for teratogenesis. Variations on the three-generation test include most of these parameters but the panel believes that increased emphases should be placed on the techniques for evaluating and interpreting intrauterine and extrauterine growth retardation, and determination of the maternal–fetal LD_{50} ratio. Certainly items 9, 10, and 11 in Table 8 are important areas for investigation because information on these subjects would both simplify and improve the applicability to man of animal tests. If the metabolic fate of a chemical and its mechanism of action are known, many empirical testing steps could be eliminated.

A multilevel teratogenicity test in animals is proposed in Table 9. The first level would consist of a teratogenicity screen employing large numbers of a readily available animal, such as rat or mouse, for the purpose of finding the embryotoxic range of dosage. A test substance causing no significant embryotoxicity at appropriate multiples of the anticipated human dose would advance to the second level of testing in which a carnivore (dog, cat, or ferret) or an ungulate (pig or sheep) would be used, depending on which showed greater similarity to man in the metabolism

TABLE 8   Factors To Be Considered in Establishing Testing Procedures for Teratogenesis

1. Exposure duration
2. Exposure level and range
3. Stage of exposure
4. Route of exposure
5. Number of control and experimental litters
6. Number of species of test animals
7. Examination of near-term fetuses
   Malformations, including internal as well as external
   Term fetal weight (presence of growth retardation)
   Intrauterine death rate (LD_{50} maternal–fetal ratio)
8. Examination of offspring following spontaneous delivery
   Structural and functional normalcy as regards growth, longevity, behavior, reproductive capacity, etc.
9. Fetal and maternal metabolism of test substance
10. Placental transport
11. Determination of mechanism of action of teratogenic substances

TABLE 9   Teratogenicity Testing Based on Multilevel Tests in Different Types of
Animals

Order of Test	Reason for Use	Suitable Species
1st Level	Find embryotoxic dose range	Rat, mouse, hamster *or* rabbit
2nd Level	Confirm or adjust above	A carnivore—dog, cat, or ferret—*or* an ungulate—pig or sheep
3rd Level	Only if 2nd level results are equivocal	Alternate to that used in 2nd level
4th Level	Only if exposure in human pregnancy is unavoidable	*Macaca* (monkey) *or* *Papio* (baboon)

NOTE: Tests would terminate at 2nd level in most situations involving environmental chemicals.

of the compound in question. Such information on metabolism could be
accumulated in the course of prior toxicological studies. The higher costs
and lower fecundity of this second test animal (e.g., dogs or pigs) would
dictate the use of smaller numbers than in the initial screen, but this
would be acceptable because the general range of effective dosage would
already have been defined. The second level test would thus be for the
purpose of confirming and revising embryotoxic dosage found at the
first level in another species that might metabolize the test substance
more like man than did the rodent-type animal, but in any event would
not have the atypical yolk sac placenta of the first-level animal.

For environmental chemicals it would ordinarily not be necessary to
proceed beyond the first or second level proposed in Table 9. If the compound being tested were found to show embryotoxicity only at, for example, 100 times or greater the level corresponding to the upper limits of
human exposure, this might be regarded as a tolerable margin of safety
and a tolerance level set accordingly. If, however, there were uncertainty
about the margin of safety between the dose that causes embryotoxicity
in either first or second level tests and the exposure level of man, or if
the compound were of a nature that might under certain conditions involve exposure of pregnant women, a third level of subprimate tests
would seem justified. A fourth level of tests using simians would be
justified only in the event that a chemical already in the environment became suspect of association with human embryotoxicity. Intensive
simian tests might help to resolve an issue of whether heroic efforts were
to be undertaken either to remove the questionable chemical from the
environment or to protect pregnant women from it.

Mutagenicity Testing

One of the central questions in studies on environmental mutagenesis is to determine ways to extrapolate data from model systems to man more reliably. Work in this area is facilitated by the fact that evaluations for certain types of genetic effects can be made directly on man himself, as well as on human cells in culture. For example, by comparing the level of effects on mammalian cells *in vitro* with the effects produced on the same cells *in vivo* as well as on human cells *in vitro*, it may be possible to predict a level of effect in man. To increase the reliability of extrapolation for gene mutations, it is useful to have experimental data collected on a variety of indicator organisms and assay systems. If the agent produces essentially the same quantitative and qualitative effects in all of these systems, then it may be assumed that this agent should constitute a hazard for the human population or some undefined portion thereof.

An important area of concern is the ascertainment of whether induced mutations accumulate within the spermatagonia throughout the reproductive life of man. It is also of importance to know whether the end result is dependent upon the specific agent or mechanism responsible for the mutation. Answers to these questions are forthcoming only from those systems that have the theoretical potential to register genetic events arising from long-term, low-level exposure to chemical mutagens.

One possible experimental approach might involve an extensive geimsa-geimsa-bank cytogenetic analysis of progeny from mutagen-exposed parents. It is conceivable that no more than 50 rodent progeny would be required for a single test compound. The small number of progeny is made possible by virtue of the high degree of resolution afforded by chromosome-banding techniques; indeed, with some mammals as many as 1000 genetic characters can be studied per single karyotype. Thus, the need for large numbers of progeny may well be negated.

INTERPRETATION

Monitoring for Developmental Defects

If the present testing procedures for teratogenicity and mutagenicity are not reliable in predicting these adverse effects in man, what measures can be taken to further reduce the risks? Better clinical surveillance is certainly one answer. A computerized monitoring program should be established at a national level and should include exhaustive coverage of (1) birth certificates with indication of the infant's physical condition,

(2) abortion and stillbirth records, (3) infant death certificates, (4) complete medical history of the pregnancy, and (5) a genetic history. This information should be analyzed so that attention would be called as early as possible to new statistical correlations and significant changes in incidence of disease. Such a program would have almost immediate benefits, and the value of such a monitoring program would increase with time as the epidemiologic methods were further refined. Measures would have to be taken to improve current levels of interest and participation by physicians and hospitals in providing such information.

The simplest manual punch-card system would have uncovered the association between thalidomide and limb malformations after less than 15 cases, rather than the several thousand that actually occurred. The establishment of clinical surveillance programs is not a new idea, but it is one that has been rather consistently ignored. In 1964 it was suggested (Brent, 1964) that

At the present time, the most reliable method of protecting the public from all harmful effects of drugs is through strict clinical surveillance programs.

Ingalls and Klingberg (1965) published the same message. Clinical monitoring is expensive, it is tedious, it will take years to educate the physician, public, and administrative agencies to comply with the regulations. But if such a program had been established in 1964 it would be fully operational today.

Thresholds as Applied to Reproduction

The concept of thresholds is a matter of major importance in relation to the safety evaluation of new chemicals and other environmental agents. The focal issue is whether the demonstration of toxic manifestations at high dosage levels signifies that the substance in question is unsafe at all levels. In other words, is there a threshold below which no manifestation of toxicity is seen (i.e., a no-effect range of dosage) or does the probability of adverse effects simply become smaller as a dosage is lowered toward the vanishing point?

In contrast to the situation in mutagenicity and carcinogenicity, where thresholds have not been proven to exist, experimental teratologists have generally assumed that all chemical agents do have a threshold below which no effect can be demonstrated. This is based on a large number of studies in animals using the easily quantitated criteria of intrauterine death and structural abnormality in near-term fetuses. When a suitable range of dosage has been given during sensitive periods of development, a no-effect range below the threshold at which embryotoxicity appears to begin has often been demonstrated. The argument that extremely large numbers of animals are necessary to establish the existence of no-effect levels may be valid under two conditions: (1) when the slope of the dose–response curve is very flat, and (2) when independent cells, rather than organisms, capable of regulation and repair are studied. As will be discussed below, dose–response curves in teratology are usually quite steep. The teratogenic response depends on the reaction of integrated groups of cells in tissues, organs, and organisms. Only in certain types of chronic toxicity, such as carcinogenesis and mutagenesis, are individual cells thought to react independently to environmental chemicals.

Thus, available evidence indicates that a dosage can always be found below which teratogenicity and embryolethality in excess of that seen in control is not produced, although the validity of this generalization has not been fully explored as regards possible alterations at the ultrastructural level. The same is almost certainly true for growth retardation, but this has not been as exhaustively studied as have death and malformation. Another area of embryotoxicity for which the existence of a no-effect range of dosage can reasonably be questioned concerns subtle functional, particularly behavioral, changes because there is little basis in direct evidence for a conclusion at this time. A definitive determination of whether small doses of adverse influences could cause permanent functional disorder would require that large numbers of animals be subjected to a comprehensive battery of physiologic tests for an extended period of time after treatment. Until such tests become practicable, the lack of evidence to the contrary permits a tentative assumption that functional disorders, like other types of developmental toxicity, have thresholds of dosage.

Typically the dose–response curve for acute embryotoxic effects has been shown to have a relatively steep slope—sometimes going from minimal to maximal effect levels by merely doubling the dose. The well-known primate teratogen, thalidomide, seems to be an exception in that initial teratogenic effects are seen during the susceptible period of the embryo at surprisingly low dosage, but many multiples of this may be required to produce total embryolethality, and maternal toxicity is exceedingly difficult to demonstrate (Wilson, 1972).

Thresholds as Exemplified by Radiation Effects A striking difference exists in the dosage of radiation required to produce different types of biological effects (Brent and Gorson, 1972). Gene mutations and, perhaps, cancer can be induced by comparatively small doses, and several investigators have argued that there may be no threshold (i.e., dosage below which no effect occurs), for the production of these effects. In contrast, malformation, growth retardation, intrauterine death, and postnatal functional deficits generally require larger dosage and are thought by most investigators to have thresholds of dosage below which these effects are not seen. Radiation effects provide excellent illustrations of the conditions which determine the presence or absence of thresholds in biological systems. Some biological effects of radiation—such as gene mutations, chromosome breaks, and possible cancer induction—may have no or a very low threshold, but most other biological effects that have been adequately studied exhibit a threshold. The difference between systems that do and those that do not exhibit a threshold hinges on whether the cells can be affected independently or whether there is a capability on the part of the organism to replace affected cells.

Effects that seem not to show a dosage threshold occur in independent or individual cells, such as germ cells, cells in culture, or when affected cells are able to react autonomously (e.g., in carcinogenesis). Effects that appear only after a threshold of dosage is reached occur in organized or associated groups of cells, such as comprise an embryo, in which replacement of damaged cells is possible. When radiation or other cytotoxic agents are applied to nonassociated cells in culture, each presumably reacts independently of what may happen in surrounding cells. The total number of cells affected—probably tantamount to the number killed (Hollaender and Stapleton, 1959)—is directly proportional to dosage and, in the case of radiation, depends on how many individual cells are "hit". The probability of hitting any one cell diminishes as dosage decreases but theoretically does not disappear as long as ionizing radiation reaches the chromatin of any cell; hence, there is no threshold to irradiation for cells in culture.

Effects in multicellular organisms (death, growth retardation, and malformation) depend on the destruction of a critical number of cells out of the total of those making up the organism or embryo. Although the initial effect may be on the chromatin of individual cells (Dewey et al., 1971), probably leading to cell death, the final effect on the embryo depends on the proportion of the total number of cells in vital parts that are destroyed. It has been reported by a number of investigators (Russell and Russell, 1954; Wilson, 1954; Brent, 1969) that irradiation of embryos prior to the beginning of organogenesis produces very few malformations but may cause embryonic death and growth retardation if the dosage is above a threshold level (25–100 R). Cells are undoubtedly killed at subthreshold doses, but embryos of all species are thought capable of tolerating the loss of a limited number of cells without lasting effect, owing to their regulative or regenerative capacity.

After organogenesis begins, different groups of cells acquire different potentialities for future development. Nevertheless, a certain number of cells may still be killed without causing a lasting effect, depending on the capacity of the tissue to regenerate. If a critical number of cell deaths occurs in a differentiating tissue, however, the organ derived from this tissue may be malformed, as has been demonstrated with chemical cytotoxic agents as well as radiations (Hicks, 1954; Ritter *et al.*, 1971). Thus the regenerative or regulative powers of the embryo make possible the repair of organ primordia up to a point beyond which repair is inadequate and malformation is likely to be the result. Such a threshold phenomenon probably exists in all organisms that have retained appreciable regenerative capacity.

There are experimental data indicating that there may not be a demonstrable threshold for mutagenesis. Whether the above explanation is applicable is not known, but, because mutagenic agents seem to act in a more or less random fashion on the DNA of individual cells, it is plausible to assume that cells are able to react independently to mutagenic agents. In this event cells exposed to a mutagen, whether in the germinal epithelium of the gonads or in some highly organized somatic tissue, would be affected in proportion to dosage. The smaller the dosage, the fewer cells would suffer damage to their heritable material; but there would be no chance to replace the damaged cells. No threshold would exist, therefore, because some cells would theoretically be affected even at minimal doses. Whether or not a mutation would be identifiable would depend on the developmental potential of the affected cells. Germ cells that were still capable of participating in fertilization would be more likely to display the damage to their hereditary material than would somatic cells, which would ordinarily have relatively few mitotic progeny in a tissue or organism composed largely of normal cells. Thresholds for other adverse effects on reproduction have not been studied, but they are assumed to be operative in organs and organisms that are capable of any degree of regulation and repair.

Levels of Testing

That all chemicals in the environment do not represent risks to reproduction is assumed and, accordingly, all do not need to be subjected to the same degree of testing. A question then arises as to what criteria will be used to determine whether tests are needed and, if they are, what degree of rigorousness it is appropriate to apply considering the estimated risk posed by the chemical in question. Criteria for approving the release of any substance into the environment will be based on considerations of social and economic benefits as opposed to the risks entailed. This judgment should also be made in the light of available alternative substances. Where a substance can be demonstrated to have a high level of benefit, a greater degree of risk may be acceptable. The panel proposes that categories of social benefit be established and incorporated as integral components of every application for regulatory approval. This would include not only the proposed purpose and likely distribution, but also a comparison with alternatives in use. This is particularly important in view of the inadequacy of current methods for evaluating risk to reproduction. Three criteria are important for the evaluation of risk: anticipated exposure (dose and distribution), presumed risk (severity, number and susceptibility of individuals at various exposure levels, specific toxicity), and reliability of testing systems.

SUMMARY

The importance of the potential hazards of environmental chemicals to the reproductive processes is presented. A review of the points of vulnerability and susceptibility of the reproductive process to chemical attack are discussed and examples given.

Mutagenic and teratogenic testing methods are critically reviewed and ways for improvement are suggested. The panel stressed the importance of data interpretation; especially as it relates to thresholds for these effects. Three criteria for evaluating risk should be used: anticipated exposure, presumed risk (severity, number of individuals and specific toxicity) and reliability of the testing system.

REFERENCES

Bateman, A.J., and S.S. Epstein. 1971. Dominant lethal mutations in mammals. In Hollaender, A., ed., *Chemical Mutagens, Principles and Methods for Their Detection.* Vol. 2. Plenum Press, New York, pp. 541–568.

Beck, F., J.B. Lloyd, and A. Griffiths. 1967. A histochemical and biochemical study of some aspects of placental function in the rat using maternal injection of horseradish peroxidase. *J. Anat.* 101:461–478.

Binns, W., C. Ceuto, B.C. Eliason, H.E. Heggestad, G.H. Hepting, P.F. Sand, R.F. Stephes, and F.H. Tschirley. 1970. Investigation of spray project near Globe, Arizona. Investigation conducted February 1970. Office of Pesticide Programs, Environmental Protection Agency, Washington, D.C.

Brambell, F.W.R. 1957. The development of fetal immunity. In Josiah Macy, Jr. Foundation. *Fourth Conference on Gestation.*

Brent, R.L. 1964. Drug testing in animals for teratogenic effects: Thalidomide in the pregnant rat. *J. Pediatr.* 64:762–770.

Brent, R.L. 1969. The direct and indirect effects of irradiation upon the mammalian zygote, embryo and fetus. In Nishimura, H., and J.R. Miller, eds., *Methods for*

Teratological Studies in Experimental Animals and Man. Igaku Shoin Ltd., Tokyo. pp. 63–75.

Brent, R.L. 1971. Antibodies and malformations. In Tuchmann-Duplessis, H., ed., *Malformations Congénitales des Mammifères.* Masson et Cie, Paris. pp. 187–220.

Brent, R.L. 1972. Protecting the public from teratogenic and mutagenic hazards. *J. Clin. Pharmacol.* 12:61–70.

Brent, R.L., and R.O. Gorson. 1972. Radiation exposure in pregnancy. In Moseley, R.D., D.H. Baker, R.O. Gorson, A. Lalli, H.B. Latourette, and J.L. Quinn. eds., *Current Problems in Radiology.* Vol. 2. Year Book Medical Publishers, Chicago. pp. 1–48.

Burns, J.J. 1970. Pharmacological aspects of teratology. In Fraser, F.C., and V.A. McKusick, eds., *Congenital Malformations.* Excerpta Medica, Amsterdam. pp. 173–179.

Butt, E.M., and D.G. Simonsen. 1950. Mercury and lead storage in human tissues. *Am. J. Clin. Pathol.* 20:716–723.

Cahen, R.L. 1966. Experimental and clinical chemoteratogenesis. *Adv. Pharmacol.* 4:263–349.

Clegg, D.J. 1971. Teratology. *Ann. Rev. Pharmacol.* 11:409–424.

Clive, D., W.G. Flamm, and M.R. Machesko. 1972. Mutagenicity of hycanthone in mammalian cells. *Mutat. Res.* 14:262–264.

Cohen, M.M., and K. Hirschhorn. 1971. Cytogenetic studies in animals. In Hollaender, A., ed., *Chemical Mutagens, Principles and Methods for Their Detection.* Vol. 2. Plenum Press, New York. pp. 515–534.

Courtney, K.D., D.W. Gaylor, M.D. Hogan, H.L. Falk, R.R. Bates, and I.A. Mitchell. 1970. Teratogenic evaluation of pesticides: A large-scale screening study. *Teratology* 3:199.

Cutting, R.T., T.H. Phuoc, J.M. Ballo, M.W. Benenson, and C.H. Evans. 1970. *Congenital Malformations, Hydatidiform Moles, and Stillbirths in the Republic of Vietnam 1960-1969.* U.S. Government Printing Office, Washington, D.C.

de Serres, F.J., and H.V. Malling. 1971. Measurement of recessive lethal damage over the entire genome and at two specific loci in the *ad-*3 region of a two-component heterokaryon of *Neurospora crassa.* In Hollaender, A., ed., *Chemical Mutagens, Principles and Methods for Their Detection.* Vol. 2. Plenum Press, New York. pp. 311–342.

Dewey, W.C., H.H. Miller, and D.B. Leeper. 1971. Chromosomal aberrations and mortality of x-irradiated mammalian cells: Emphasis on repair. *Proc. Natl. Acad. Sci.* (USA) 68:667–671.

Drake, J.W. 1970. *The Molecular Basis of Mutation.* Holden-Day, San Francisco.

Dyban, A.P., V.S. Baranov, and I.M. Akimova. 1970. Basic methodic approaches to testing chemicals for teratogenic activity. *Arkh. Anat.* 59(10):89–100.

Everett, J.W. 1935. Morphological and physiological studies of the placenta in the albino rat. *J. Exp. Zool.* 70:243–282.

Fave, A. 1971. Tecniques du controle toxicologique dans le domaine de la reproduction. In Tuchmann-Duplessis, H., ed., *Malformations Congénitales des Mammifères.* Masson et Cie, Paris. pp. 293–312.

Ferm, V.H. 1965. The rapid detection of teratogenic activity. *Lab. Invest.* 14:1500–1505.

Ferm, V.H. 1966. Congenital malformations induced by dimethyl sulphoxide in the golden hamster. *J. Embryol. Exp. Morph.* 16:49–54.

Fish, S.A. 1966. Organophosphorus cholinesterase inhibitors and fetal development. *Am. J. Obstet. Gynecol.*, 96:1148–1154.

Fishbein, L., W.G. Flamm, and H.L. Falk. 1970. *Chemical Mutagens; Environmental Effects on Biological Systems.* Academic Press, New York.

Food and Drug Administration. Advisory Committee on Protocols for Safety Evaluations. 1970. Reproduction studies in the safety evaluation of food additives and pesticide residues. Report of the Panel on Reproduction. *Toxicol. Appl. Pharmacol.* 16:264–296.

Fox, B.W., and M. Fox. 1967. Biochemical aspects of the actions of drugs on spermatogenesis. *Pharmacol. Rev.* 19:21–57.

Fraser, F.C. 1963. Methodology of experimental mammalian teratology. In Burdette, W.J., ed., *Methodology in Mammalian Genetics.* Holden-Day, San Francisco. pp. 233–246.

Frohberg, H., and H. Oettel. 1966. Method of testing for teratogenicity in mice. *Ind. Med. Surg.* 35:113–120.

Generoso, W.M. 1973. Evaluation of chromosome aberration effects of chemicals on mouse germ cells. *Environ. Health Perspect.* (Experimental Issue No. 6). pp. 13–22.

Gibson, J.P., R.E. Staples, and J.W. Newberne. 1966. Use of the rabbit in teratogenicity studies. *Toxicol. Appl. Pharmacol.* 9:398–408.

Gottschewski, G.H. 1965. Können Tierversuche zur Lösung der Frage nach der teratogenen Wirkung von Medikamenten auf den menschlichen Embryo beitragen? *Arzneimittelforschung* 15:97–104.

Harada, Y. 1968. Infantile Minamata disease. In Study Group of Minamata Disease. Kumamoto University, Japan. *Minamata Dis.* pp. 73–91.

Harris, S.B., J.G. Wilson, and R.H. Printz. 1972. Embryotoxicity of methyl mercuric chloride in golden hamsters. *Teratology* 6:139–142.

Hemsworth, B.N. 1968. Embryopathies in the rat due to alkane sulfonates. *J. Reprod. Fertil.* 17:325–334.

Hicks, S.P. 1954. The effects of ionizing radiation, certain hormones, and radiomimetic drugs on the developing nervous system. *J. Cell. Comp. Physiol.* 43 (Supplement 1):151–178.

Hollaender, A. 1971. *Chemical Mutagens, Principles and Methods for Their Detection.* Vols. 1, 2. Plenum Press, New York.

Hollaender, A., and G.E. Stapleton. 1959. Ionizing radiation and the living cell. *Sci. Am.* 201:94–100.

Ingalls, T.H., and M.A. Klingsberg. 1965. Implications of epidemic embryopathy for public health. *Am. J. Public Health* 55:200–208.

Kalter, H. 1971. Correlation between teratogenic and mutagenic effects of chemicals in mammals. In Hollaender, A., *Chemical Mutagens, Principles and Methods for Their Detection.* Vol. 1. Plenum Press, New York. pp. 57–82.

Kalter, H., and J. Warkany. 1959. Experimental production of congenital malformations in mammals by metabolic procedure. *Physiol. Rev.* 39:69–115.

Karnofsky, D.A. 1965. Mechanisms of action of certain growth-inhibiting drugs. In Wilson, J.G., and J. Warkany, eds., *Teratology: Principles and Techniques.* University of Chicago Press, Chicago. pp. 185–213.

Khera, K.S., and D.J. Clegg. 1969. Perinatal toxicity of pesticides. *Canad. Med. Assoc. J.* 100:167–172.

King, C.T.G., S.A. Weaver, and S.A. Narrod. 1965. Antihistamines and teratogenicity in the rat. *J. Pharmacol. Exp. Ther.* 147:391–398.

Kučera, J. 1968. Exposure to fat solvents: A possible cause of sacral agenesis in man. *J. Pediat.* 72:857–859.

Lee, I.P., and R.L. Dixon. 1972. Antineoplastic drug effects on spermatogenesis studied by velocity sedimentation cell separation. *Toxicol. Appl. Pharmacol.* 23:20–41.

Lorke, D. 1963. Method for the investigation of embryotoxic and teratogenic effects on rat. *Naunyn-Schmiedebergs Arch. Pharmakol. Exp. Pathol.* 246:147–151.

Lucey, J.F., and R.E. Behrman. 1963. Thalidomide: Effect upon pregnancy in the rhesus monkey. *Science* 139:1295–1296.

Malawista, S.E., H. Sato, and K.G. Bensch. 1968. Vinblastine and griseofulvin reversibly disrupt the living mitotic spindle. *Science* 160:770–772.

Matsumoto, H., G. Koya, and T. Takeuchi. 1965. Fetal Minamata disease. A neuropathological study of two cases of intrauterine intoxication by a methyl mercury compound. *J. Neuropathol. Exp. Neurol.* 24:563–574.

McKusick, V.A. 1968. *Mendelian Inheritance in Man*, 2nd ed. Johns Hopkins Press, Baltimore.

McLaughlin, J., Jr., E.F. Reynaldo, J.K. Lamar, and J.-P. Marliac. 1969. Teratology studies in rabbits with captan, folpet, and thalidomide. *Toxicol. Appl. Pharmacol.* 14(No. 72):641.

Meselson, M.S., A.H. Westing and J.D. Constable. 1970. Background material relevant to presentations at the 1970 annual meeting of the AAAS. Revised January 14, 1971. Herbicide Assessment Commission, American Association for the Advancement of Science, Washington, D.C.

Mortimer, R.K., and T.R. Manney. 1971. Mutation induction in yeast. In Hollaender, A., ed., *Chemical Mutagens, Principles and Methods for Their Detection*. Vol. 1, Plenum Press, New York, pp. 289–310.

Nishimura, H. 1964. *Chemistry and Prevention of Congenital Anomalies*. Charles C Thomas, Springfield, Ill.

Nomura, T. 1969. Management of animals for use in teratological experiments. In Nishimura, H., and J.R. Miller, eds., *Methods for Teratological Studies in Experimental Animals and Man*. Igaku Shoin Ltd., Tokyo. pp. 3–15.

Padykula, H.A., J.J. Deren, and T.H. Wilson. 1966. Development of structure and function in the mammalian yolk sac. I. Developmental morphology and vitamin B_{12} uptake of the rat yolk sac. *Dev. Biol.* 13:311–348.

Palmer, A.K. 1969. The relationship between screening tests for drug safety and other teratological investigations. In Bertelli, A., ed., *Teratology; Proceedings of Symposium on Teratology at Como, Italy*. Excerpta Medica, Amsterdam. pp. 55–72.

Palmisano, P.A., R.C. Sneed, and G. Cassady. 1969. Untaxed whiskey and fetal lead exposure. *J. Pediat.* 75:869–872.

Rapport fram en expert grupp. 1971. Fenoxisyror, granskuing av aktuell information. Giftnämnden, Stockholm.

Ritter, E.J., W.J. Scott, and J.G. Wilson. 1971. Teratogenesis and inhibition of DNA synthesis induced in rat embryos by cytosine arabinoside. *Teratology* 4:7–14.

Robens, J.F. 1969. Teratologic studies of carbaryl, diazinon, norea, disulfiram, and thiram in small laboratory animals. *Toxicol. Appl. Pharmacol.* 15:152–163.

Robertson, D.S.F. 1970. Selenium—a possible teratogen? *Lancet* 1:518–519.

Robson, J.M. 1970. Testing drugs for teratogenicity and their effects on fertility. The present position. *Br. Med. Bull.* 26:212–216.

Russell, L.B., and W.L. Russell. 1954. An analysis of the changing radiation response of the developing mouse embryo. *J. Cell. Comp. Physiol.* 43(Supplement1): 103–150.

Schumacher, H.J., J.G. Wilson, and R.L. Jordan. 1969. Potentiation of the teratogenic effects of 5-fluorouracil by natural pyrimidines. II. Biochemical aspects.
Teratology 2:99–105.

Smith, R.H., and H.R. vonBorstel. 1971. Inducing mutations with chemicals in
habrobracon. In Hollaender, A., ed., *Chemical Mutagens, Principles and Methods
for Their Detection.* Vol. 2. Plenum Press, New York. pp. 445–460.

Snyder, R.D. 1971. Congenital mercury poisoning. *New Eng. J. Med.* 284:1014–
1016.

Spyker, J.M., and M. Smithberg. 1972. Effects of methylmercury on prenatal development in mice. *Teratology* 5:181–189.

2,4,5-T Advisory Committee. 1971. Report submitted May 7, 1971, to William D.
Ruckelshaus, Administrator. Environmental Protection Agency, Washington,
D.C.

Thiersch, J.B. 1962. Effects of acetamides and formamides on the rat litter *in utero.
J. Reprod. Fertil.* 4:219–220.

Tuchmann-Duplessis, H. 1972. Teratogenic drug screening. Present procedures and
requirements. *Teratology* 5:271–285.

Tuchmann-Duplessis, H., and L. Mercier-Parot. 1964. Repercussions des neurolep-
tiques et des antitumoraux sur le developpement prenatal. *Bull. Schweiz. Akad.
Med. Wiss.* 20:490–526.

VanLoosli, R., and E. Theiss. 1964. *Methodik und Problematik der medikamentos-
experimentellen Teratogenese.* Schwabe and Co., Basel.

Vogel, F., and G. Röhrborn, eds. 1970. *Chemical Mutagenesis in Mammals and Man.*
Springer-Verlag, New York.

Warkany, J. 1971. *Congenital Malformations; Notes and Comments.* Year Book
Medical Publishers, Chicago.

Watanabe, G., S. Yoshida, and K. Hirose. 1968. Teratogenic effect of benzol in
pregnant mice. In *Proceedings of the Congress of the Anomalies Research Association of Japan, Eighth Annual Meeting.* Tokyo. p. 45.

Wilson, J.G. 1954. Differentiation and the reaction of rat embryos to radiation.
J. Cell. Comp. Physiol. 43(Supplement 1):11–38.

Wilson, J.G. 1966. Effects of acute and chronic treatment with actinomycin D on
pregnancy and the fetus in the rat. *Harper Hosp. Bull.* 24:109–118.

Wilson, J.G. 1970. Embryotoxicity of the folic antagonist methotrexate. *Anat. Rec.*
166:398.

Wilson, J.G. 1971. Use of rhesus monkeys in teratological studies. *Fed. Proc.*
30:104–109.

Wilson, J.G. 1972. Abnormalities of intrauterine development in non-human primates. In Diczfalusy, E., and C.C. Stanley, eds. *The Use of Non-Human Primates
in Research on Human Reproduction.* World Health Organization. Research and
Training Center on Human Reproduction, Stockholm. pp. 261–292.

Wilson, J.G. 1973a. *Environment and Birth Defects.* Academic Press, New York.

Wilson, J.G. 1973b. Present status of drugs as teratogens in man. *Teratology* 7:3–15.

World Health Organization. 1967. *Principles for the Testing of Drugs for Teratogenicity.* ITS Tech. Rep. Ser. No. 364. Geneva.

Yerganian, G., and K.S. Lavappa. 1971. Procedures for culturing diploid cells and
preparation of meiotic chromosomes from dwarf species of hamsters. In
Hollaender, A., ed., *Chemical Mutagens, Principles and Methods for Their Detection.* Vol. 2. Plenum Press, New York. pp. 387–410.

Zimmermann, W. 1964. Methoden für experimentelle Untersuchungen am Kaninchen während der frühen Embryonalentwicklung. *Zentralbl. Bakt. Parisitenkd. Abt. I. Orig.* 194 A:255-266.

SUGGESTED READINGS

Brent, R.L. 1970. Implications of experimental teratology. In Fraser, F.C., and V.A. McKusick, eds., *Congenital Malformations.* Excerpta Medica, Amsterdam. pp. 187-195.
Fishbein, L., W.G. Flamm, and H.L. Falk. 1970. *Chemical Mutagens; Environmental Effects on Biological Systems.* Academic Press, New York.
Hollaender, A. 1971. *Chemical Mutagens, Principles and Methods for Their Detection.* Vols. 1, 2. Plenum Press, New York.
Warkany, J. 1971. *Congenital Malformations; notes and comments.* Year Book Medical Publishers, Chicago.
Wilson, J.G. 1973. *Environment and Birth Defects.* Academic Press, New York.

XI

Effects on Behavior

Among the vexing problems that confront industry and regulatory agencies in setting safe exposure levels of environmental chemicals is the question of subtle behavioral impairment and its early detection. Heavy metals, such as lead and mercury are notorious for presenting a collection of vague, nonspecific, often subjective complaints.

Actually, lead encephalopathy may begin like any other encephalopathy, with decrease in alertness, orientation, memory, affect and perception . . . after a period of months to weeks, or even days or hours, these early changes may progress to mania, delirium, partial or complete blindness, transitory aphasia, paralysis, mental obtundation of any degree and finally seizures, either focal or generalized, isolated, repeated or continuous (Whitfield, Ch'ien, and Whitehead, 1972, p. 794).

Many chemicals involved in human intoxications produce similar vague signs and symptoms. Thus, behavioral assessment is an important component in the evaluation of chemically induced adverse effects. Since behavior represents an integrated response of the organism, an impairment in the functioning of nearly any system may be reflected as a behavioral change. As a result, sensitive behavioral measures might serve as indicators that some, as yet covert, toxic action has occurred.

Behavioral processes are also important in themselves. Deficits in sensory sensitivity, motor performance (particularly skilled performance), and complex intellectual processes are exceedingly disadvantageous to an organism.

These considerations imply two major roles for behavioral toxicology in the assessment of chemicals with an environmental impact:

- selection of animal test systems to reveal behavioral toxicity; and
- monitoring and evaluation of behavioral effects in exposed humans.

The most reasonable approach to toxicology, including behavioral toxicology, is to follow a progression of questions that permit, at any step in the progression, a decision about rejection, acceptance, or continuation of the assessment.

SEQUENTIAL ASSESSMENT OF TOXICITY

General Strategy

The sequence of decisions that seem important in behavioral evaluations is presented schematically in the form of a flow diagram (Figure 8). This diagram illustrates the principles of an evaluation sequence; not all parts of the sequence are invariably followed. The circumstances under which exposure is expected to occur will dictate the actual sequence adopted.

As emphasized in previous chapters (Chapters II and VI) the depth to which a compound is studied depends upon the ultimate use and the known effects. If no adverse behavioral effects are observed in the preliminary screen, the compound will undergo a normal sequence of testing procedures (Chapter VII, VIII, IX and X), that is, acute to subchronic, chronic, reproductive, and carcinogenesis testing. In all of these animal test procedures, behavior must be an important component of the observations. The basic premise of the flow diagram is that there are certain critical choice points in the progression of decisions that either require rejection of the compound, lead to a decision that no further testing for central nervous system effects is needed, or provoke a more detailed, sensitive, and comprehensive study of such effects.

Although the flow diagram emphasizes single exposures for the sake of clarity, the same general sequence of operations and decisions is followed for substances with different anticipated use patterns. The most relevant assessment procedures will mimic the natural conditions of exposure. Route, duration, and frequency are the three basic parameters, and their values will also modify the relative emphasis given to the various steps in the sequence. For example, adverse effects at high doses will be more

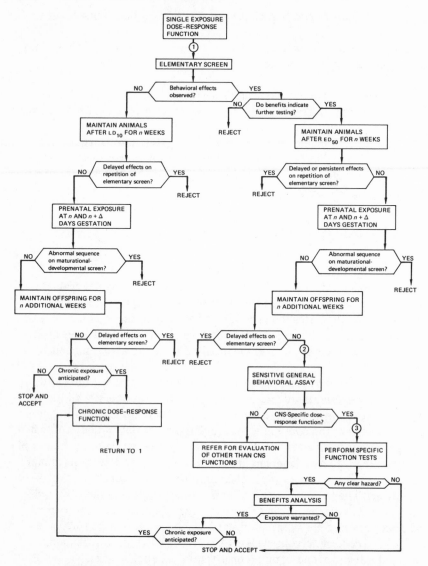

FIGURE 8   Flow diagram for decision sequence in behavioral evaluation.

acceptable if they are reversible than if they linger, so that certain steps in the sequence may be repeated if adverse effects occur. The more lasting the exposure, the greater the proportion of population exposed, and the greater must be the depth of the testing.

It is reasonable to continue extensive testing of behavioral effects beyond the early, elementary screen only if some special benefit is offered by the new agent. A fabric softener, for example, may hardly warrant any permissible CNS effects at less than lethal dosage levels because of its minor, marginal benefits. An organic solvent that could replace a currently used, indispensable, but highly toxic substance could be worth pursuing in depth if there is a chance that it would prove to be less toxic.

Preliminary Screening

The first step with any agent is to obtain dose–response functions for readily observable CNS effects. Concern with the total environment probably requires observations on one or more mammalian and one or more nonmammalian organisms (e.g., fish, in particular, seem useful target species; *see* Appendix D).

The acute toxicity studies (Chapter VII, Acute and Subchronic Effects) include observations exemplified by the following list.

1. *Activity Changes*—locomotion of a standard distance in standard time, gross movements, excitement or depression in spontaneous, exploratory locomotion, presence of abnormal locomotion, such as circling, etc.

2. *Objective Signs*—tremors, ptosis, salivation, lacrimation, defecation, convulsions, abnormal postural changes, etc.

3. *Reflex Changes*—hyper- or hypo-reflexia, such as corneal, pinna, righting, placing, etc.

4. *Elicited Responses*—grasping, response to nose or tail pinch, handling or noise-induced convulsions, orientation, etc.

5. *Body Weight Changes*—Immediate and brief weight losses and failure to gain weight when compared to normal growth curves

This list is obviously not exhaustive, but typifies procedures used in the pharmaceutical industry to screen for CNS activity. Observations should be made "blind" in order to eliminate observer bias (i.e., the observers are unaware of which are the treated animals). Observations should be repeated at intervals that will permit an assessment of effects that might occur after a period of time necessary for absorption and metabolism of the potentially toxic agent. The observations should continue throughout the postdosing period to determine whether delayed or residual effects occur. Alkylating agents, for example mustards, may produce overt neurological effects and morphological changes in brain tissue detectable only after several months since the exposure. If delayed behavioral changes are observed in the acute or subchronic studies, special attempts should be made to ascertain low level effects.

Any delayed effect is good reason to reject a compound for consideration. It most likely reflects an underlying pathological process that by then has progressed far enough to be expressed as a functional impairment. Even if the overt effects prove to be reversible, the underlying damage may still not have been repaired. One example of such an agent is methylmercury. It does not produce immediate CNS effects. With human exposures to toxic levels, the observable consequences typically do not appear for several weeks. The recent disaster in Iraq from contaminated grain (Bakir *et al.*, 1973) was one such insidious and widespread phenomenon. Although recovery of function may occur, it is not due to repair of the affected cells in the brain, but to the assumption of these functions by remaining viable cells in the CNS. However, the damage remains, making it less likely that the individual will be capable of withstanding further CNS destruction or deterioration, as might result from natural phenomena such as aging.

Sensitive General Behavioral Assay

If CNS effects are revealed by the preliminary screening, then a sequence of questions is asked. The fact that CNS effects have been observed now makes it necessary to characterize them more precisely and with more sensitive criteria. It is useful to use one or more of the relatively simple, yet sensitive indicators, in order to describe the dose range within which such effects can be found. One such variable is spontaneous motor activity, which can be determined with untrained animals and which requires a minimum of instrumentation. Baselines provided by stabilized avoidance performance are also useful.

This step in the sequence, No. 2 in the flow diagram, is used mainly to provide guidance for the more specific procedures. These have been categorized under sensory processes, motor processes, complex functions, and phylogenetically determined performances (step No. 3).

Functional Analysis of Behavior

Results of behavioral tests are influenced by a number of factors, all of which must be considered in evaluating their significance. The most important influences include the consequences of various responses that organisms perform during the tests (Skinner, 1969), the housing and testing environments that constrain and shape their behavior (Marler and Hamilton, 1966), past experience in laboratory and natural settings (Hinde, 1970), and the adaptive significance and evolutionary history of the behaviors chosen for observation (Eibl-Eibestfeldt, 1970). Behavioral test procedures, like other toxicological test procedures, must be executed by adequately skilled personnel, and the sensitivity and reliability of the methods must be calibrated periodically by standard treatments whose effects are known.

Sensory functions Many agents affect sensory systems, sometimes in subtle ways. For example, aspirin, certain antibiotics, and certain diuretics can impair hearing under certain conditions. Carbon monoxide elevates the threshold for light detection. Methylmercury induces deficits in tactual sensitivity and visual function.

Although observed changes in sensory sensitivity may sometimes be attributable to factors not directly related to CNS function, the overwhelming importance of sensory information for all life activity requires the careful evaluation of potential toxic effects on sensory processes. This entire domain of issues has been virtually ignored by traditional toxicologic methodology. Moreover, considerable data strongly support the argument for behavioral, rather than physiologic or structural, studies of sensory systems: For example, the "intactness" of the visual system can not be judged by examination of the retina alone (fundascopically); nor will histopathological studies reveal deficits in function. Any test of visual function in any organism must involve the entire receptor-processing-response system, which, in the last analysis, involves behavior.

The measurement of sensory processes (e.g., vision, audition, olfaction, somesthesia) in laboratory animals is of special relevance for prediction of potential behavioral toxicology, since many measurement techniques can be applied to humans and animals with equal facility. In each instance, the organism's response (detection of signal) can be calibrated against an energy source specified in physical terms. The range of sensitivity to environmental stimuli that characterizes the primary sensory systems commends sensory changes as an unusually precise barometer of the functional capacity of the organism. Human and animal psychophysics provide a compelling illustration of the sensitivity range of sensory systems and the accuracy of the measurement techniques available (Stebbins, 1970).

An illustration of the occurrence of a preventable toxic effect is the induction of red–green color blindness in patients treated with pheniprazine, an MAO inhibitor, used in the treatment of depression. In most cases, neither the patients nor their physicians were aware of their steadily decreasing color sensitivity, even though the exposure periods often spanned many months. Normal visual function was recovered in no more than a fraction of the affected patients. It was only some time after the drug's introduction into practice, unfortunately, that clinical investigators became aware of this unpredicted drug effect—emphasizing the necessity for monitoring the sensory capacities of exposed human populations (Jones, 1961).

This particular decrement in color sensitivity could also be demonstrated in pigeons (Hanson *et al.*, 1964). Using a narrow bandwidth monochrometer as a light source, pigeons were trained to respond by pecking a translucent disk illuminated by the monochrometer. The birds were reinforced with grain only when they pecked in the presence of two of five selected wavelengths (green and orange) and not for responding to the other wavelengths (blue, yellow, and red). The birds rapidly learned to discriminate between the stimulus wavelengths. After a month or more of daily administration, pheniprazine produced a loss of discrimination; that is, the birds responded equally to all wavelengths. After withdrawal of the compound, the original discrimination was recovered.

Experimental approaches to the evaluation of sensory processes include both behavioral and physiological measures. Such techniques can be used with almost any species, but most research has been done with primates. It is reasonable to assume that studies of this complexity will be performed with either primates or dogs since these organisms have very real advantages for systematic routine monitoring and evaluation of other physiological parameters and are conveniently long lived.

Although behavioral techniques have been emphasized in this section, physiological techniques also possess some potential for sensory system assessment. Averaged evoked potentials probably make the most sense (Regan, 1972) since they lend themselves to chronic experiments. For example, the response of the monkey visual system might be studied by recording, through skull electrodes, the brain's electrical response to repeated flashes of a checkerboard pattern. Unfortunately, the analytical techniques available for quantitative evaluations are still rather primitive compared to those applicable to behavioral situations. Physiological techniques are also inappropriate for determinations of fine discriminations, such as distinguishing between visual stimuli of different shapes.

Motor Control It is apparent that motor control is involved in any behavioral measurement since all existing techniques require a motor response to indicate sensory discrimination or detection. Beyond this aspect of motor function is the need to study specific impairments in motor function itself. In its simplest form, measurement may consist of simple observations of walking or running or postural adjustments to various conditions. Although the motor behavior involved is unlearned, it does involve the complex integration of many physiological systems and as such is an important expression of the general state of the organism.

Many techniques of varying complexity are available for finer examination of motor function. For example, "rotarod" procedures are slightly more complex than simple observation but demonstrably sensitive to many pharmacological agents (Watzman and Barry, 1968). These procedures—primarily useful with rodents—test an experimental animal's ability to balance on a slowly revolving cylinder and, in this way, monitor vestibular control, coordination, and muscular strength. At the other extreme of complexity are behavioral techniques that measure a rat or monkey's ability to maintain a certain preset manual pressure on a specially designed force transducer in order to avoid shock or gain food reward. These latter techniques require extensive instrumentation and would be employed only when subtle motor effects were suspected of playing a significant role.

Devices are available for measuring tremor, particularly in small animals, but these are probably more useful as an aid to quantification than as primary detectors of neuromuscular impairment.

Electrophysiological techniques are more useful for motor than for sensory assessment. Electromyography is an attractive alternative to the direct measurement of tremor in untrained animals; again, however, behavioral methods are unsurpassed for questions aimed at functioning of the total organism and for measurement of subtle effects.

Complex Processes   One of the most useful and sensitive indices of chemical effects on behavior is the frequency and distribution in time of a specific class of responses (Kelleher and Morse, 1968). An example of use of this behavioral methodology to examine the gradually increasing consequences of mercury vapor exposure employed a multiple fixed-ratio, fixed-interval reinforcement schedule (Armstrong *et al.*, 1963).

These examples of how to employ and interpret what is called "operant" behavior reflect only a minute facet of an immense literature. Operant technology has been applied to a great range of drugs and situations, and is the core of the discipline of behavioral pharmacology.

Phylogenetically Determined Performances   Behavioral characteristics that have evolved as a consequence of selective environmental pressures play a central role in maintaining wild populations. A wide range of such crucial behaviors can be affected by toxic substances. Changes in such behaviors can impair the survival of species when, for example, sexual or parental behaviors are disrupted.

Certain adaptive specializations are particularly useful for detecting toxic actions that cause nothing more significant than a general malaise at low doses. The rat, for example, cannot vomit and avoids new food substances. If rats are fed a relatively novel food that is not toxic and then receive a toxic agent that causes noxious consequences, they subsequently avoid the novel food. If no toxic effects occur after novel food ingestion, the initial "bait shyness" disappears. This avoidance specialization in rats can be used to test for a variety of subtle toxic actions.

Efficient and reliable procedures exist for assessing a wide variety of phylogenetically determined animal behaviors. Documented examples for various classes of behavior include, for sexual behavior, Young (1961, 1969), Schein and Hale (1965), Michael and Zumpe (1971); for aggressive behavior, Tedeschi *et al.* (1959), Horovitz *et al.* (1966), Scott (1966), Charpentier (1969); for ingestive behavior, Falk (1971); for thermoregulatory behavior, Weiss and Laties (1961), (Satinoff (1964), Carlisle (1970); and for circadian rhythms, Richter (1959).

Phylogenetically specialized behaviors may be particularly helpful for assessing long-term risks. These distinctive patterns are resistant to modification with repeated experience (Breland and Breland, 1966; Lehrman, 1970). Changes in such stable baselines can detect delayed effects of substance exposure (Joffe, 1968), insidious effects of repeated exposure (Vogel and Leaf, 1972), and withdrawal effects after establishing dependence (Lister, 1970). All of these situations involve detection of small, progressive, or cumulative effects.

Protocols for compounds that may reach significant environmental levels or have long persistence should assess adequate samples of phylogenetically determined behavior in at least one terrestrial mammalian species. Sexual behaviors in both sexes should be studied in at least one species. Significantly inpaired sexual or ingestive behavior at dose levels within an order of magnitude of those expected in the environment should be classified as extremely serious hazards.

Tolerance and Dependence   In addition to the effects of chemical agents on sensory and motor processes and complex functions, a complete protocol should consider other aspects of cumulative effects that can be described as tolerance and physical dependence. Tolerance refers to the fact that increasing doses of an agent are required to produce a constant effect. Tolerance does not necessarily develop to all effects of a substance, and may develop at different rates for different effects. Tolerance may therefore cause changes over time in the predominant pattern of effects caused by exposure to an agent. Such effects can be measured by many of the behavioral techniques referred to elsewhere. The time course of induction of tolerance can vary from a single dose, as in the case of morphine, to a gradual change in effect, as is usually observed with alcohol. The persistence of tolerance is difficult to measure unambiguously since testing necessarily involves readministration of the tolerance-producing agent.

Physical dependence refers to the cluster of biological signs that occur within some hours or days following removal of a chronically administered agent. Although physical dependence is usually induced as a function of prolonged exposure, there is evidence that physical dependence can be very rapidly induced (several days) under certain conditions (Goldstein, 1972). The persistence of physical dependence remains a controversial issue, but it has been shown that a biological "memory" for an addictive process may persist as long as 6–9 months (Cochin and Kornetsky, 1964; Goldberg and Schuster, 1969).

The relevance of the concepts of *tolerance* and *physical dependence* to toxicology resides in their practical consequences for assessing chemical effects on the central nervous system. Although these concepts are usually associated with self-administration of chemical agents, scheduled administration of the same agents can produce equivalent effects. Chronic chemical exposure has been known to lead to physical dependence. The effects of chronic exposure to nitroglycerin on production workers is a classic example of such an effect.

Prenatal Exposure

Since behavior is at least as susceptible to prenatal chemical influence as other developmental mechanisms, it is essential that observations made during the reproductive studies (Chapter X) include behavior. At times, subtle behavioral effects may not be readily evident and may require special tests. Furthermore, a morphological or biochemical lesion may remain dormant and not manifest itself until later in life as a functional impairment or behavioral disorder. To determine long-term or delayed effects of particular chemical exposures on biological and behavioral functions requires longitudinal research designs. Assessment of behavioral effects must continue throughout gestation and the offspring's life span.

Since it is extremely difficult to predict what types of subtle or delayed effects will be seen following a particular prenatal treatment, or when, it is essential to utilize a variety of maturational and behavioral measures at various periods of the lifespan. Test results will depend on the nature and potency of the environmental chemical in question, its specificity of action, the stage of development when the organism is exposed, the genetic predisposition of the organism, and maternal–offspring interactions. Changes may be seen at one developmental stage and not at another; one form of behavior may be affected and not another. Furthermore, it is possible to find alterations in behavior that appear as improvements in performance, as well as behavioral defects.

The discriminative power of any behavioral analysis increases as a function of the range of behavioral end points examined. The following categories are frequently included in developmental assessment.

1. *Morphological and Physical Characteristics*—congenital defects, sex, age of eye opening, age of pilage, physical appearance (ptosis of eyelid, tremor, abnormal postural changes, etc.), survival time;

2. *Growth*—weight at birth, weaning, and other age periods (frequently used as best index of general health);

3. *Specific Responses, Reflexes, and Sensory–Motor Capacities*—righting reflex, tactual placing reflex, corneal reflex, grasping, orienting, etc. (especially during first few weeks of life to assess maturation);

4. *Activity Levels*—spontaneous activity in home cage at various ages, open-field performance, measures of exhaustion;

5. *Neuromuscular Ability*—tests (of coordination, strength, speed, endurance, agility), locomotor performance, gait evaluation, varying degrees of difficulty (Spyker *et al.*, 1972);

6. *Learning Measures*—simple classical conditioning to complex operant behavior;

7. *Measures of Emotionality* (to assess role of autonomic nervous system);

8. *Sexual Development*—mating behavior, reproductive efficiency, maternal behavior; and

9. *Physiological Rhythms*—maturation of homeothermic temperature regulation, circadian rhythm.

The evaluation should be done during the early stages of the animals' lifespan—for example, in the mouse, birth through puberty (3–4 weeks) and into young adulthood (2–6 months). If no deviations are detected during the developmental screen, offspring should be maintained for longitudinal testing and biological and behavioral functions periodically assayed to determine if delayed effects can arise from prenatal exposure to the chemical in question.

One important precaution must be observed. In mammals, any experimental maternal treatment producing prenatal effects (i.e., chemical effects on the fetus directly via placental transfer or indirectly by interfering with placental function) must also be considered capable of affecting offspring postnatally. Maternal residual (postnatal) chemical effects may be mediated, directly by the milk of the nursing mother or indirectly through maternal neglect of offspring and other early experience factors (e.g., aberrant maternal retrieving, grooming, and activity). For this reason, cross-fostering is essential.

EVALUATION OF HUMAN TOXICITY

Perspectives on Human Exposure

Studies on the toxic effects of drugs in humans are often justified by the research for more effective therapeutic agents. A lesser advantage accrues to the chemical manufacturer producing an agent that might be a more effective dry cleaner. Given the present position of FDA and the medical research community, and the justifiable restrictions imposed on human experimentation, it is rather unlikely that extensive data on human toxicity will be available before a new agent is introduced into the environment. For this reason, the burden placed on testing in nonhuman subjects is multiplied manifold.

Every opportunity for human testing should be exploited, however, despite the numerous difficulties this presents. Besides the obvious reason—setting standards on the basis of the target organism—human data also present the chance to validate the predictive value of laboratory animal test methods.

Three exposure situations are available for human testing: occupational exposure, environmental exposure, and laboratory exposure. Methods employed to assess toxicity will vary from one setting to another, since some measures are relevant and possible in one situation that do not apply to others. For example, occupationally exposed groups are better populations than environmentally exposed groups for determining early symptoms of chronic exposure. Environmentally exposed populations may be more useful for certain epidemiological questions because of the large samples or wide age ranges that may be required for such work. Experimental exposures in the laboratory, if used at all, will be to determine acute effects at low dose levels.

Environmental Exposure Invariably, certain groups will have been exposed, in the course of daily living, to potentially toxic materials. To be most useful, body burden measures should be derived that reflect exposure to and absorption of the chemicals. In addition, certain groups will be exposed accidentally to a chemical and can be viewed as subjects in a "natural" experiment.

Examples of such nonoccupationally exposed groups include individuals and families residing near point sources of industrial pollution, such as smelting and metal-refining operations and petroleum and petrochemical plants; groups in heavily industrialized areas; individuals in central metropolitan areas exposed to vehicle exhaust and numerous fuel additives; groups residing in areas that provide natural sources of potentially toxic materials, such as high concentrations of certain minerals in drinking water.

Occupational Exposure   Workers exposed to a substance in the course of its production provide the clearest source of chronic human toxicity data. Such data are especially crucial to the task of characterizing the early symptoms of exposure.

Once a procedure is validated in an occupationally exposed population, it can then be redirected, perhaps in modified form, towards monitoring the impact of the substance on the community at large.

Laboratory (Experimental) Exposures   When animal research cannot provide the required information, and when exposure to the chemical agent is consistent with the safety of volunteer subjects, experimental exposures of humans can be used to answer such questions as the following: What is the function relating aversiveness of smell to concentration? Are there subjective effects at concentrations too low to produce overt effects? Are there subtle changes in sensory, motor, or complex performance functions detectable only by precise psychological techniques?

Applicable Methodology

The scope of possibilities for damage that arises from an agent with wide environmental distribution argues for simultaneous observations from three data sources: behavioral surveys based on functioning within the community; assessments of psychological problems from community or occupational samples; and laboratory analysis of specific behavioral functions.

Behavioral Surveys   It can be anticipated that community studies of the behavioral impact of environmental chemicals will be extremely difficult and would only be feasible in a limited geographic area where exposure levels to a specific agent are distinctively high. Provided adequate controls are available, an evaluation survey might be constructed to determine whether the inhabitants of that area are experiencing difficulties expressed as behavioral or neurologic disorders. Such a survey might include the following measures: unemployment rates; school attendance; mental hospital admissions; incidence of cerebral palsy, epilepsy, and similar neurological aberrations; referrals by school psychologists; suicide incidence; and rate of diagnosed alcoholism.

Any such community or area will surely be the focus of a broadly based epidemiologic survey. Since such surveys tend to focus on mortality and overt morbidity, the committee simply emphasizes the utility of including items that may yield clues to the intrusion of less well-defined adverse effects. Such data are especially useful in the context of a prospective research design.

Within occupational contexts similar questions can be asked, sometimes with more precision. Such a limited population, with its greater homogeneity, is probably more useful, however, for asking questions of greater specificity and depth.

Assessment of Psychological Problems The epidemiologic survey is a crude method if the relevant effects focus mainly on such problems as heightened irritability, emotional lability, and depression. It makes more sense, if an adequately defined sample can be extracted from the community or manufacturing plant (defined, perhaps, by body burden measurements), to subject such a sample to in-depth analyses.

A number of instruments are available for assessing those behavioral disorders short of frank psychoses requiring inpatient treatment. Interviews by psychiatrists or psychologists guided by a set of explicit criteria are one possibility, but are rather expensive, time-consuming, and probably not sufficiently reliable for monitoring purposes (Alexander, French, and Pollock, 1968). Another possibility is to use one of the standardized inventories designed for "personality" assessment, especially one that can be self-administered. Most of these, however, focus on stable, long-standing behavior patterns (traits) rather than changes in behavior.

The most promising kind of tool for this kind of survey is one that would be especially sensitive to shifts in symptom constellations. Several currently used instruments might fit such a criterion. Among those that are largely self-administered are the Minnesota Multiphasic Personality Inventory (Dahlstrom *et al.*, 1972) and the Goldberg General Health Questionnaire (Goldberg, 1972).

Any such instrument must be used with considerable precautions (too lengthy to discuss here) in administration, scoring, and interpretation. It would make its optimal contribution, of course, in a prospective study that permits a longitudinal assessment of change.

Laboratory Experiments and Measurements Laboratory studies in humans can serve two functions: First, they could provide toxicity data before an agent is released for general use, especially for acute exposures;

second, they can be carried out in a monitoring context, such as following a sample of workers whose occupational exposures should provide clues about what may happen to the general population.

Useful guidelines can be derived from research in psychopharmacology. Procedural variables play a major role in securing reliable human data. If exposure is to take place in the laboratory, both subject and technician should, within the limits of informed consent, be unaware of which observations are made with a control preparation and which with the active agent. Especially with nonscientist subjects, it is necessary to maintain the subjects' cooperation: Unless a subject is cooperative, any variations in performance cannot be interpreted simply as a response to a chemical agent. Monetary payoffs are useful here, especially if based on performance. Procedures for ensuring attention are also essential, and can be derived from situations used in animal work (Mello, 1971).

The range of effects that might be expected from a single agent, given the experience of behavioral pharmacologists with CNS drugs, is rather broad. Amphetamines provide an excellent example of such breadth (Weiss and Laties, 1962); their effect in several areas are listed below.

- Physical Strength and Endurance—Enhance athletic performances ranging from swimming to shot-putting.
- Motor Coordination and Control—Enhance some reactions and depress others (e.g., reaction time and hand steadiness).
- Vigilance Performance (detecting infrequent stimuli)—Enhance, even after sleep loss.
- Performance on Simple, Monotonous Intellectual Tasks—Enhance, but no effect is seen on complex tasks.
- Subjective Fatigue—Reduced, but the magnitude of such an effect is not well correlated with performance effects.

Psychodietetics provides several examples of how important it is to examine patterns of change (Brozek, 1970). For example, severe, prolonged caloric restriction—enough to reduce body weight by 25 percent—does not produce changes on test scores of intellectual functions, but greatly reduces the number of self-initiated intellectual activities. Strength and endurance may undergo a dramatic loss after chronic starvation, but acute starvation and thiamine deficiency impair coordination without diminishing strength.

Laboratory studies can draw on a vast repertoire of techniques from experimental psychology. Under some conditions a study may focus on a single "critical" function, such as color vision, selected either by biological considerations and prior experience with similar compounds, or occupational considerations. Where the chemical may affect several aspects of behavior, a broader spectrum of functions must be covered, selected on the basis of earlier animal studies, clinical reports, or general considerations. Although some of the subjective symptoms of toxicity might be uncovered by questionnaire inventories of the type alluded to above, many kinds of deficits will not be revealed except under the controlled conditions of the laboratory setting. A good example is provided by carbon monoxide. At carboxyhemoglobin levels of 4 percent, there is significant impairment of brightness discrimination (McFarland *et al.*, 1944). O'Hanlon (in press) found deficits in vigilance performance at levels of about 7 percent. Such relatively low levels are unlikely to produce clear subjective, much less overt, symptoms.

Even considerable impairment of color vision is likely to remain undetected except under laboratory conditions or in the hands of a skilled opthalmologist. As pointed out earlier, the M A O-inhibitor pheniprazine produced such an effect in patients, but it went unrecognized for a long time (Gillespie *et al.*, 1959; Jones, 1961; Highman and Maling, 1962; Maling *et al.*, 1962; Palmer, 1963; Simpson *et al.*, 1963).

Special problems are presented by the evaluation of toxic effects in children, just as in animal research, because of the introduction of developmental variation. The recent task force report on research designed to evaluate and detect the existence of subtle impairments of sensory and motor function provides a compendium of approaches that have been used, for the most part, with only minimal success (Chalfant and Scheffelin, 1969). The problems faced in attempting to specify reliable behavioral indices of the complex phenomena of "minimal brain dysfunction" in children share many features in common with the attempt to analyze toxic effects in exposed adults. The behavioral effects may be extremely subtle and involve several integrative systems in addition to simple visual, auditory, and motor functions: For example, even if the reception of a specific sensory signal is adequate, the processing and integration of the signal with consequent appropriate behavior may be somehow impaired. This phenomenon has been referred to as a dysfunction in the "synthesis" of sensory information. A second general category of dysfunctions may occur in processes involving auditory language, reading, and writing as well as acquisition of quantitative (mathematical) language skills. The extent to which impairments in such processes may characterize the vaguely defined syndrome of minimal brain dysfunction, as well as CNS toxic effects, has to be determined through further research

SUMMARY

A sequence of decisions that are of importance in behavioral evaluation is presented. The depth to which a compound is studied is dependent upon ultimate use and known effects. Emphasis is placed on the importance of behavior as a component of the observations made in other toxicity studies.

Advances in behavioral science equal to the task of monitoring changes due to minimal pollutant exposure will require extensive basic research. Until our understanding of the central nervous system mechanisms controlling all aspects of behavior has progressed substantially beyond its current level, accurate behavioral assays of all potentially toxic agents will not be available. If resources for behavioral toxicology are equally distributed between examinations of high-risk exposed populations with the best tools available, and basic research in neurobehavioral science, the goals of evaluating pollutants should be rapidly achieved.

REFERENCES

Alexander, F., T.M. French, and G.H. Pollock, eds. 1968. *Psychosomatic Specificity. Vol. I. Experimental Study and Results.* University of Chicago Press, Chicago.

Armstrong, R.D., L.J. Leach, P.R. Belluscio, E.A. Maynard, H.C. Hodge, and J.K. Scott. 1963. Behavioral changes in the pigeon following inhalation of mercury vapor. *Am. Ind. Hyg. Assoc. J.* 24:366–375.

Bakir, F., S.F. Damluji, L. Amin-Zaki, M. Murtadha, A. Khalidi, N.Y. Al-Rawi, S. Tikriti, H.I. Dhahir, T.W. Clarkson, J.C. Smith, and R.A. Doherty. 1973. Methylmercury poisoning in Iraq. *Science* 181:230–241.

Breland, K., and M. Breland. 1966. *Animal Behavior.* Macmillan Co., New York.

Brozek, J. 1970. Research on diet and behavior. *J. Am. Diet. Assoc.* 57:321–325.

Carlisle, H.J. 1970. Thermal reinforcement and temperature regulation. In Stebbins, W.C., ed., *Animal Psychophysics: The Design and Conduct of Sensory Experiments.* Appleton-Century-Crofts, New York. pp. 211–229.

Chalfant, J.C., and M.A. Scheffelin. 1969. *Central Processing Dysfunctions in Children, Review of Research.* National Institute of Neurological Diseases and Stroke. NINDS Monogr. No. 9. U.S. Government Printing Office, Washington, D.C.

Charpentier, J. 1969. Analysis and measurement of aggressive behavior in mice. In Garattini, S., and E.B. Sigg, eds., *Aggressive Behaviour.* Excerpta Medica, Amsterdam. pp. 86–100.

Cochin, J., and C. Kornetsky. 1964. Development and loss of tolerance to morphine in the rat after single and multiple injections. *J. Pharmacol. Exp. Ther.* 145:1–10.

Dahlstrom, W.G., G.S. Welsh, and L.E. Dahlstrom. 1972. *An MMPI Handbook. Vol. I: Clinical Interpretation,* rev. ed. University of Minnesota Press, Minneapolis.

Eibl-Eibesfeldt, I. 1970. *Ethology, the Biology of Behavior.* Holt, Rinehart and Winston, New York.

Falk, J.L. 1971. Determining changes in vital functions: Ingestion. In Myers, R.D., ed., *Methods in Psychobiology, Vol. I: Laboratory Techniques in Neuropsychology and Neurobiology.* Academic Press, New York.

Gillespie, L., Jr., L.L. Terry, and A. Sjoerdsma. 1959. The application of a monoamine-oxidase inhibitor, 1-phenyl-2-hydrazinopropane (JB-516), to the treatment of primary hypertension. *Am. Heart J.* 58:1–12.

Goldberg, D.P. 1972. *The Detection of Psychiatric Illness by Questionnaire.* Oxford University Press, London.

Goldberg, S.R., and C.R. Schuster. 1969. Nalorphine: Increased sensitivity of monkeys formerly dependent on morphine. *Science* 166:1548–1549.

Goldstein, D.B. 1972. Relationship of alcohol dose to intensity of withdrawal signs in mice. *J. Pharmacol. Exp. Ther.* 180:203–215.

Hanson, H.M., J.J. Witoslawski, and E.H. Campbell. 1964. Reversible disruption of a wavelength discrimination in pigeons following administration of pheniprazine. *Toxicol. Appl. Pharmacol.* 6:690–695.

Highman, B., and H.M. Maling. 1962. Neuropathologic lesions in dogs after prolonged administration of phenylisopropylhydrazine (JB-516) and phenylisobutylhydrazine (JB-835). *J. Pharmacol. Exp. Ther.* 137:344–355.

Hinde, R.A. 1970. *Animal Behavior: A Synthesis of Ethology and Comparative Psychology,* 2nd ed. McGraw-Hill Book Co., New York.

Horovitz, Z.P., J.J. Piala, J.P. High, J.C. Burke, and R.C. Leaf. 1966. Effects of drugs on the mouse-killing (muricide) test and its relationship to amygdaloid function. *Int. J. Neuropharmacol.* 5:405–411.

Joffe, J.M. 1968. *Prenatal Determinants of Behavior.* Pergamon Press, New York.

Jones, O.W., III. 1961. Toxic amblyopia caused by pheniprazine hydrochloride (JB-516, Catron). *Arch. Ophthalmol.* 66:55–62.

Kelleher, R.T., and W.H. Morse. 1968. Determinants of the specificity of behavioral effects of drugs. *Ergeb. Physiol. Biol. Chem. Exp. Pharmacol.* 60:1–56.

Lehrman, D.S. 1970. Semantic and conceptual issues in the nature–nurture problem. In Aronson, L.R., E. Tobach, D.S. Lehrman, and J.S. Rosenblatt, eds., *Development and Evolution of Behavior: Essays in Memory of T.C. Schneirla.* W.H. Freeman and Co., San Francisco. pp. 17–52.

Lister, R.E. 1970. Detection of potential to produce drug dependence. In Paget, G.E., ed., *Methods in Toxicology.* F.A. Davis Co., Philadelphia. pp. 215–257.

Maling, H.M., B. Highman, and S. Spector. 1962. Neurologic, neuropathologic, and neurochemical effects of prolonged administration of phenylisopropylhydrazine (JB-516), phenylisobutylhydrazine (JB-835), and other monoamine oxidase inhibitors. *J. Pharmacol. Exp. Ther.* 137:334–343.

Marler, P.R., and W.J. Hamilton. 1966. *Mechanisms of Animal Behavior.* John Wiley & Sons, New York.

McFarland, R.Á., F.J.W. Roughton, M.H. Halperin, and J.I. Niven. 1944. The effects of carbon monoxide and altitude on visual thresholds. *J. Aviat. Med.* 15:381–394.

Mello, N.K. 1971. Alcohol effects on delayed matching to sample performance by rhesus monkey. *Physiol. Behav.* 7:77–101.

Michael, R.P., and D. Zumpe. 1971. Patterns of reproductive behavior. In Hafez, E.S.E., ed., *Comparative Reproduction of Nonhuman Primates.* Charles C Thomas, Springfield Ill. pp. 205–242.

O'Hanlon, J. (In press.) Preliminary studies of the effects of carbon monoxide on vigilance in man. In Weiss, B., and V.G. Laties, eds., *Behavioral Toxicology.* Appleton-Century-Crofts, New York.

Palmer, C.A.L. 1963. Toxic amblyopia due to pheniprazine. *Br. Med. J.* 1:38.

Regan, D. 1972. *Evoked Potentials in Psychology, Sensory Physiology and Clinical Medicine.* John Wiley & Sons, New York.

Richter, C.P. 1959. Lasting after-effects produced in rats by several commonly used drugs and hormones. *Proc. Natl. Acad. Sci.* (USA) 45:1080–1095.

Satinoff, E. 1964. Behavioral thermoregulation in response to local cooling of the rat brain. *Am. J. Physiol.* 206:1389–1394.

Schein, M.W., and E.B. Hale. 1965. Stimuli eliciting sexual behavior. In Beach, F.A., ed., *Sex and Behavior.* John Wiley & Sons, New York.

Scott, J.P. 1966. Agonistic behavior of mice and rats: A review. *Am. Zool.* 6:683–701.

Simpson, J.A., J.I. Evans, and I.D. Sanderson. 1963. Amblyopia due to pheniprazine. *Br. Med. J.* 1:331.

Skinner, B.F. 1969. *Contingencies of Reinforcement.* Appleton-Century-Crofts, New York.

Spyker, J.M., S.B. Sparber, and A.M. Goldberg. 1972. Subtle consequences of methylmercury exposure: Behavioral deviations in offspring of treated mothers. *Science* 177:621–623.

Stebbins, W.C., ed. 1970. *Animal Psychophysics: The Design and Conduct of Sensory Experiments.* Appleton-Century-Crofts, New York.

Tedeschi, R.E., D.H. Tedeschi, A. Mucha, L. Cook, P.A. Mattis, and E.J. Fellows. 1959. Effects of various centrally acting drugs on fighting behavior of mice. *J. Pharmacol. Exp. Ther.* 125:28–34.

Vogel, J.R., and R.C. Leaf. 1972. Initiation of mouse killing in non-killer rats by repeated pilocarpine treatment. *Physiol. Behav.* 8:421–424.

Watzman, N., and H. Barry, III. 1968. Drug effects on motor coordination. *Psychopharmacologia (Berlin)* 12:414–423.

Weiss, B., and V.G. Laties. 1961. Behavioral thermoregulation. *Science* 133:1338–1344.

Weiss, B., and V.G. Laties. 1962. Enhancement of human performance by caffeine and the amphetamines. *Pharmacol. Rev.* 14:1–36.

Whitfield, C.L., L.T. Ch'ien, and J.D. Whitehead. 1972. Lead encephalopathy in adults. *Am. J. Med.* 52:289–298.

Young, W.C. 1961. The hormones and mating behavior. In Young, W.C., ed., *Sex and Internal Secretions,* 3rd ed. Vol. II. Williams and Wilkins Co., Baltimore. pp. 1173–1239.

Young, W.C. 1969. Psychobiology of sexual behavior in the guinea pig. In Lehrman, D.S., R.A. Hinde, and E. Shaw, eds., *Advances in the Study of Behavior.* Vol. 2. Academic Press, New York.

SUGGESTED READINGS

Thompson, T., and C.R. Schuster. 1968. *Behavioral Pharmacology.* Prentice-Hall, Englewood Cliffs, N. J.

Weiss, B., and V.G. Laties. 1969. Behavioral pharmacology and toxicology. *Ann. Rev. Pharmacol.* 9:297–326.

Weiss, B., and V.G. Laties, eds. (In press.) *Behavioral Toxicology.* Appleton-Century-Crofts, New York.

Young, R.D. 1967. Developmental psychopharmacology: A beginning. *Psychol. Bull.* 67:73–86.

Part Four

NONHUMAN BIOLOGICAL EFFECTS

XII

Introduction to Nonhuman Biological Effects

The concern shown by Americans for subtle effects of chemicals on human health may appear excessive to a population faced with short-term dangers of epidemic insect-borne disease or starvation. The parallel concern of this committee for the well-being of plants and animals in the environment seems frivolous even to some Americans. Nonetheless, it seems prudent to increase our understanding of chemical effects on populations and ecosystems in order to guard against the possibility that unforeseen future changes may have serious impact on species of central importance in the natural and cultivated ecosystems upon which we depend.

Environmental toxicology, unlike human toxicology, is primarily concerned with populations rather than individuals. Natural competition eliminates individuals whose life processes are impaired, and their loss is not necessarily evident as long as the population as a whole is healthy and producing a surplus of young. For this reason, although the study of environmental effects can use knowledge and techniques from human health oriented toxicology, it requires its own set of principles and assessments. Further, environmental studies need special techniques because they are concerned with great variation in sensitivity between species groups.

In Chapters XIII, XV, and XVI these techniques and special considerations are discussed as they apply to nonhuman organisms and levels of

219

increasing biological complexity—from single species studied in the laboratory to field studies of populations, communities, and ecosystems. In Chapter XIV consideration is given to simulated systems, both physical and mathematical, that may permit tentative predictions regarding the fate and effects of toxic chemicals in ecosystems.

Levels of Biological Organization

A decrease in predictability typically occurs in the progression from laboratory toxicology experiments on single species to field studies of community and ecosystem response to chemicals. The decrease is related to a shift in the degree and type of biological organization involved.

Characteristic types of organization exist at cellular, tissue, and organ levels with new characteristics emerging at each higher level of complexity. The various mechanisms and processes at these fundamental levels are coordinated within the individual organism and are refined as a whole by natural selection acting to improve the fitness of the individual, which is the unit of selection. But a major change in organization occurs between the level of the individual and that of the population. Each individual of a population is to a greater or lesser degree competing with other individuals of that population and with individuals of other species.

Populations have characteristics—such as age structure, mortality rate, and replacement rate—that are not relevant to the organization within an individual. The effects of natural selection acting over many generations are such that each individual organism grows as fast, as large, and produces as many young as possible in the environment in which it finds itself. The higher trophic levels depend on this "excess" production of living tissue as a resource base.

A community or ecosystem has additional characteristics of structure (i.e., diversity) and of function (i.e., energy transfer, nutrient cycling) not exhibited by populations. Ecosystems studied to date appear to be aggregates of many alternative pathways of energy and nutrient transfer and many contrasting age structures and life spans. It appears that a community of few species in which most species have similar life spans is likely to be unstable, whereas one containing many species—some with very long and others with very short life spans—is likely to suffer few conspicuous changes. This redundancy appears to be one of the chief characteristics of "successful" ecosystems and may in part be responsible for the resiliency of natural systems, but in practice it means that there are so many partially independent subsystems aggregated in what is called one ecosystem that analysis into functional parts may be more an art than a science.

Effects of Chemicals at Different Levels

The effects of toxic chemicals at cellular and tissue levels are similar among a wide range of test organisms, but special phenomena appear at population and community levels. A chemical may be directly toxic only to individuals in a particular age group, or it may in some manner alter an individual's competitive ability, thus resulting in premature death. Thus, the effects of a chemical may in some cases be detectable only in changes in a population's mortality rate or reproductive rate, reflected in measurable changes in its age structure.

In the same way that toxic effects on populations result from effects on individuals, the effects of chemicals on ecosystems reflect differential effects on populations. If sensitive species decrease, the structure of a community is changed by a decrease in diversity. If the populations involved are numerous, the chemical may affect the functioning of the community, including the fixation and transfer of energy and nutrient cycling.

Need for Testing at Each Level

In addition to the need for determining chemical effects at the cellular, tissue, and organ levels, tests are needed for subtle effects on individuals and populations. At present, many chemical contaminants are found in plants and animals, but the biological implications of these body burdens are largely unknown. Attention should be given to possible effects on such life functions of the individual as metabolic rate, adaptability, reproduction, and life span. Thus, an important stage in testing should involve use of graded dosages, measurement of the resulting body burdens, and a multigeneration follow-up for effects.

Such information could be additionally useful for biological monitoring. For example, interference with certain biochemical activities and organ systems—reproduction, nerve transmission, liver and kidney—has been shown in some cases to be correlated with body burdens of chemical contaminants and with the levels of these contaminants in the environment. Thus, physiological responses and levels of chemicals in the tissues may be useful as indicators of the level of hazard to the population.

Tests are needed also for interspecific effects such as biomagnification and alteration of energy pathways and nutrient cycles. Simple simulated ecosystems are being studied in which known densities of known species can be observed in closed systems under controlled conditions. It is still not clear, however, to what degree it is possible to generalize from studies on rapidly growing, short-lived organisms to populations of large, long-lived, slowly growing organisms. Other tests are needed in seminatural, simplified systems such as ponds, stream diversions, field enclosures, or agro-ecosystems in which a limited number of factors are subject to natural variation and out of the control of the experimenter. In these experiments however, an added major complexity is that the test systems are no longer closed and may be subject to movement of organisms and chemicals into and out of the systems.

Finally, field studies of populations and ecosystems on the broadest scale (Chapters XV and XVI) are needed to detect unforeseen effects of chemicals released into the environment. The value of field surveillance is its ability to detect progressively more subtle but ecologically pervasive effects. For example, certain species in natural communities are apparently unusually sensitive to chemicals because of inherent responses or because of their place in the structure of an ecosystem. This is especially true of species at the top of long food chains. The species concerned are often valuable not only for their symbolic value in human society, but as useful indicators of changes in complex systems.

Because natural ecosystems are open systems and organisms and materials move from one to the next to a greater or lesser degree, chemical effects upon any one system tend to diffuse through neighboring systems. Many interacting and poorly known forces are aggregated at the organizational level of the ecosystem and, as a result, it is frequently difficult to predict the results of observed changes in structure. Furthermore, responses run the gamut from slight changes in population size or growth rate, or small changes in diversity, to massive changes—expressed as shifts in species responsible for primary productivity or in such species as blue-green algae that are unpalatable to most forms of life. Ecosystem characteristics thus supply a sensitive alarm system to detect unpredicted effects.

The following chapters expand these principles extensively.

XIII

Environmental
Toxicology

INTRODUCTION

The test procedures discussed in this chapter are limited to investigations of the effects of chemicals on preselected test organisms in which the environmental variables are reasonably well controlled, thus excluding most studies of natural ecosystems. The results of these investigations will serve as aids in determining the need for additional testing and as guides to planning these more elaborate tests.

With present limited knowledge, it is very difficult to predict whether the release of a new chemical into the environment will have a beneficial or harmful effect, or any effect at all, on the biota; however, similarities in structure to known compounds are helpful in establishing priorities for testing. Initial laboratory studies should be designed to reproduce on a very small scale what could occur on a large scale if the chemical were widely released.

Test systems available include phytotrons, greenhouses, field plots and cages for the study of terrestrial organisms, and aquaria and artificial ponds and streams for experiments with aquatic species. Sealed chambers of various designs have been used to study the toxicity of gases and aerosols.

The Dose–Response Curve

The main objective of this kind of testing is to obtain some kind of dose–response relationship (i.e. a relationship between the amount of the chemical to which the organism is exposed and a quantitative measure of its effect on the test organism). In studies of air pollutants and in tests on aquatic organisms, the chemical under investigation is normally mixed with or dissolved in the test medium (air or water), and the exposure level is often expressed in units of concentration times the duration of the exposure. In such studies, the amount absorbed is unknown unless specifically measured.

The ranges of responses that might be measured are extremely varied. If an absorbed substance interferes with the chemical processes sustaining life, it may cause death. Animals might also suffer sublethal adverse effects on growth, behavior, reproductive capability, sensory perception, and the regulation of body temperature or water. In plants, absorbed chemicals can cause tissue damage, reduced growth or yield, or impaired reproductive capacity. In some cases where the mechanism of the effect is known, sensitive biochemical techniques may be used to measure response. Generally speaking, the degree of response exhibited by the organism is proportional to the amount of active chemical. In practice, however, an individual organism is not tested more than once: Tests are carried out on groups of organisms at various levels of exposure. The dose–response curve thus obtained is a measure of the fraction of the population exhibiting a specific response at each exposure level. It can thus be used to predict the level of chemical that represents a dose of low risk to an average organism in the population (Chapter V).

Sources of Variability

The results of laboratory toxicity studies are subject to several kinds of variability. In experiments where the test organism is exposed to a known concentration of the chemical in the test medium and not injected directly, the amount absorbed may vary. The amount actually absorbed (i.e., the dose), which may sometimes be determined by radioactive tracer studies, does not necessarily produce identical responses on every occasion the dose is applied. The degree of response may be influenced by a constellation of intrinsic factors—such as age, genetic constitution, and nutritional, seasonal and reproductive state—as well as exposure to other stresses. Variability in soil and water chemistry and in atmospheric climatology is also extremely important.

It is thus necessary to determine some form of average response over the whole range of variability exhibited by individuals of the test species. In establishing limits for environmental exposure, it is necessary to consider whether any important stage in the life history (e.g., juveniles, reproductive individuals) is significantly more sensitive than another. Ideally, testing should take place in the natural environment where all of these sources of variability are operating; however, rather elaborate testing procedures would be required for this kind of testing, and, as a first approximation, more rapid and less costly testing can be done on simpler systems.

GENERALIZED SEQUENCE OF TESTING

Figure 9 presents a suggested scheme for laboratory studies to evaluate chemical threats to the biological components of man's environment. This scheme, which incorporates a feedback mechanism for returning to earlier steps, has five stages: (1) characterization of the chemical; (2) preliminary assessment of hazard; (3) short-term tests on individuals; (4) tests for chronic effects on individuals; and (5) tests for interspecies effects. A discussion of these elements follows.

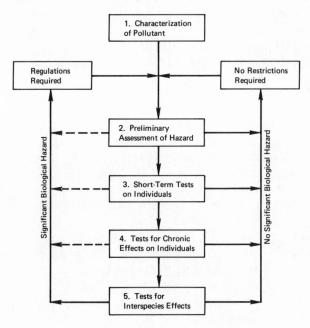

FIGURE 9 Flow diagram for laboratory investigations of toxicity.

Characterization of the Chemical

The characterization of a chemical should include a thorough review of its physical and chemical properties and an examination of the available data on its toxicity. As indicated in Chapter IV, physical and chemical characteristics are useful in predicting where the chemical is most likely to be found in the environment and at what concentration. Those organisms likely to be exposed to the highest concentration of the chemical would logically be considered first in toxicity tests. Environmental factors—such as temperature, pH, water quality (for aquatic organisms), and soil types—which can influence the biological availability of the chemical, should also be considered at this time.

It is possible that a substantial amount of toxicity data for occupational exposure will be available at the time when environmental effects are being considered—especially in the case of existing chemicals, previously used only in contained systems, which might be proposed for a new use involving dispersal into the environment. Similarity in chemical structure to known compounds might also be used as an indication of potential toxicity.

Tests conducted in the laboratory on living cells, microorganisms, tissue slices, or organ cultures may also be used as a rough guide to the toxicity of a substance. Tests carried out on these materials generally use biochemical and cell structure response criteria. They may give misleading results if the substance is metabolized *in vivo* to a less toxic or more toxic form before reaching the target cells or organs.

Preliminary Assessment of Risk

At this stage, an initial and tentative decision should be made as to the degree of testing for effects on the biota to be required. It is possible that existing regulations and controls for the purpose of protecting human health will be adequate to ensure the integrity of the environment as well. If there are no controls, or if existing controls appear inadequate, testing will then be required. It would be helpful to classify the chemical according to its anticipated biological impact and dispersal in the environment. Such a classification (Table 10) would indicate priorities among various chemicals that might be tested and in determining the extent of testing required. The intensity of the biological impact can be thought of in terms of the factors listed in Table 11. In both these tables, the lower numbers indicate greater significance. Thus, from Table 10, a chemical with a high biological impact that is proposed for a use involving widespread dispersal with the release of large quantities to

TABLE 10 Scheme for Classification of Chemicals According to Biological Impact and Dispersal

Chemical Dispersal	Biological Impact		
	High (1)	Medium (2)	Low (3)
(1) Widespread, high release	1	2	3
(2) Widespread, low release	2	4	6
(3) Localized, high release	3	6	9
(4) Localized, low release	4	8	12

NOTE: Low number indicates high priority.

the environment would have high priority and required extensive testing for biological effects.

The elements of biological impact listed in Table 11 are not meant to be all-inclusive, but they are indicative of the complexity of environmental problems. Table 10 reflects national or regional problems and priorities. In dealing with highly localized release of chemicals, several other factors might be considered:

- What receptors are close to the source?
- Which are the most sensitive?
- How important are they as a group?

Short-Term Tests on Individuals

Experiments of relatively short duration—from a few hours to perhaps 1 or 2 weeks—using high concentrations of the test chemical would be undertaken at this stage to determine the acute toxicity of a chemical

TABLE 11 Factors Contributing to Biological Impact

Factor	Level of Importance		
	(1)	(2)	(3)
Toxicity	high	medium	low
Receptor importance	high	medium	low
Type of effect	Interference with ecosystem functioning	Chronic effects at the level of the individual	Acute effects at the level of the individual
Availability to organism	high	low	
Potential for biomagnification	high	low	
Stability and persistence	high	low	

NOTE: Low number indicates high significance.

and its tendency for accumulation in organisms. At least a crude method of measuring residues of the chemical in plant and animal tissue should be available for studies of accumulation.

The most common end point of acute toxicity determinations is death; however, more subtle measures of the well-being of the test organism might also be used. For example, experiments with terrestrial plants can be devised to measure the effects of chemicals on seed germination, photosynthesis, and transpiration. With animals, changes in the rate of ventilation, heartbeat, or oxygen consumption might be used as indicators of the effects of chemicals. Considerable caution should be exercised in interpreting the results of tests for sublethal acute effects because not all change is necessarily adverse or beyond the limits of compensation.

Short-term bioassays can sometimes give helpful information on the rate of degradation of a toxic compound: For example, a decrease with time in the observed toxicity of a test solution to fish would indicate removal of the toxicant by degradation or some other means. Similarly, an increase in toxicity could indicate the formation of a more toxic material as part of the degradation process. Only actual analysis over time, however, can give reliable information on the rates of degradation and transformation.

Analysis of body burdens of the test chemical before and after exposure would reveal a tendency for bioaccumulation, even at concentrations that do not produce adverse effects.

If the chemical is rapidly degraded, if the decomposition products and the original compound are of low toxicity, and if bioconcentration is minimal, then additional testing may be unnecessary unless the anticipated use of the chemical under study would involve widespread dispersal in large quantities. Additional testing should be required for toxic chemicals or their toxic decomposition products that are persistent, tend to accumulate within an organism, or are of high toxicity.

Tests for Chronic Effects on Individuals

Long-term tests for chemical effects can use more sensitive indicators than are possible in short-term tests (e.g., weight gain, food consumption, longevity, behavioral response, and reproductive success in animals, and growth, yield, effects on reproductive systems, and changes in populations for plants). Acute toxicity tests may show that a chemical is harmful in large amounts, but may fail to detect the effects of exposure to the lower levels likely to be encountered in the environment.

Some chemicals accumulate slowly until a critically toxic level is reached (e.g., cadmium ingested in microgram quantities daily will often reach toxic levels in mammalian kidney by late middle age of the species checked). Accumulative chemicals can be sequestered harmlessly in storage sites but may be released at toxic levels on remobilization of the store (e.g., DDT stored in body fat can be remobilized under starvation stress; lead stored in bone can be remobilized with calcium stress during pregnancy–lactation). Some chemicals applied transiently to a young organism affect the progeny (e.g., diaplacental poisons).

Tests for Interspecies Effects

The direct effects of chemicals as indicated by tests on individual organisms has been the only method of testing discussed thus far. Experience with persistent toxic chemicals, which accumulate and are magnified in the food chain, however, has shown that simple tests on individuals can be woefully inadequate. If the chemical under study or its metabolites or decomposition products are stable, toxic, and accumulative—and if the anticipated use of the chemical will lead to widespread release in large quantities—then tests for ecological effects are indicated. Effects studied should include plant–plant interactions, productivity, plant–animal relationships, transport through food chains, and alteration of the chemical as a result of chemical, photochemical or microbial activity.

Transport through the food chain may be followed conveniently through the use of radioisotopes. The simplest studies to determine the effects of biomagnification involve feeding organisms that have accumulated the toxic compound to their natural predators. More elaborate studies can be devised using test plots, artificial ponds, and laboratory microcosms containing several species at different trophic levels (Chapter XVI, Simulated Systems). By far the most expensive, but perhaps the most thorough, method for determining ecological effects are the full-scale field studies of ecosystems discussed in Chapter XV.

SUMMARY

A generalized scheme for a laboratory evaluation of the potential acute, chronic, and ecological effects of a chemical is presented in Figure 9 and discussed in the body of this chapter. The planning of laboratory studies of the effects of a chemical involves a consideration of its expected behavior in the environment and its toxicity, as indicated by its physical and chemical properties and by preliminary experiments. A method for establishing the depth of testing required is given by the classification shown in Table 10, which uses the anticipated biological impact of the chemical and its pattern of dispersal for establishing priorities.

Appendix F contains a list of terrestrial species suggested for laboratory studies, an example of a sequence of tests for terrestrial species, and a similar example for aquatic organisms. The list of suggested readings that follows should provide adequate initial guidelines and background for high quality toxicity testing.

SUGGESTED READINGS

American Public Health Association. 1971. *Standard Methods for the Examination of Water and Wastewater.* 13th ed. APHA, New York. 874 pp.

Betts, J.L., T.W. Beak, and G.G. Wilson. 1967. A procedure for small-scale laboratory bioassays. *J. Water Pollut. Control Fed.* 39:89–96.

Heagle, A.S., D.E. Body, and W.W. Heck. (In press.) An open-top field chamber to assess the impact of air pollution on plants. *J. Environ. Qual.*

Heck, W.W., J.A. Dunning, and H. Johnson. 1968. *Design of a Simple Plant Exposure Chamber.* Access No. PB 195191. National Technical Information Service, Springfield, Va. 24 pp.

Heck, W.W., and D.T. Tingey. 1972. Ozone: Time-concentration model to predict acute foliar injury. In H.M. Englund and W.T. Beery, eds., *Proceedings of the Second International Clean Air Congress.* Academic Press, New York. pp. 249–255.

Henderson, C., and C.M. Tarzwell. 1957. Bioassays for control of industrial effluents. *Sewage Ind. Wastes* 29:1002–1017.

Marking, L.L. 1969. Toxicological assays with fish. *Bull. Wildl. Dis. Assoc.* 5:291–294.

Maugh, T.H. 1972. Polychlorinated biphenyls: Still prevalent, but less of a problem. *Science* 178:388.

Metcalf, R.L., G.K. Sangha, and I.P. Kapoor. 1971. Model ecosystem for the evaluation of pesticide biodegradability and ecological magnification. *Environ. Sci. Technol.* 5:709–713.

Mrak, E. 1969. *Report of the Secretary's Commission on Pesticides and Their Relationship to Environmental Health.* U.S. Dept. of Health, Education, and Welfare, Washington, D. C. 677 pp.

Pimentel, D. 1971. *Ecological Effects of Pesticides on Nontarget Species.* Report to Office of Science and Technology, Executive Office of the President. U.S. Government Printing Office, Washington, D. C. 220 pp.

Sprague, J.B. 1969. Measurement of pollutant toxicity to fish: I. Bioassay methods for acute toxicity. *Water Res.* 3:793–821.

Sprague, J.B. 1970. Measurement of pollutant toxicity to fish: II. Utilizing and applying bioassay results. *Water Res.* 4:3–32.

Sprague, J.B. 1971. Measurement of pollutant toxicity to fish: III. Sublethal effects and "safe" concentrations. *Water Res.* 5:245–266.

Warner, R.E. 1967. Bioassays for microchemical environmental contaminants. *Bull. World Health Organ.* 36:181–207.

XIV

Simulated
Systems

The function of simulated systems is to bridge the gap between the artificially simplified laboratory test systems and the complexity of the more diverse field systems of the real world. In the context of this study, tangible or conceptual models were used to predict the response of natural ecosystems to chemical stresses, on the basis of limited knowledge of the effects of the chemicals on representative species or groups of species under controlled conditions. The first stage in testing the adequacy of such models was to compare their behavior with the observed behavior of stressed ecosystems: Only models which passed this initial test were deemed of value for predictive purposes.

Two very different types of simulated systems were considered:

Laboratory and Field Microcosms—These simulate the behavior of systems of a small number of species or a small area under more or less controlled physical and chemical conditions. They include bench-top systems and small field plots and ponds.

Theoretical Models—These model the behavior of ecosystems or subsystems by means of mathematical equations. Some of the simpler models are amenable to mathematical analysis, but most models—especially those of complete ecosystems—are designed for computer simulation.

Within each of these two categories there are models of varying degrees of complexity. At the simplest level, models are required simply to investigate the effect of a chemical on individual organisms as functional systems in themselves, and from there to populations of single species. Changes that may be explored include not only reproductive rates, biomass, photosynthesis, respiration productivity, behavior, etc., but changes in intragroup properties as well—age structure, turnover, genetic composition, competitive interactions, spatial distribution, and social hierarchies. At the next level, models are used to investigate the effect of stresses on two-species systems, including predator–prey relations and competition for resources. More complex models investigate three or more species systems or branched food webs. This hierarchy of models approaches the simulation of ecosystems by building up through progressively more complex subsystems.

An alternate strategy of model-building is to start with a simple model of an entire ecosystem and break it down into progressively finer detail. In the first stage in such a hierarchy of models, the species are aggregated into such functional groups as trophic levels and the physical environment is aggregated into relatively large parcels. This type of simplification in theoretical models corresponds, to some extent, to the use of a small number of species and a controlled environment in laboratory microcosms. Progressive development of such models involves the inclusion of increasingly fine detail in the environment and progressively more subdivisions of the trophic web. The most successful models of this type have been concerned primarily with the transport of chemical nutrients and their effects on simplified biological systems. There is still a significant gap between these aggregated models of biological communities and the detailed models of interspecific interaction within the communities. It is not yet clear to what extent the fine detail of intraspecific and interspecific interactions may influence overall system properties and their relevance to the decision-making process.

Models of one type or another are inherent in all descriptions of ecological processes. Other panels have dealt with models to describe environmental transport of chemicals, pharmacodynamics, population turnover, and structural and functional properties of ecosystems. All of these models overlap with those considered in this chapter. However, the Panel on Simulated Studies has tried to isolate for review those models of chemically stressed systems that are designed as microcosms of much more complex systems. Comparatively few models specifically of this kind have been designed and investigated.

LABORATORY MICROCOSMS

Few toxicological studies in the laboratory have treated a single-species population as the unit of study. One example by Cairns *et al.* (1967) gave the unexpected result that a toxic stress increased reproductive success by reducing cannibalism by adult fish on their young. An example of a two-species system is the work of A.S. Cooke (1971), who found that a predator selectively took intoxicated prey. Another is that of Mosser *et al.* (1972), who found effects of a chemical on competition between phytoplankton species at levels below those required to show effects on either. Reinert (1967) measured bioaccumulation in a three-species food chain. Such systems appear promising as a sensitive test for ecosystem effects, but at present are in the research stage.

One of the most elaborate of controlled microcosms is the seven-species system described by Metcalf (1974) designed to model the ecological processes involved in a coupled terrestrial–aquatic ecosystem. The model includes a plant, an herbivorous insect, an alga, a crustacean, a snail, an aquatic insect, and a fish, maintained under controlled conditions for a 30-day period. The system has been used primarily to trace the transport, metabolism, and bio-accumulation of relatively persistent chemicals. However, some effects of various chemicals on sensitive species have been noted. The system has obvious potential for extension to measure dose–response relations of these sensitive species to chemicals under food web conditions of exposure, including effects of the chemicals on the routes and rates of uptake.

Despite the relative complexity of Metcalf's system, some functionally important groups, such as soil organisms and benthic fauna, are not included. The best reason for confidence in the validity of the system is the similarity of the behavior of chemicals in it to that in large-scale field tests, such as those conducted by Meeks (1968). Other multispecies microcosms include models of sewage treatment plants and multispecies microbial systems reviewed by G.D. Cooke (1971). These microcosms have the advantage of higher species diversity (one system mentioned by Cooke contains 19 species) but are limited in the number of functional groups, especially consumers. They have been used primarily to study community and ecosystem properties.

Another category of controlled microcosm is the laboratory stream reviewed by G.D. Cooke (1971) and Warren and Davis (1971). These continuous-flow systems have the advantage of permitting wide variation in physical and chemical parameters while maintaining a limited number of species. One limitation is the difficulty of maintaining a realistic level of downstream immigration and emigration. Another disadvantage is their relatively high cost. Comparatively few experiments specifically designed to evaluate the effects of toxic chemicals have been carried out in laboratory streams, but Warren and Davis (1971) quote several cases in which chemicals had adverse effects on fish at levels lower than those required to cause comparable effects in aquarium tests.

A final category of experimental microcosm is the test plot in which a small enclosed portion of a natural ecosystem is treated with a toxic chemical under otherwise uncontrolled conditions. Examples include the grassland plots studied by Barrett (1968) and the experimental ponds studied by Hurlbert et al. (1972). These systems, in general, contain a large (and unknown) number of species, and the number of toxic effects and species interactions that can be studied is limited only by the time and resources available to the experimenter. One of their greatest advantages is the ability to study the effects of chemicals on functional groups within field ecosystems. For example, Barrett (1968) found effects of an insecticide on the rate of decomposition of litter, and Hurlbert et al. (1972) found that poisoning of zooplankton led to a proliferation of phytoplankton species. The greatest disadvantages of these systems are probably their size and cost.

The microcosms discussed above form a hierarchy of increasing complexity and cost. Considered as a research tool, the entire hierarchy of experiments is required to contribute to knowledge of the ecosystem effects of chemicals. For the purposes of this conference the microcosms of intermediate complexity offer the best promise as test systems: They provide the best compromise between the complexity of interspecific interactions in real ecosystems and the advantages of dealing with known species in controlled conditions.

Selection of species for laboratory microcosms still must be largely *ad hoc*, and these choices will be modified in the future as ecologists gain better understanding of the ways in which communities are organized in nature, especially the relative importances of species in that organization. Quite separately, the question of scaling—in terms of area, heterogeneity, number of species, and individual densities—is not an easy one to settle.

MATHEMATICAL MODELS

The prototype mathematical models for time-varying processes are systems of ordinary differential (or difference) equations, which relate the time rate of change of the concentration (or abundance, biomass, etc.) of each component of the system to some function of the state of the system, time, and external parameters. The components of the system may include species abundances and chemical concentrations; the parameters of the system include thermal variations and levels of nutrients and toxins. For ecosystem considerations it often makes more sense to seek coherent ways to cluster or "lump" species into functional categories (e.g., decomposers, primary producers, and consumers). The implicit assumption in such a procedure is that the fine details of the interspecies interactions are of less importance to the ecosystem than the overall interactions between clusters of species, and that variations in species densities within clusters are of little importance if the overall biomass of the cluster is relatively constant. Such a simplification, while powerful, must of course be exercised with great care and may not always be justifiable.

Models of the type described above will in general predict a unique future for any given set of starting conditions and, in theory, could predict the response of any ecosystem component to particular stresses.

Species or chemicals distributed patchily over space may be treated within the above framework, but continuous distributions require recourse to partial differential equations. Passive diffusion and active transport by biological species, wind, and water are major considerations in assessing the impact of chemicals in ecosystems and may well require the use of partial differential equations. Of course, models of this type come in varying degrees of complexity. In some, attention is focused on the rather specific interactions between a small number of species, as in prey–predator, host–parasite, and host–parasite–hyperparasite systems. Such subsystems may be the direct objects of interest, or also may be the results of simplifying much more complex systems. Rosenzweig (1971) and Smith (1969) adopt the latter approach in examining three and four trophic level systems. In one of Smith's models, for example, the individuals at each trophic level are divided into a feeding portion and an anabolizing portion, providing for eight independent variables. Adding the densities of the free resource and the detritus provides a system of ten differential equations—still a rather cumbersome assemblage, but a great deal more tractable than an accounting of every species—chemical and biological—in the system would be.

A number of still more complex models have been described, but most of these have been concerned primarily with computing changes in physical and chemical parameters, and include relatively few biological variables. One example, the model of Chen and Orlob (1972) summarized in Appendix F, includes 16 physical and chemical variables, but only seven biological variables (representing functional groups of species).

Systems of equations of the types described can only rarely be exactly solved, although it is often possible to say much of an analytical nature about systems that are not too large. Such possibility of analysis is one of the major justifications for these simplifications and lumpings. Formal analysis of such systems generally emphasizes computations of steady states and evaluation of stability. The stability analysis most often employed is linear and relevant to "small disturbances" of population densities or of external parameters, but generally does not address itself to the critical (nonlinear) threshold problem: When is a disturbance no longer a "small disturbance"?

Most mathematical models have been explicitly designed for computer simulation. Some advantages and disadvantages of these methods are listed in Appendix E. Very few attempts have been made to use mathematical models of the type described here specifically for the problem of primary concern to this conference, prediction of the effect of toxic chemicals on ecosystems. One of the only analytic solutions available is the classic result of Volterra (1931): In a simple predator–prey model, an agent that increases the mortality rate of both species increases the numbers of the prey and decreases those of the predator. Extensive work in computer simulation has been carried out on the effect of increased nutrients, including prediction of eutrophication effects (e.g., Smith, 1969; Chen and Orlob, 1972). The most successful use of such models appears to be in describing and predicting transport of chemicals (a topic discussed in depth in Chapter IV).

Prospects for the future use of mathematical models in the prediction of effects of toxic chemicals are a matter of some dispute. In principle, the models used to predict the effects of nutrient chemicals on aggregated groups of biological organisms can very simply be extended to predict the effects of general toxins. However, real chemicals have selective effects, and these cannot be included in a model unless many more biological variables are included. The information required for such extended models would include (1) rate coefficients for uptake, metabolism, and excretion, (2) lethal thresholds and sublethal effects on growth, and (3) other functions *for each species.* Such information can only be derived empirically, a lengthy process, which would offset the main advantage of the computer model: speed. In the immediate future, the best promise offered by models of this type is therefore the quick prediction of the likely range of ambient concentrations for which toxicity measurements are required.

In the more distant future, it is possible to envisage a role for mathematical models as part of adaptive control systems for management of ecosystems after release of toxic chemicals. Such control systems require continuous updating as new information becomes available on toxicity of specific chemicals on specific organisms. Their weaknesses currently lie in the area of biological interactions where the laboratory microcosms and test plots or ponds should be of greatest value.

CONCLUSIONS

From this survey, a number of conclusions can be drawn:

- Although ecosystem modeling is in a very active phase of development, comparatively few studies have been made specifically of chemically stressed systems.
- Computer modeling has been of greatest value in describing transport and accumulation of chemicals; knowledge of toxic effects is, so far, primarily empirical.
- Most models of biological communities have been simple subsystems of from one to three species (laboratory tests), or of highly generalized aggregated systems (test plots and mathematical models). The most promising intermediate system [the multispecies microcosm of Metcalf (1974)] has not yet given easily generalizable results.
- Most models—at least those of subsystems—have been primarily of value in illustrating single mechanisms of action (e.g., effects on growth, competition, or cannibalism). The importance of each mechanism in the functioning of the entire ecosystem is poorly understood.

In brief, development of simulated systems is still at the experimental stage, where alternative models of phenomena and mechanisms observed in the field are being tested for the plausibility of their behavior. Their use in prediction of otherwise unknown effects is still in doubt. Nevertheless, there are some useful empirical generalizations about the behavior of stressed ecosystems. For example, Woodwell (1970) has pointed out that several kinds of stress—chemical, physical, or radiological—produce similar effects on ecosystems: a simplification in structure, reduction in diversity, size shift in dominant species towards a less complex life form, and loss of nutrients into adjacent systems. These empirical generalizations are encouraging with respect to the ultimate development of useful predictive models.

A final warning should be given about the potential misuse of simulated systems. The usefulness of models is limited not only by their inherent assumptions but also by the competence of their practitioners. Results from models—whether mathematical models or microcosms—should be carefully evaluated before they are used as a basis for decision making.

SUMMARY

The function of simulated systems is to bridge the gap between the artificially simplified laboratory or field test systems and the complexity of the real world. Two types of simulated systems are considered, experimental microcosms and mathematical models.

Experimental microcosms range in complexity from one-, two-, or three-species test systems, through controlled microsystems, to test plots and experimental ponds under seminatural conditions. There is a corresponding increase in cost and realism, but a decrease in knowledge and understanding of detail. A controlled microcosm of seven species appears to offer a reasonable compromise and offers promise of development into a useful test system for ecosystem effects.

In principle, mathematical models permit a similar range in complexity, but in practice most models are highly aggregated with only 1–7 biological variables. They have been developed most fully for studies of the transport and effects of nutrient chemicals, and their best promise for application to toxic chemicals is probably in studies of transport and bioaccumulation. Few have been used specifically to study toxic effects, and their usefulness for this purpose is limited by the scarcity of empirical information on the toxicity of specific chemicals to specific organisms. In the immediate future, the most important role of simulated systems in toxicology will probably be in explaining the general functioning of ecosystems and of the action of selective toxins on them.

REFERENCES

Barrett, G.W. 1968. The effects of an acute insecticide stress on a semi-enclosed grassland ecosystem. *Ecology* 49:1019–1034.

Cairns, J., Jr., N.R. Foster, and J.J. Loos. 1967. Effects of sublethal concentrations of dieldrin on laboratory populations of guppies, *Poecilia reticulata* Peters. *Proc. Acad. Nat. Sci. Phila.* 119:75–91.

Chen, C.W., and G.T. Orlob. 1972. *Ecologic Simulation for Aquatic Environments.* OWRR Rep. No. C-2044. Report to the U.S. Department of the Interior. Water Resources Engineering, Inc., Walnut Creek, Calif. 156 pp.

Cooke, A.S. 1971. Selective predation by newts on frog tadpoles treated with DDT. *Nature* 229:275–276.

Cooke, G.D. 1971. Aquatic laboratory microsystems and communities. In J. Cairns, Jr., ed., *The Structure and Function of Freshwater Microbial Communities.* Res. Div. Monogr. 3. American Microscopical Society Symposium, Virginia Polytechnic Institute and State University, Blacksburg. pp. 47–85.

Hurlbert, S.H., M.S. Mulia, and H.R. Willson. 1972. Effects of an organophosphorus insecticide on the phytoplankton, zooplankton, and insect populations of freshwater ponds. *Ecol. Monogr.* 42:269–299.

Meeks, R.L. 1968. The accumulation of ^{36}Cl-ring labeled DDT in a freshwater marsh. *J. Wildl. Manage.* 32:376–398.

Metcalf, R.L. 1974. A laboratory model ecosystem to evaluate compounds producing biological magnification. *Essays Toxicol.* 5:17–38.

Mosser, J.L., N.S. Fisher, and C.F. Wurster. 1972. Polychlorinated biphenyls and DDT alter species composition in mixed cultures of algae. *Science* 176:533–535.

Reinert, R.E. 1967. The accumulation of dieldrin in an alga (*Scenedesmus obliquus*), daphnia (*Daphnia magna*), guppy (*Lebistes reticulatus*) food chain. Ph.D. Dissertation, University of Michigan, Ann Arbor. 85 pp.

Rosenzweig, M.L. 1971. Paradox of enrichment: Destabilization of exploitation ecosystems in ecological time. *Science* 171:385–387.

Smith, F.E. 1969. Effects of enrichment in mathematical models. In *Eutrophication: Causes, Consequences, Correctives*. National Academy of Sciences, Washington, D.C. pp. 631–645.

Volterra, V. 1931. *Leçons sur la Théorie Mathématique de la Lutte Pour la Vie.* Gauthier-Villars, Paris. 214 pp.

Warren, C.E., and G.E. Davis. 1971. Laboratory stream research: Objectives, possibilities and constraints. *Ann. Rev. Ecol. Syst.* 2:111–144.

Woodwell, G.M. 1970. Effects of pollution on the structure and physiology of ecosystems. *Science* 168:429–433.

XV

Field Studies of Populations

The type of field studies discussed here are done out-of-doors on naturally occurring species populations of plants or animals not contained by laboratory walls or pens. Such populations may occupy areas ranging in size from an acre to a continent, and the principles discussed apply to populations of plants or animals on land, in soil, in fresh or saltwater, or in various combinations of these.

The field biologist needs certain information before planning a study on the effects of a chemical on field populations. He needs to know where the chemical is likely to be encountered in the environment and at what levels and what its tendency to accumulate in the tissues of organisms is (Chapter IV). He also needs to know the chemical's toxicity, including its effects on the laboratory animals used in evaluating hazards to human health (Chapters VI–XI) and its environmental toxicity from tests on controlled groups of plants and animals (Chapters XIII and XIV).

The productivity of a continuing dialogue between the field populations specialist and those doing studies in controlled environments cannot be overemphasized, both at the stage of screening tests to assess environmental or human health hazards, and at a later stage to work out details of the biological activity of the chemical in question. Slight additions to the screening process suggested by the field man, such as data on the levels of the chemical in the tissues of laboratory rodents, may make crucial differences in the planning of his field studies. Regulatory agencies must insist on this dialogue.

WHEN SHOULD FIELD POPULATION STUDIES BE MADE?

Extensive field studies may not have to be planned for every new chemical proposed for introduction into the environment. However, field tests at some level are indicated when the chemical is toxic and especially when it is persistent. When the initial toxicology data and estimates of exposure levels carry no evidence of effects in the field, no field studies should be planned specifically for that chemical. This judgment will often be wrong, and there are general field surveys designed to look for such unexpected effects. Such general surveys will also often fail to identify effects, but they offer an alternative to field population studies, which are often expensive and time-consuming and—if done routinely on all new chemicals—would consume more skilled man-years than are economically justified.

When there is evidence of potential harmful effects from initial toxicology, such as biological accumulation, or from exposure level estimates, such as very wide dispersion, then some level of field population studies should be required. This initial evidence will often not be strong enough to warrant halting the release of the chemical. In these cases, a form of provisional release should be arranged in which a limit would be placed on the total amount released or on the places where it would be used, or on the time period of initial release. Consequent release would then be conditional on the results of field population studies designed to follow up the hints from the initial screening process.

When the initial screening gives very strong indication of unacceptable field effects, then clearly the chemical would not be released and no field studies done.

When a chemical has already been released and evidence of effects appear in the field, population studies should be undertaken at once. Here, again, a close liaison between the population biologist and laboratory toxicologists must be maintained so that hypotheses about relationships between the chemical and population effects may be rapidly refuted or confirmed by controlled experiment.

There are three considerations to be balanced simultaneously in decisions of when to do field population studies on a particular chemical. These considerations are the degree (1) of anticipated population risk as suggested by preliminary data, (2) of stringency of control of the provisional release of the chemical, and (3) of anticipated social benefit of the chemical. For example, anticipated great social benefit would increase the degree of risk acceptable in provisional release and increase the scale of the population studies undertaken. Within this context, there are a series of nodal points for the decision maker:

1. general release with no field study indicated;
2. general release, but with field studies required;
3. conditional release, but with field studies required;
4. general release withheld pending satisfactory results of field trials (deliberate exposure of the chemical to populations); and
5. no release.

Finally, in spite of the knowledge that is and will become available from field studies of populations, regulatory agencies should openly assume that they will often be wrong in trying to predict population effects of new chemicals. Population ecology involves such complex multivariate situations that no other assumption is justified. Populations of organisms have great variability within species, and even greater variability in sensitivity exists between species (e.g., relative toxicity of pesticides to insects and mammals). Much of this variability cannot be anticipated. Reducing the frequency of being wrong in this situation is a difficult task. The principles set out here are aimed at the attainment of this goal.

SELECTING A POPULATION

Choosing a Site

The study site with the highest probability of damage to population should be chosen bearing in mind the likely environmental characteristics of the chemical and the exposure level data. Factors in this choice are the likely occurrence of very high local concentrations of the chemical, or of lower concentrations spread over long periods or wide areas. Experience with chlorinated hydrocarbons, however, underlines the truism of population biology: Long-term subacute effects, such as reproductive impairment, spread widely through a population's range, are much more damaging than complete elimination of individuals in a small part of the species' range—a disaster from which most populations, well equipped through evolution, recover.

Choosing Populations Within a Site

There are a number of population characteristics that should guide the choice of populations, bearing in mind, again, the environmental behavior of the chemical in question (e.g., whether it is soluble in water, attached to some organic material, or concentrated in an organism's food, or whether it is moved by air or by water). Not all of these have to be included in one situation:

1. susceptibility to magnified exposure levels (e.g., by being high on a food pyramid, by some behavior pattern, by high metabolic rate, etc.);
2. high economic or human social importance as a food, amenity, or resource, or as an endangered or rare species;
3. sensitivity to the kind of chemical in question (i.e.. observations of the species composition of a community exposed to the chemical may reveal the disappearance of one species or the increase of another and thus call attention to species that are suitable to assess the effect);
4. appropriate short or long generation time (depending on, for example, whether the chemical accumulates with organism age, or whether there is need to complete the study in a very short time—utilization of invertebrates with short generation time, for example, certain insects, as a useful short-cut to obtaining impact data or, on the other hand, use of species with long lifespans to assess another type of chemical impact); and
5. minimal avoidance capability.

Because of the variation in environmental behavior of chemicals combined with the enormous variability in sensitivity of species in the regional flora and fauna, it is impossible to be more specific. Beyond this, one must rely on the experience and judgment of a good population biologist.

ASSESSING THE EFFECT OF A CHEMICAL ON A POPULATION

The Population Approach

The main objective of this approach is to demonstrate in the field whether the chemical in question is having any effect, beneficial or harmful, on the population selected for the study. This is best done by attempting to establish a dose–respone relationship between environmental levels of the chemical under investigation and its effects on the biological performance of the selected population. In some economically utilized species, the criterion will be that of utilization of the species. Populations have special characteristics not shared by individual organisms such as age structure, reproductive and mortality rates, dispersion, recruitment, oscillation, and interindividual activities that may betray chemical effects not manifest in individuals.

It is widely recognized that it is much easier in such studies to measure the prevailing chemical burden than it is to quantify biological performance. Serious sampling problems arise from such factors as variability in age, genetic constitution, and seasonal behavior of individual organisms within a population. The sampling process itself may often disturb the population, especially when the population is small in size or when the sampling disrupts the habitat. These problems are aggravated by fluctuations in the biological success of a population that are a result of natural phenomena alone, such as droughts and food shortages. Above all, there is no simple quantitative measure of biological performance for gauging the response of a population; therefore, situations arise where a small but possibly important biological response to a chemical (signal) may remain undetected, being swamped by the background variability (noise) of the population. It is thus unsafe to conclude that what cannot be measured does not exist and, when embarking on population studies in the field, it is important to realize that a negative result does not necessarily indicate that no biological effect has occurred.

Estimating the Chemical Dose to a Population

This step involves estimating prevailing levels and flux rates of the chemical in a population under study and in its supportive environment. Care is needed in interpreting the data because of the many problems which can arise. The following indicate some of the difficulties.

- Chemicals released to the environment sporadically (e.g., rare usage or as the result of accidental spillage) and rapidly degraded chemicals (e.g., cyanides, organophosphate pesticides) may escape detection or be underestimated. Knowledge of chemical release times to the environment and decay rates (half life) in water, soil, and relevant biota is essential.
- Chemical concentrations may not truly reflect their biological activity because a chemical may be selectively concentrated at metabolically active sites within an organism, thereby increasing its effect, or a chemical may be adsorbed onto surfaces (e.g., sediments, soils, aerosols), thus altering its availability to the target population. The release of experimental doses of the chemical into a field trial area, especially of radioactivity-labeled material, may be particularly useful in determining the transient pathways and sites of activity.
- Molecular transformations may increase toxicity (e.g., methylation of mercury) or environmental persistence (e.g., oxidation of aldrin to dieldrin).
- Co-action of chemicals may potentiate (e.g., low pH increases

toxicity of SO_2 to plants) or antagonize one another (e.g., high Ca^{2+} in water reduces heavy metal toxicity to fish and plant life). Similar synergistic effects occur between chemical effects and stress (e.g., starvation).

Some of these problems can be reduced if suitable standard bioassay species, plants (e.g., mosses), or animals (e.g., fish) are introduced into the test environment to act as convenient integrators of prevailing chemical levels in a more reproducible manner.

Thus, although prevailing chemical levels are a useful guide to dosage, a truer reflection of the burden to a population is the product of frequency of release, amount released, persistence, toxicity, and input–output dynamics within the population.

Estimating the Response of a Population

Attention has already been drawn to the difficulties and advantages of the use of populations in quantifying biological response to a chemical. The criteria adopted below for defining biological performance in a population are substantially those evolved by population ecologists who have used them to create a classical picture of the dynamic structure of populations of wild plants and animals. Although the objective of the present study is somewhat different, experience and discrimination are necessary in using the following criteria to arrive at the best possible quantitative estimate of biological response.

Productivity, Biomass, and Growth Rate of a Population These are often easily measurable and may frequently be responsive to chemical influence.

Size and Distribution of Populations Many populations of plants, invertebrates, birds and other higher animals, and microorganisms are known to decrease in number or geographical range under chemical influence. Populations at the edges of a species' normal geographical range appear to be especially sensitive. Vanishing or endangered species are a special instance where census work may be important. Bird populations have often proved comparatively easy to count.

Specific Population Characteristics Reproductive success, life expectancy, mortality, age structure, and migration in and out of the population all contribute to population size but may be easier to measure than population size. Species that are producing more offspring than are needed to replace adult mortality can be expected to maintain their numbers in the presence of a hazardous chemical. But an early indication of any long-term trend may be given dependably by a change in age structure of the population.

Pathology   Many populations may respond to chemical burdens by succumbing more readily to pathogenic organisms. Knowledge of the relation of known body burdens to sensitivity to pathogens or other types of stress could be a useful tool in quantifying population response.

Additionally, just as introduced bioassay species were suggested for use as standardized assessors of prevailing levels (dosage) of a chemical in the environment of a population, so introduced sentinel species specially sensitive to specific chemicals may be used as a standard for assessing the effects (response) of a population (e.g., *Gladiolus* sp., sensitive to fluorine, *Nicotiana* sp., sensitive to SO_2, *Sinapis alba* sensitive to heavy metals.)

Behavioral Response   Chemicals can have direct and often subtle impacts on behavior that influence the species' competitive success and even survival. Small changes in courtship or mating rituals induced by chemicals may lead to mating failure. Similarly, learning, dominance, maternal behavior, swarming, and other behavior-centered responses could be likewise affected by chemicals. The ability of a species to search for and select its food, or to detect and catch prey, or to avoid predators or parasites as influenced by chemicals in amounts far below lethal values could in a very subtle way reduce competitive ability or survival success. Many extremely promising lines of approach can be found here.

Phenology   Such local perturbations in the seasonal timing of biological phenomena as flowering and leaf emergence in plants, arrival of migrating birds and insects, and pupation of insects may be used as indicators of chemical effects.

Experimental Design

In selecting these criteria for study, it should be recognized that the most effective use of field investigations can be achieved by linking them closely with supportive laboratory experiments. There is an invaluable, mutually beneficial interaction between field and laboratory studies, where field results can be taken into the laboratory for validation, and in turn the laboratory findings serve as the starting point for a new level of penetration of the problem in the field.

A special difficulty already touched upon is the problem of separating *signal* from *noise* in these complex systems. It should be emphasized that one way of minimizing this difficulty is to ensure that as many "response" observations are taken in control situations as are made in chemically affected environments, ranging from low dosage to high dosage. This makes the use of the necessary multivariate statistical techniques much easier in identifying the most likely cause–effect relationships and in separating interactions from random effects.

A special difficulty with some population studies is that they normally take so long to carry out that it is not possible to make a second test contingent on the results of the first, and so on, in a time sequence. This is not true of microbial and some invertebrate populations. A more practical method is to collect the field data pertinent to a hierarchical range of tests at one and the same time, but to order the manipulations and analysis of the data in a cascading manner so that data treatment of a second-stage test is contingent on the results of the data analysis from the first-stage test. After systematic studies of chemical impact on field populations are undertaken on a widescale basis, a background of experience will develop that will make possible a sound strategy of practical field testing.

Additional Supportive Studies

It is also particularly valuable to collect and store samples of biological material, soils, sediments, and other relevant environmental samples from the study sites in case back reference is needed at some future time when new information coming to light necessitates a new approach to the problem. In this context, existing herbarium and museum materials fulfill a valuable function in furnishing chemical baseline data for substances hitherto suspected to be either absent from the environment or present in extremely low amounts. This historical analysis can usefully be extended to peat profiles, tree rings, and any other materials accumulating in a time sequence. In the same way, representative and extensive samples of study populations should be preserved frozen as a valuable baseline resource for the future.

CONTINUING STUDIES AND DETECTION OF CHEMICAL EFFECTS

Rationale

However efficient the design and implementation of population studies tailored to elucidate the effects of chemicals introduced into the environment, these studies cannot be expected to reveal all such effects, especially those which are subtle or unusual. In fact, in recent history many first indications of chemical effects have originated from general studies conducted for other reasons, or from observations of competent natural-ists (e.g., the effects of DDT on eggshells or mercury on seed-eating birds, changes in bee fauna of apple orchards and robin populations on college campuses, fish kills, and fish contamination). Although many of these early warnings did not show a cause and effect relationship, they did provide the trigger for more detailed observations and experimentation. Because natural communities are so complex and so little understood, monitoring of natural populations is necessary to warn of abnormal or unusual modifications of population characteristics, which may be related to man-induced changes, including those produced by the use of chemicals.

Study Sites

Location An array of study sites should be involved that would provide a gradient of risk of exposure to chemicals. One such gradient could be provided by an array of ecosystems with varying intensities of land management (e.g., urban–industrial complex with associated market gardening, agriculture with or without irrigation, range or pasture lands, and forested lands or wilderness). Gradients of other variables in the in-tensity of man's modification of ecosystems, such as rivers and lakes with variable chemical loads might be formulated.

Character Considerable control over the study sites would be required, particularly in terms of permanence, stability of land management, and access. This control would be necessary for a period of at least several decades. A number of favorable study sites displaying the required gradient, permanence, and stability may be already under control for other purposes (e.g., military reservations, protected water supply water-sheds, wildlife preserves, national forest lands, recreational areas, and agricultural reserve acreage).

Nature of Studies Decisions about the specific populations within a com-munity and the population characteristics studied would be guided by the principles set forth earlier under Selecting a Population. An array of study sites as described here will also be quite useful to studies of chemi-cal effects on ecosystem dynamics. In many instances, the same data would be useful to both.

Use of Ecological and Population Surveys

A number of surveys covering wide areas are conducted annually by both amateur and professional groups. These include counts of birds, game animals, and endangered species and phenological surveys of plants. For example, the Breeding Bird Survey provides an index of the populations of many songbirds; the North American Nest Record Card Program provides an index of bird productivity; and the several waterfowl surveys give indices of breeding and wintering populations of exploited ducks and geese. In many cases, only small additions to staff in existing agencies would be needed to stimulate, standardize, and coordinate such surveys and examine their data for population changes that may relate to chemical use.

At least some of these surveys include the collection of biological samples, for example, the collection of wings of gamebirds shot by hunters. Other surveys might be encouraged to do so. These biological samples should be exploited as material for chemical analysis, since they come from what are often well-designed sampling procedures, and since they would be needlessly expensive to duplicate for reasons of chemical study alone. Gamebird wings have already proved useful in this regard. Such work should include the permanent storage of subsamples for future chemical reference. Results of chemical analyses from these widespread annual surveys could prove useful as tests of general models estimating exposure levels in the environment, and as measurements of the changes of these exposure levels with time. Of course, these same results may also be used to relate biological effects to chemical levels in the individual populations being surveyed.

Use of Manipulated Ecosystems

Signals of possible chemical impact may also be revealed by data coming from the closely monitored man-manipulated agro-ecosystems and from lakes, rivers, and estuaries in suburban and urban areas. These clues should be followed up by observations and possibly by field studies in other ecosystems.

SUMMARY

Field studies on naturally occurring populations of plants or animals should not be done routinely before the release of every chemical, but only when initial toxicology or exposure level estimates indicate a problem. In many cases, however, a chemical's continued or more widespread use should be contingent on results of population studies.

Population studies should be done at least at one site where the probability of damage is highest or at a similar site, and on those populations which are most likely to be at risk or have greatest social value.

Assessing the effects of a chemical on a population is best done by establishing a dose–response relation. The dose is a product of frequency of chemical release, amount released, persistence, toxicity, and input–output dynamics. The response is a change in the biological performance of a population, largely measured by the techniques of classical population ecology.

Apart from such studies aimed at the effects of a known chemical on particular populations, monitoring of natural populations for unsuspected changes that may relate to chemical use is necessary because prediction of chemical effects on natural populations is often inaccurate. Continuing studies for this purpose should be started on controllable sites graded by risk of chemical exposure. In addition, many existing population surveys done for other purposes could, with slight amendment, provide data on the distribution or effects of chemicals already released into the environment.

There is an invaluable, mutually beneficial interaction between field and laboratory studies, where field results can be taken into the laboratory for validation and, in turn, laboratory data can serve as an initial point for new studies in the field to further elucidate effects of chemicals on natural populations of organisms.

SUGGESTED READINGS

Allee, W.C., A.E. Emerson, O. Park, T. Park, and K.P. Schmidt. 1949. *Principles of Animal Ecology.* W.B. Saunders Co., Philadelphia. 837 pp.

Lack, D.L. 1954. *The Natural Regulation of Animal Numbers.* Oxford University Press, New York. 343 pp.

Rudd, R.L. 1964. *Pesticides and the Living Landscape.* University of Wisconsin Press, Madison. 320 pp.

Slobodkin, L.B. 1962. *Growth and Regulation of Animal Populations.* Holt, Rinehart and Winston, New York. 184 pp.

Wynne-Edwards, V.C. 1962. *Animal Dispersion in Relation to Social Behavior.* Hafner Publ. Co., New York. 653 pp.

XVI

Field
Studies
of
Ecosystems

The preceding sections have outlined approaches for examining the environmental effects of chemicals on progressively more complex (and less controllable) systems. This chapter considers the search for effects on large-scale systems. As many of the techniques to be used have been already identified in previous chapters, only general summarization is given here.

The primary purpose of ecosystem field studies is to identify possible subtle and indirect effects that might be unanticipated or undetected in studies of individual organisms, populations, or simplified simulated systems. Although most chemicals will be adequately screened by the methods discussed in Chapters XIII, XIV and XV, for others it might be necessary to permit the release of known amounts of a chemical to simulate environmental exposure, and to follow these releases with monitoring and ecosystem field studies. Such field studies are more expensive than laboratory tests and should be required for only a limited number of releases.

A secondary purpose of ecosystem field studies is to utilize the scientific opportunity presented when massive spills of substances occur through accidents or other mechanisms. These incidents make it possible to study the effect of lethal or high sublethal exposures to the ecological system. Evaluation of ecosystem recovery after such stress conditions is of particular importance because these studies present test situations on a scale that cannot be duplicated in the laboratory.

WHICH ECOSYSTEMS SHOULD BE TESTED?

A chemical entering some portion of the biosphere may have a very limited distribution if it is retained by adsorption onto colloidal materials or by other mechanisms, or if it is subjected to negligible dispersion. On the other hand, many chemicals are widely dispersed by application, by leaching through soil into groundwater, by soil erosion, or by translocation by movements of air or water.

Thus, a chemical may be of concern only in a small area, its impact may be felt in a larger but still limited region, or it may affect organisms living in most of the biosphere (Miller and Berg, 1969). These considerations were discussed in greater detail in Chapter IV.

Ideally, the impact of a chemical should be assessed in each distinctly different type of ecosystem into which it might enter, but this, clearly, is not possible. The number of test ecosystems must be reduced to a group that can be readily, economically, and adequately investigated. Unfortunately, little attention has been given to developing small prototype ecosystems that can be used in such screening programs. Such proposals should be encouraged, but as first approximations, which can and should be replaced by more valid prototypes that may come from future research.

Individual chemicals need not be tested in all types of ecosystems if it is clear through estimation of exposure levels that distribution will be limited. If, however, the potential mobility of the chemical is unsure, and if other tests indicate that it is likely to cause significant effects on ecosystems, it is essential to examine its impact on systems of probable entry.

Three major classes of environments—terrestrial, freshwater, and marine—should be examined in evaluating a chemical expected to have widespread distribution. There are special subsystems of these which may be of unique importance because of their intrinsic value as buffer zones, because of their fragility, or because they may provide a controllable subsystem amenable to experimental manipulation. Examples are agroecosystems or test plots (terrestrial), test ponds and small streams or lakes (freshwater), and estuaries and salt marshes (marine) [see Chapter XIV]. A special but very important ecosystem is the biological sewage treatment plant. Its function can be destroyed by release of toxic chemicals, and any serious disturbance of this man-made ecosystem might have serious consequence to man, wildlife, and the environment.

The only means by which it will be possible to reduce the large number of ecosystems that might theoretically be tested is by finding suitable prototypes. Thus, a major obstacle to satisfactory protocols for ecosystem testing is the absence of "standard" terrestrial, freshwater, or marine habitats. On the basis of the experience of environmental engineers, it appears that a reasonable standard model sewage treatment plant microecosystem can be established (Hawkes, 1963). In the case of the terrestrial, freshwater, and marine ecosystems, one must make an approximation based on the best available evidence as to what would constitute a proper sample to include representative animal, plant, and microbial communities and physical and chemical properties that are typical of a high percentage of natural habitats.

In addition to testing chemicals for ecosystem effects, continuous monitoring of sample natural ecosystems would provide an early warning system of unanticipated effects (Wilson and Matthews, 1970). More importantly, perhaps, it would be desirable to have a system in which consideration and response could be given to reports of ecological changes or chemical pollution hot spots located or identified by biologists not associated with monitoring schemes.

WHICH CHEMICALS SHOULD BE TESTED?

There are three major characteristics of each pollutant that must be understood before the possible impact or hazard of its release to the environment can be evaluated: the quantities produced which may reach the environment, the toxicity of the pollutant to organisms and to man if it will reach him in his food, and the persistence of the pollutant in the environment. Our knowledge is incomplete, sometimes with regard to all three of these essential characteristics of pollution.

Chemicals enter natural ecosystems in many ways. Some, such as pesticides, are deliberately introduced because they serve useful functions. Others are released deliberately after they have been used for the purpose for which they were designed (e.g., detergents in municipal wastes). Many substances are discharged as by-products or wastes of manufacturing activities, as a result of cleaning or flushing operations, and through the burning of fossil fuels. Finally, a number enter waters, soil, or the atmosphere inadvertently because of leakages from machinery and spills from barges or trucks.

The fates of these chemicals are diverse. Some remain in place and persist, largely or wholly unchanged, for many months or even years. Some are not appreciably modified but are transported to adjacent or distant localities by physical processes. Others are immobilized and not dispersed beyond the immediate area of contamination. The mobile compounds are of particular concern with regard to protocols for assessing effects of chemicals on ecosystems.

Of particular importance is the fact that many chemicals are converted to other compounds by natural processes. Some chemicals are rapidly degraded to carbon dioxide, water, and other simple, innocuous compounds. If conversions do not result in accumulation of intermediate degradation products, then only the parent molecule need be tested.

In identifying those substances that should be tested, and in establishing a protocol for testing ecosystems, it is necessary to consider the following points, some of which were discussed in greater detail in Chapter IV but merit repeating here.

- A chemical may be present in the ecosystem into which it is introduced for a very short period, perhaps less than one day, or it may persist for many years.
- Potential effects may be different from those expected on the basis of laboratory tests because the chemical is rendered less active through conjugation reactions or sorption on colloids or sediments. A small amount of the chemical may still be slowly available, for long periods of time, as it is released from the sorbed or conjugate state. It is also possible for chemicals to be stored gradually and released suddenly, as is the case with zinc entering highly alkaline waters which may become acidic suddenly for short periods of time.
- A chemical which disappears from the environment into which it is initially introduced is not necessarily destroyed because it may be transported to a new site where, however, it usually will be present in a lower concentration.
- A chemical in an ecosystem may be present in low concentration, but because of bioaccumulation and biomagnification the level to which some populations are exposed may be considerably higher than analysis of environmental samples indicates.
- A proper assessment of the potential hazard of a chemical must include measurements of the influence of products formed from it during biodegradation and from microbiological, chemical, and photochemical processes that do not wholly convert the initial substance to innocuous products. Some of these products will be generated *in situ* in the test ecosystem, but others will in nature reach an ecosystem in which they are not generated, because of any one of several environmental transport mechanisms.
- Translocation from one organism to another (different from biological magnification) may be important under some circumstances.

CHARACTERISTICS OF ECOSYSTEMS AND
ECOLOGICAL IMPACTS OF CHEMICALS

As stated in the introduction to this section, the principal objectives of
ecosystem field studies are (1) to detect and evaluate sublethal effects of
chronic exposure of a chemical on ecosystem processes, and (2) to evaluate the impact on and recovery of an ecosystem resulting from sudden
spills that precipitously introduce large amounts of chemicals into the
environment.

Sublethal effects are especially important, may develop slowly, and
be unrecognized in their early stages. These include bioaccumulation,
biomagnification, and impact on productivity, energy flow, nutrient
cycling, and diversity, as well as a number of indirect or secondary effects
(Wilson and Matthews, 1970). It is important that these be considered
in protocols for evaluating ecosystem effects.

Bioaccumulation and Biomagnification

The process by which a chemical becomes more concentrated in an organism than it is in the environment is known as bioaccumulation and can
be evaluated in laboratory tests. In some cases, as organisms are eaten by
predators at higher trophic levels, body burdens of chemicals may
progressively increase in a process known as biomagnification. Also, the
body burden may increase with size or age of the animal, as has been
shown to be the case with mercury content of fish. Because of the complex structure of food webs in nature, it is generally not possible to
duplicate the entire process of biomagnification in simplified systems,
but its effects can be detected in the field.

Productivity, Energy Flow, and Nutrient Cycling

The productivity of ecosystems varies from place to place and from time
to time, depending upon a variety of environmental factors including the
season, availability of light and essential plant nutrients, and the import
or export of various materials into or out of the system. It should be emphasized that a high rate of productivity is not necessarily an indication
that the ecosystem is healthy or of value to man. For example, weeds in
terrestrial systems or noxious algae in aquatic systems may have high
productivity but little human value or they may be detrimental to human interests.

Ecosystem functioning is based, in part, on recycling of elements
essential to biological productivity. Unlike energy, which follows a path

from its fixation in photosynthesis to its ultimate dissipation as heat, nutrients are returned to the system as a result of decomposition and can be used repeatedly (Odum, 1971). The productivity of an ecosystem is frequently limited by the lack of nutrients. Various types of pollution of water bodies—such as domestic or food processing wastes—enrich the waters with nutrients and, when present in excessive amounts, can result in the replacement of the typical plant populations with noxious species. This process, *cultural eutrophication,* changes the entire biotic structure of the ecosystem (NAS, 1969). Air pollution with SO_2 or soil contamination with elements or salts may similarly alter terrestrial communities toward simple ones characteristic of lower life forms.

Certain biogeochemical cycles in soils or water may be especially sensitive, for example, nitrification. Enzymatic processes can be poisoned by chemicals and critical parts of the cycle could be broken with long-term detrimental effects. It would be unrealistic to attempt studies of all chemicals on these processes, but the impact would generally be readily apparent in field studies with proper controls.

One essential plant nutrient, phosphorus, is commonly blamed for excessive enrichment of surface waters. This indictment of phosphorus is justified only when it is established by experiments to be the critical element in short supply relative to plant needs. Such experiments generally are done using natural waters introduced into confined systems under controlled laboratory conditions.

Diversity

A wide variety of indices has been developed to evaluate the diversity of ecosystems by relating the number of different species to the total abundance of organisms (Brookhaven National Laboratory, 1969). Natural and undisturbed ecosystems have different characteristic degrees of diversity often correlated with degrees of natural stresses on the system. In general, ecosystems with high diversity are the most stable ones, perhaps because there are large numbers of pathways for the transfer of nutrients and energy from one part of the system to another.

Pollution, or any other man-made modification of the environment, amounts to a stress imposed on the ecosystem and will tend to eliminate some species while favoring the forms that are more resistant and tolerant to that stress. The disappearance of species and the consequent decrease in diversity may be the first indication of ecologically significant change in the environment. However, before diversity can be used as an indicator of change, the natural diversity of the environment being studied must be known.

Prediction of impacts on diversity based upon laboratory tests with standard test organisms may not be possible. This is because the test organisms may not be the most sensitive species in the ecosystem. Indeed, the sensitive organisms may not be amenable to laboratory culture. Their disappearance from the ecosystem can be determined by field tests, however.

Where particular species are affected, it will be necessary to determine whether or not they are critical to the maintenance of ecosystem structure and function. For example, some predators fill an important role in maintaining prey diversity in an ecosystem. Although a species may not be vital to the integrity of the ecosystem, it may have special economic or symbolic value to man (e.g., whales, lobsters, eagles, or butterflies).

Behavior of Organisms

Chemicals affect plants and animals in many ways: directly, by affecting growth-regulating mechanisms in plants and the nervous systems of animals; or, indirectly, by affecting the reception of chemical clues from the environment (Klopfer, 1962). The growth of plants is strongly affected by chemicals in the environment. For example, high concentrations of SO_2 in the atmosphere have marked effects on growth, photosynthesis, and reproduction of plants. Because plants establish the habitat for animals, the effects of chemicals on their growth and functions can have extensive ecosystem effects.

The behavior of many species of animals is mediated by chemical stimuli that can act at very low concentrations. The homing of salmon and other anadromous fishes to the stream of their birth is, in part at least, a response to the unique chemical character of the water. Breeding activities of insects are stimulated by sex hormones which attract the male to the female. Many feeding activities of terrestrial and aquatic animals are triggered by chemicals released to the environment.

Chemicals may also have a direct effect on the action of the nervous system of animals, especially those animals showing complex behavior patterns. Chemical effects should be looked for in an animal's ability to react to such environmental stimuli as those which influence its ability to find and catch prey, its ability to escape predators, and its interactions with members of its own species. Each of these influences on the behavior of particular animal species will affect the ability of a population to survive and to perform its role in ecosystem structure and function.

Potential for Recovery

Very little is known about the ability of ecosystems to recover if stresses imposed by man are modified or removed. Although various man-made modifications are irreversible, removal of some sources of pollution permits recovery of an ecosystem. The familiar example of old field succession illustrates the ability of some communities to re-establish themselves once a stress has been removed. Much could be gained from the facilitation of these processes.

In aquatic systems polluted over many years, a large reservoir of toxic materials may form in sediment, and the system may take years to recover. For pollutants remaining in solution, the recovery time will be a function of the flushing time of the system.

Inadvertent destruction of parts of or even all of ecosystems can result from an accidental spill or release of toxic materials. The damage may be widespread and persistent, but if refuges where the species can survive are available, the ecosystem may return to normal. Field studies of such accidental releases should be encouraged so that we can develop the ability to predict recovery rates. These rates will differ widely, depending upon the persistence of the chemical in the environment, the sizes of the populations involved, their reproductive rates, and dispersal mechanisms, among other things.

Alteration of the Environment

An environmental problem of major consequence is the impact of chemicals released in the environment on the physical and chemical characteristics of an ecosystem. This problem is especially important in aquatic systems when spills occur through accidents or other mechanisms (Warren, 1971). For example, a substance discharged into an aquatic system may alter the pH of the water, may create surface films and thus affect light transmission and gaseous transfer, and may significantly alter the dissolved oxygen concentration in the water.

One of the most significant of these problems is oxygen depletion. Assessment of potential impacts involves simultaneous measurements of dissolved oxygen and the concentration of the chemical because toxicity stress and stress caused by oxygen depletion are often inter-related. For materials causing these problems, it is necessary to know the theoretical oxygen demand (i.e., quantity of ultimate oxygen demand per quantity of substance) and rate function for the demand. The technology for determining oxygen demand and demand rates is well established in the waste treatment field, and suitable test procedures can be adapted for substances that may be discharged locally, in large quantity, to an ecosystem. The decision hierarchy for selecting appropriate tests should identify those materials that are discharged in quantity from domestic, industrial, or other sources or which are shipped in bulk commerce. Information on oxygen demand and oxygen demand rate should be provided for these materials.

The potential magnitude of the problems discussed above should additionally be assessed by measuring the biodegradability of the substance. Determination of biodegradability is therefore a high priority requirement in evaluating the effects of a substance or its transformation products in the environment. At this time, greater efforts toward definition and standardization of methods are probably needed more for measuring biodegradation than for any other testing procedure.

PREDICTION OF ECOLOGICAL IMPACTS

The impact of a chemical or its transformation products on an ecosystem is not a phenomenon which can be quickly and precisely measured or predicted. There are, however, a variety of test procedures of different levels of precision, difficulty, and expense that, when coupled with expert knowledge of ecosystems, can give considerable insight into potential impacts. The test procedures discussed in Chapters XIII, XIV and XV, together with tests for biodegradability and oxygen demand, can serve as screening mechanisms to determine which substances should be examined by higher order testing of ecosystems. The results of animal studies to determine possible effects on human health should also be considered. Even the most extensive of these tests, however, are not infallible, and the scientific community must be continually alert for unique substances or transformation products that interfere in unexpected ways with ecosystem functions.

Pilot Ecosystem Studies

Pilot ecosystem studies are defined as experiments conducted in natural systems of up to a few square kilometers in land or water area. In assessing the potential environmental impact of a chemical, tests of this magnitude may be deemed necessary on the basis of information derived from the various tests discussed above. Pilot studies are contrasted to simulated systems and test plots or small ponds, on one hand, and the evaluation of macrosystems, such as watersheds or estuaries, on the other.

Pilot studies should, of course, be used to determine effects that can be observed only at the ecosystem level. These include biomagnification, productivity, nutrient cycling, energy flow, and changes in community diversity.

Large-Scale Ecosystem Studies and Monitoring Programs

After pilot experiments on ecosystems have been completed and a chemical has been released for use, ecosystems into which the chemical enters should be studied and monitored for unanticipated effects. In this way deleterious impacts can be detected promptly and corrective action taken. The scale of ecosystem studies could range from the evaluation of a single river basin to nationwide monitoring, depending on the extent of the distribution of the chemical in the environment. There frequently is a "scale effect" characteristic of most natural ecosystems, and if too small an area is studied some ecosystem attributes will not be perceived (e.g., population dispersion, successional changes, and gene drift in response to selective pressures).

It should also be noted that if an ecosystem is adversely affected by a chemical, adjacent ecosystems not contaminated by the chemical may suffer "spinoff" effects. Natural ecosystems are not generally self-contained and patterns of biological imports from and exports to an affected area may thus affect other systems.

SUMMARY AND CONCLUSIONS

The objectives and purposes for evaluating the environmental impacts of chemicals through field studies of ecosystems have been defined as detecting and evaluating sublethal effects of chronic exposure of a chemical on ecosystems, and evaluating the impact on and recovery of an ecosystem resulting from sudden discharges of large volumes of chemicals into the environment. The range of types of ecosystems which should be studied has been discussed, as have the mechanisms by which chemicals enter ecosystems and their potential significant impacts.

The need for field studies to determine the ecological impact of a chemical will depend on its expected behavior in the environment and on the outcome of studies of toxicity under controlled conditions. Chemicals with limited distribution or mobility may not need to be studied in all three major classes of environments (terrestrial, freshwater, and marine). Ecosystem studies would be indicated for potentially toxic chemicals, which are introduced in large quantities, highly mobile, persistent and likely to be concentrated by physical, chemical, or biological processes. Chemicals that are capable of altering physical and chemical characteristics of the environment, such as pH, dissolved oxygen, and surface properties of water, should also be considered candidates for study at the ecosystem level.

No attempt has been made to specify particular methodology for assessing ecosystem effects because of the wide range of descriptive literature on ecosystems and the lack of standardized or certified testing procedures. Ecosystem studies should examine the possibility of bioaccumulation and biomagnification and effects on productivity, energy flow, nutrient cycling, and the behavior of organisms—all of which could affect the overall structure and function of ecosystems.

Since the number of ecosystems is finite and replacement is not possible, an appropriate management plan is mandatory for ecosystem testing. All large-scale ecosystem tests involving substantial application of hazardous materials should be outlined in considerable detail and reviewed by a competent panel before being authorized. Perhaps this process should be accompanied by impact hearings for the very large-scale tests. There should be guarantees that these investigations, once initiated, will be completed in terms of stated objectives unless a rigorous review deems this unnecessary.

Ecosystem evaluations are the most expensive in funds, talent, and time and should therefore not be used except where potential hazards cannot be delimited with other techniques. Regular feedback for additional laboratory tests will often hasten the acquisition of needed information, reduce costs, and help perfect the integration and effectiveness of assessing effects on all components of the ecosystem.

REFERENCES

Brookhaven National Laboratory. 1969. *Diversity and Stability in Ecological Systems.* Brookhaven Symposia in Biology, No. 22. Access No. BNL-50175. Clearinghouse for Federal Scientific and Technical Information, Springfield, Va. 264 pp.

Hawkes, H.A. 1963. *The Ecology of Waste Water Treatment.* Pergamon Press, Oxford, England. 203 pp.

Klopfer, P.H. 1962. *Behavioral Aspects of Ecology.* Prentice-Hall, Inc., Englewood Cliffs, N.J. 171 pp.

Miller, M.W. and G.G. Berg. 1969. *Chemical Fallout.* Charles C. Thomas, Publ., Springfield, Ill. 560 pp.

National Academy of Sciences. 1969. *Eutrophication: Causes, Consequences, Correctives.* Proceedings of a Symposium. National Academy of Sciences, Washington, D.C. 661 pp.

Odum, E.P. 1971. *Fundamentals of Ecology,* 3rd ed. W.B. Saunders Co., Philadelphia. 574 pp.

Wilson, C.L., and W.H. Matthews, eds. 1970. *Man's Impact on the Global Environment: Assessment and Recommendations for Action.* M.I.T. Press, Cambridge. 319 pp.

Warren, C.E. 1971. *Biology and Water Pollution Control.* W.B. Saunders Co., Philadelphia. 434 pp.

SUGGESTED READINGS

Cook, L.M., ed. 1969. *Cleaning Our Environment: The Chemical Basis for Action.* Committee on Chemistry and Public Affairs, American Chemical Society, Washington, D.C. 249 pp.

Goodman, G.T., R.W. Edwards, and J.M. Lambert, eds. 1965. *Ecology and the Industrial Society.* Br. Ecol. Soc. Symp. No. 5. John Wiley and Sons, Inc., New York. 395 pp.

Inger, R., *et al.*, eds. 1972. *Man in the Living Environment.* Report of the Workshop on Global Ecological Problems, Institute of Ecology. University of Wisconsin Press, Madison. 288 pp.

International Biological Program. 1969–1972. *IBP Handbooks.* Nos. 1–24. F.A. Davis Co., Philadelphia.

McKee, J.E., and H.W. Wolf. 1963. *Water Quality Criteria,* 2nd ed. State Water Qual. Control Board Publ., No. 3-A. Resources Agency of California, Sacramento. 548 pp.

National Academy of Sciences. (In press.) *Water Quality Criteria, 1972.* U.S. Government Printing Office, Washington, D.C.

Singer, S.F., ed. 1970. *Global Effects of Environmental Pollution.* Symposium sponsored by AAAS, Dallas, 1968. Springer-Verlag, New York, 218 pp.

VanDyne, G.M., ed. 1969. *The Ecosystem Concept in Natural Resource Management.* Symposium of the Annual Meeting of the American Society of Range Management, Albuquerque, 1968. Academic Press, New York. 381 pp.

XVII

Episodic
Exposures

The major thrust of study has been directed toward substances discharged into the environment on a more or less continuous basis and generally found in the environment at relatively low concentrations. In addition to those discharges there are annually thousands of short-term discharges creating much higher concentrations in very localized geographic areas; therefore, it was deemed appropriate to give special consideration to the situations created by large spills of concentrated chemicals and to examine the applicability of methods and priorities established primarily for prolonged exposure to relatively low levels. The spill situation may generally be categorized as involving a sudden release (accidental or deliberate) of a substance to the environment resulting in dangerous concentrations. The spill may involve any one or more of the segments of the atmospheric, aquatic, or terrestrial environments.

In examining the problems created by spills, the Panel on Episodic Exposures confined its evaluation to determining those unique conditions of the spill situation that differentiated the resulting pollution from that associated with continuous discharges. Attention was then given to the requirements for test data prior to the episode, the priorities to be established for acquiring such data, and the monitoring and ecosystem evaluation to be conducted after the spills occurred. Control and safety actions to be taken with regard to spills were not considered because of the existence of extensive contingency control plans.

SPILL VERSUS AMBIENT POLLUTION

Spill pollution differs from background pollution in several important ways.

1. There is no specific advance knowledge with regard to when or where a spill may occur, the kind or amount of material involved, the resulting concentration, the size of the affected environment, and the duration of the episode. All of this basic information is gathered during and after the crisis.

2. Spills generally involve much higher environmental concentrations than found in background pollution. However, these high concentrations may not last as long and may be in a more limited area.

3. Preventive measures can do much to reduce the frequency and size of spills but spills cannot be totally eliminated. Available data indicate that the present rate of transportation accidents involving spills and near-spills is much higher than generally realized.

4. Perhaps the most important difference between spill and background pollution situations lies in the need for immediate action to evaluate the hazard of a spill and to institute control measures.

APPROACH TO THE PROBLEM

The basis data required to evaluate the effects of chemicals on man and his environment under the spill situation are generally the same as are required for the evaluation of continuous discharges. These descriptors of the spill include time, place, material, quantity, physical and chemical properties, ecosystems at risk, and toxicity.

Much of these data can be acquired in advance of a spill and stored for ready access at the time of the emergency. Priorities for collecting such data should be based upon (1) the likelihood of a spill as indicated by transportation patterns and (2) the potential for significant environmental damage (i.e., toxicity). The Chemical Transportation Emergency Center (CHEMTREC) system of the Manufacturing Chemists Association and the Chemical Hazards Response Information System (CHRIS) of the U.S. Coast Guard are good steps in this direction. CHEMTREC is a national center for providing information on hazardous materials involved in spills and for notification of the shipper that an emergency exists (Manufacturing Chemists Association, 1971). CHRIS is a system of field manuals and central computer data being developed by the U.S. Coast Guard to upgrade response to hazardous material accidents (Arthur D. Little, Inc., 1972).

The methods for using test data are not necessarily the same for the spill situation as for the continuous discharge situation, and some modification of the management system may be required. The priority and emphasis given certain data are not the same when evaluating potential harm from spills versus potential harm from continuous discharges. The environmental concentrations resulting from spills frequently approach or exceed those producing significant acute toxic effects on man or the biota inadvertently exposed, as well as those involved in control and cleanup of the spill.

Following a spill, it will be necessary not only to predict the distribution of the material but also to monitor its dispersal into the environment until such time as dilution, degradation, or other mechanisms have reduced the contamination to a safe level. When spills do occur advantage should be taken of the prime research opportunities they present to measure the effect of large massive doses of substances on ecosystems. No intentional testing at such levels could ever be reasonably contemplated. These studies are particularly valuable for estimating potential acute effects and the recovery of ecosystems after stress. The contingency plans mentioned earlier might well include field research teams to take full advantage of these situations.

Hazards, such as fire and explosion, associated with the release of the material are also important. Information on these hazards is needed, but the specifications for particular test methods are available elsewhere and are not presented here (National Research Council, 1964; Hazardous, etc., 1971).

HUMAN HEALTH EFFECTS

Primary information needed to protect the population from the immediate effects of the spilled material includes acute and subacute toxicity data for exposure through inhalation, skin contact or ingestion of the material, or the contamination of food and drinking water. Information on sublethal, disabling concentrations are particularly important for the protection of those involved in controlling and cleaning up spilled chemicals. The more subtle effects of substance—for example, chronic toxicity, carcinogenesis, and effects on reproduction and behavior—may also be important under certain circumstances.

For ethical reasons it is not possible to obtain experimental data on human exposure to toxic materials at acute or high level subacute exposures. Information on such exposure is normally extrapolated from exposure tests conducted with experimental animals (Chapter V); however, human exposure data is often obtained as a result of the exposure of humans to accidental spills. The value of such information can be very substantial, and efforts should be made to collect it at the time of the emergency.

ENVIRONMENTAL CONSIDERATIONS

A primary environmental parameter is acute toxicity as it relates to organisms found in an ecosystem. Disabling sublethal effects are important but to a lesser degree than for human exposure.

In the aquatic system the oxygen demand characteristics of a substance are often of equal or greater significance than the acute toxicity. Generally, in spills involving materials whose acute toxicity is greater than 5 mg/l, oxygen demand will be of greater concern than toxicity. Thus, the laboratory determination of oxygen demand and the rate of oxygen demand becomes highly significant with regard to spills.

The concentration and movement of a substance in the environment is a function of its chemical and physical properties. Data on geometry, wind and flow data, and other environmental parameters are needed almost instantly in the spill situation. These data appropriately have a higher order priority under the spill situation than under the continuous flow situation.

ANALYSIS AND MONITORING

Spills require a very different type of analysis and monitoring than that required for continuous discharges. Quick analytical techniques for field use must be ready and available on short notice, and monitoring equipment must be mobile to follow the spilled substance as it moves through the environment. Although fixed sophisticated monitoring systems are of questionable value under the spill situation, real-time computer collected and analyzed data on meteorological conditions, stream flow, and other environmental parameters could prove invaluable.

Tagging of spills with fluorescent dyes on other material for which analysis is more rapid and accurate than for the spilled material may become a useful practice.

Transport models for spills can be relatively unsophisticated because approximations must be made quickly with only limited data. Steady-state models developed for continuous discharges, and other sophisti-

cated models requiring substantial input data are inappropriate for
spills.

CONCLUSIONS

It is essential to understand that the problem of potential spills is distinctly different from that of continuous discharges and that substantially different priorities exist for the acquisition of information
regarding the properties of a chemical substance and the effect of the
substance on living organisms. Appropriate data on chemicals and
environmental systems will materially aid control of spill situations
in the aquatic environment.

Toxicity data for aquatic species and oxygen demand data needed for
substances shipped in quantity in commerce should be included in test
protocols.

Emphasis should be given to methods for rapid acquisition of
meteorological, stream flow, and other environmental data relative
to predicting routes and fates of spilled chemicals.

A more extensive toxicity information data base should be established
and made available regarding chemicals that might be spilled. This
should include the effects on major target organisms by all routes of
exposure (contact, ingestion, and inhalation). The collection of truly
complete toxicity data on all chemicals is probably an impossible and
never-ending task. However the magnitude of the problem warrants a
reasonable commitment of time, money, technical skills, and facilities
to achieve a good data base.

Spill situations should be exploited to gain the greatest possible
knowledge of effects from exposure to chemicals. Primary emphasis
should be placed on effects on human health. Field studies should be
undertaken to determine effects on the biota and the ability of damaged ecosystems to recover.

Special attention should be given to development of analytical and
biological measurement techniques for use in the spill situation. Relatively simple mathematical models should be developed for predicting
the movement and concentrations of hazardous materials in those
ecosystems likely to be subjected to spills. These models, together
with information on the effects of exposure, can be utilized to determine whether a hazard exists.

REFERENCES

Arthur D. Little, Inc. 1972. Preliminary system development. Chemical Hazards
Response Information System (CHRIS). Access Nos. AD-757472, AD-757473,

and AD-757474. National Technical Information Service, Springfield, Va. (Includes Appendixes I–VII.)

Hazardous substances: Definitions and procedural and interpretative regulations. 1971 rev. In *Code of Federal Regulations Title 21*, Part 191, Subchapter E, "Hazardous Substances." U.S. Government Printing Office, Washington, D.C. pp. 10–46.

Manufacturing Chemists Association. 1971. *CHEMTREC: Chemical Transportation Emergency Center.* Manufacturing Chemists Association, Washington, D.C.

National Research Council. Committee on Toxicology. 1964. *Principles and Procedures for Evaluating the Toxicity of Household Substances.* National Academy of Sciences, Washington, D.C. 29 pp.

Part Five

INANIMATE SYSTEMS

XVIII

Effects of Chemical Wastes on the Atmosphere

The present and potential future influence of pollution upon the atmosphere, particularly upon the earth's temperatures, clouds, and precipitation is the subject of this chapter. Of concern are the local, regional, and global effects. Consideration of the directly toxic effects of air pollution, which are treated elsewhere in this report, is excluded here. Rather, the atmospheric processes that may be affected by pollutants with subsequent impacts on weather and climate are discussed, along with criteria by which chemicals may be classified according to their effects upon atmospheric processes, and control criteria and monitoring. Summarizing conclusions and recommendations are also given for possible future air pollutants as they may affect weather and climate.

Many important topics are mentioned only briefly in this chapter. Detailed supporting arguments are contained in six appendices.

ATMOSPHERIC PROCESSES

The principal agents by which man-induced atmospheric pollutants affect weather and climate are aerosols. They operate chiefly by influencing cloud structures, precipitation, and radiation balance between the sun and earth, thereby affecting atmospheric temperatures. The effects of man-made pollutants on global climate are still

271

a matter of debate, but they might already be quite large. On the local scale, however, man's present influence on the weather is unmistakable. Even small cities generate "heat islands" several degrees above the mean temperatures of their surrounding countrysides, and precipitation patterns appear to have been markedly altered downwind of certain industrial facilities.

The localization of present weather influences by man's activities justifies concern for the sources of pollution, their dispersion, and the sinks of chemicals vented into the atmosphere. The potency of aerosols requires explanation of the dynamics of their formation and decay. Cloud-seeding and radiation-transfer effects are emphasized. This section concludes with further discussion of the influence of trace airborne chemicals upon local weather and speculation about present and future influence upon the global climate.

Atmospheric Dispersion Cycle of Pollutants

The dispersion cycle of a pollutant through the atmosphere depends on the nature of the source, its dilution and dispersion by atmospheric motions, and the removal or scavenging of the pollutant by atmospheric and surface processes.

Source Factors   The evaluation of a new material as a potential source of air pollution should consider the material at several stages in its manufacture and disposal. The initial stage is during production, where a lack of adequate emission control may vent a significant amount of material into the atmosphere. The production phase may also be a significant source of environmental pollutants: In fact, by-product emissions constitute a large fraction of current industrial air pollution problems (e.g., SO_2 from smelters or chemical aerosol particles from Kraft paper mills). After manufacture, a material may become an air pollutant as a result of its use (e.g., additives in fuel). Usage sources may be further divided on the basis of whether or not combustion is involved because combustion provides a mechanism to change the compounds, usually by oxidation. The last stage of the cycle is the final disposal of the actual material or an item of which it is a part. Incineration is probably of most concern, but volatilization of certain materials could also provide a source of air pollution.

For meteorological purposes, sources should also be classified according to their geometry. An isolated source, such as an industrial stack, is a *point source* and may cause relatively high concentrations of pollutant emissions in local areas downwind of the source. Turbulence in the atmosphere disperses a point-source emission both laterally and vertically relative to the average wind, and this achieves a relatively rapid dilution of the emission with distance downwind. Another type of source geometry that is important for this protocol discussion is the *area source,* which is usually considered to be made up of a large number of small sources distributed more or less uniformly over a large given area. Vehicle exhausts or home heating emissions are typical examples of sources that may be considered components of an area source. Here, the magnitude of the source is the integrated sum of the individual sources. Because of the size of an area source, dispersion in a crosswind direction is generally ineffective in diluting the effluent cloud, and thus, the reduction in concentration downwind must be accomplished by vertical mixing processes. Decisions whether to classify a given source as a large point source or a small area source should be made on the basis of whether or not crosswind dispersion is an effective factor in diluting the plume.

Atmospheric Dispersion Factors   Once the source is defined, atmospheric diffusion models may be applied to estimate the downwind concentration field. [*See* Appendix F, Sources and Dispersal of Atmospheric Pollution.] For estimates related to protocol decisions, rather simple models can generally be used. These models will differ in some features as the area of concern expands outward from the source. In areas close to a point source, the height of the emission plays a role in the concentration pattern. At distances represented by significant travel times, both point and area sources can be considered by the same model, and the long-range wind trajectory becomes the controlling factor in estimating exposure levels. Estimates of global concentration fields can be developed through the successive application of modeling schemes and with the appropriate climatological data. The simpler modeling schemes can be modified to include various atmospheric processes that tend to scavenge the materials from the atmosphere, if such additional sophistication is considered necessary.

Temperatures in cities are commonly 2–3 °C and, occasionally, as much as 10 °C higher than in neighboring rural areas. Although this effect, referred to as the urban *heat island,* is not due to chemical emissions, it is mentioned here because it can play a role in the dispersion of pollutants in cities. The urban heat island is produced primarily by the large areas of concrete and asphalt in cities, which absorb and store heat better than vegetation or soil. This effect is compounded by the enormous quantities of heat injected into the air in cities from combustion processes and air conditioners. On the other hand, in some cities the heat-island effect reduces fuel requirements in winter and may melt light snowfalls.

Cities also affect winds due to channeling by streets and the increased "roughness" of the surface topography. On average, the winds measured in downtown areas are about 10 percent less than at airports on the outskirts of the city. In light winds (less than about 8 knots), however, the reduction can be as high as 40 percent: Moreover, since light winds often accompany synoptic situations conducive to air pollution, reductions in their speeds produced by buildings in cities is especially harmful.

Pollutant Removal Factors   Once pollutants are emitted to the atmosphere, transformations and scavenging processes begin to affect the materials, and act in concert with the previously discussed dispersion factors to produce dilution. These transformation or scavenging processes include both chemical reaction processes and direct removal mechanisms. Since the direct scavenging processes are related to meteorological factors, they are considered here.

Precipitation provides the major mechanism by which pollutant materials are removed from the atmosphere. Although gaseous materials may be dissolved in cloud and raindrops, aerosol particles are especially susceptible to precipitation scavenging mechanisms. Small particles can be incorporated in cloud droplets and ultimately in rain by providing initial condensation or freezing nuclei. At later stages in the precipitation growth process, particles may be brought by Brownian motion into contact with cloud droplets or ice crystals. If the pollution and precipitation particles are in the proper size range, the precipitation particles may also capture the pollutants as they fall to the ground. Studies of nuclear bomb fallout have shown that precipitation scavenging processes account for about 90 percent of the atmospheric aerosol removal in regions with moderate rainfall.

The particles usually considered to represent an air pollution problem are generally too small to be significantly affected by gravitational settling: however, a process of nonprecipitation deposition is active as a scavenging mechanism. The particulate deposition rate can be related to the concentration of particles in the air through the *deposition velocity*. This factor is a function of the particulate size to some extent, but it is also apparently strongly dependent on the nature of the ground surface and aerodynamic factors of the atmospheric flow over the surface. Once a pollutant particle is deposited on the ground it is usually not resuspended in the atmosphere and thus should be considered as entering soil or water transport systems.

Aerosol Dynamics

Some of the earth's aerosol burden is injected into the air directly (e.g., smoke, from volcanoes, and wind-scoured dust). In addition, however, many complicated processes can generate aerosol gas-to-particle conversions, and the particles can then grow by surface chemistry and physical accretion. [*See* Appendix F, Gas-to-Particle Conversions.] Photochemical reactions of gaseous species, especially of the nitrogen oxides, promote oxidation of naturally occurring forest terpenes and waste industrial organic molecules, which produces the hygroscopic and polymeric species of smog. [*See* Appendix F, Photochemical Reactions in the Atmosphere.] Sulfur dioxide from smelting wastes and fuel combustion—again, with the assistance of nitrogen oxides—oxidizes to sulfur trioxide, which hydrolyzes to sulfuric acid mists and ammonium sulfate aerosols. The number and surface densities of the resulting aerosol populations increase markedly at the small end of their size spectra, that is, at radii much less than $0.1 \mu m$ (about the threshold for appreciable interaction of the aerosol particles with light). Consequently, most of the primary gas-to-particle conversions are also concentrated among the smallest particles. At the large end of the size spectrum (radius $1 \mu m$), particles begin to settle out by gravitational sedimentation and, with increasing efficiency, to be washed out by clouds and rain. Intermediate populations are maintained in a quasi steady state by coagulation kinetics.

Additionally, particles grow and shrink in response to local humidities. Particle multiplication processes (perhaps shattering) may occur in evaporating clouds. Surface active chemicals, such as fatty acids and alcohols, alter coagulation kinetics and may "stabilize" the large particles by impeding their growth. Coagulation effects resulting from electric fields have been demonstrated; many effects of trace gaseous species have been postulated, and some confirmed—for example, the influence of ammonia vapor upon sulfur dioxide oxidation and the production of sulfate particles in the presence of liquid water in clouds.

The complexity of processes affecting aerosol kinetics and the resulting populations of particle sizes and types enhances the possibilities for minor atmospheric constituents to amplify effects, possibly augmented by positive feedback. For example, aerosols may influence the vertical temperature structure of the atmosphere, which in turn influences mixing and dispersion and buildup and concentration of aerosols. For this reason, great care should be taken, now and in the future, to assess the potential influence of prospective chemical discharges into the air, upon the dynamics of aerosol formation, growth, dispersal and washout.

Cloud and Precipitation Processes

Perhaps the most sensitive processes in the atmosphere that can be affected by air pollutants are those involved in the development of clouds and precipitation. [*See* Appendix F, Clouds and Precipitation.] Experiments carried out over the past 30 years on the deliberate "seeding" of clouds have shown that the structure of clouds with temperatures below 0 °C (i.e., cold clouds) can be modified and, under certain conditions, precipitation from them altered by particles which are termed *ice nuclei.* Since only a few special substances are effective as ice nuclei—these often have crystallographic structures similar to that of ice and are virtually insoluble in water (e.g., AgI and PbI)—the concentrations of natural ice nuclei in the air are very low (about 1 particle per liter): That is, 1 in 10^8 of airborne particles are ice nuclei. Consequently, particles that are injected into the atmosphere, which are effective as ice nuclei at temperatures above about -15 °C have the potential for modifying the structure of clouds and the development of precipitation. If the concentrations of the anthropogenic ice nuclei are about 1 per liter they will tend to enhance precipitation, while if they are greatly in excess of 1 per liter they may "overseed" cold clouds and reduce precipitation. Certain steel mills have been identified as sources of ice nuclei. Also of concern is the possibility that emissions from automobiles may combine with trace chemicals in the atmosphere to produce ice nuclei.

Precipitation from clouds that have temperatures above 0 °C (i.e., warm clouds) may be modified by particles that serve as cloud condensation nuclei (CCN). Efficient CCN are hygroscopic particles with sizes in excess of a few tenths of a micrometer. A source that produces comparatively low concentrations of very efficient CCN will tend to increase precipitation from warm clouds, while one which produces large concentrations of somewhat less efficient CCN might decrease precipitation. Modifications in the structure of clouds and precipitation have been observed many miles downwind of fires of various kinds and pulp and paper mills, both of which have been shown to emit CCN into the air.

Apart from effects on precipitation processes, inadvertent modification of clouds from water to ice by ice nuclei, and of cloud droplet size distributions by CCN, affect the radiative properties of clouds. Such changes could have profound effects on temperature distributions in the atmosphere and on global climate.

Radiation Balance

Atmospheric radiation transfer and its influence upon the energy balance and temperature distribution of the air is considered at greater length later. [*See* Appendix F, Radiation Transfer.]

That radiation transfer is only indirectly the dominating mechanism in control of heat transfer in the atmosphere should be emphasized. Particularly in the troposphere, most of the energy flow is conducted by wind, with a tremendous assist from the latent heat of condensation of water in clouds. Moreover, even approximate formulations of heat transfer in the atmosphere must realistically be very nonlinear. Consequently, the problem does not permit rigorous separation into individual effects which may be discussed one at a time, although this is attempted below.

Parcels of air may absorb radiation through the excitation of electronic, rotational, and vibrational molecular energy, and—by subsequent intramolecular coupling and intermolecular collisions—they may redistribute the absorbed energy into heat. The absorption may occur both for individually dispersed molecules and for molecular aggregates dispersed as aerosols.

Many molecules absorb strongly in limited parts of the spectrum, particularly in the infrared: For example, H_2O, CO_2, and O_3 each significantly affect the heat transfer of outgoing thermal radiation from the earth's surface. The infrared is a minor part of the incoming solar power, however, which peaks at wavelengths near 0.5 μm. Only two atmospheric molecules (gases) normally occur around this wavelength in concentrations sufficient for their molecular absorptions to significantly affect the atmospheric heating rate—ozone (O_3) and nitrogen dioxide (NO_2).

Ozone absorbs strongly in the ultraviolet, with a maximum cross section of 10^{-21} m^2 at 0.25 μm. This absorption is responsible for the ultraviolet shield which protects protoplasm at the earth's surface. At longer wavelengths, absorption by ozone is weaker, and near the earth's surface it produces average heating rates less than 10^{-3} °C/d in dense urban smog, ozone concentrations occasionally approach 1 ppm, with the result that direct heating rates may approach 0.1 °C/d. Even the larger of these rates is negligible compared to advective heat transfer upwards from the hot surface of the earth. Ozone is, therefore, not a significant direct agent for energy input to the lower atmosphere. However, ozone is intimately associated with aerosol formation in photochemical smogs. [*See* Appendix F, Photochemical Reactions in the Atmosphere.] Later in this section, the significant effects of aerosols on radiation transfer in the atmosphere will be discussed.

Nitrogen dioxide absorbs strongly in the visible, with a richly structured spectrum of mean cross section 2×10^{-23} m^2 between 0.30 and 0.55 μm. Integrated over the solar spectrum, the mean mixing fraction* of 3 ppb of NO_2 in the remote troposphere produces a heating rate of 0.06 °C per 12-hour day at the earth's surface. Mixing fractions greater than 1 ppm have been observed in Los Angeles, and greater than 0.5 ppm and 0.25 ppm occur there for short durations, with an average expectancy of 3 and 39 d/yr, respectively. The greater of these values results in heating rates of 1 °C/h, a very significant contribution.

Heating rates are especially sensitive to the imaginary part of the aerosol's index of refraction and to the particle size distribution. In the troposphere, remote from large cities and industries, an aerosol burden of about 10^{-8} kg/m^3 produces a heating rate corresponding to 0.5 °C per 12-hour day. In urban conditions, on the other hand, the heating rate may exceed 1 °C/h, although this neglects multiple scattering. Such a heating rate will profoundly influence the vertical temperature distributions and stabilities above smoggy cities.

In the troposphere, the main mechanism by which a parcel of air cools is by adiabatic expansion during lifting. The dominating manner in which a parcel loses energy is by infrared radiation in the numerous molecular bonds of water vapor and carbon dioxide, and by grey-body thermal emission from water clouds. Below and in Appendix F, the "greenhouse" and radiation effects of CO_2, and the possible consequences of rising global CO_2 levels, on the radiation balance of the earth are discussed.

Arguments are presented (Appendix F, Radiation Transfer) that no atmospheric constituent at concentrations less than 1 ppm will contribute significantly to cooling the air by direct molecular emissions, and that even in dense aerosols near cities, cooling by grey-body radiation can be neglected. From these arguments, the Panel on Atmosphere concluded that any new trace chemicals introduced into the atmosphere are unlikely to affect the heating or cooling of the air through direct molecular contributions. However, aerosols, ozone, and nitrogen dioxide have been observed to be significant contributors to the heating of the

---

*The mixing fraction of component X is defined as the number of moles of X divided by the total number of moles in the mixture.

air at the present time. As these interact chemically, any trace chemical which interacts with O_3 or NO_2 has the potential for altering the radiation balance of the earth. The panel emphasizes that consideration be taken of possible interactions with aerosols, when assessing possible consequences of future chemical venting into the atmosphere. Alterations may affect the radation balance, especially near cities where feedbacks may occur to amplify air–basin stagnancy.

Of great importance to the problem of predicting effects on atmospheric motions is the observation that, for aerosol spatial distributions that are initially more or less uniform below a critical altitude (as is frequently the case below inversions), heat deposition by aerosol absorption may be concentrated just below that critical altitude with the result that the inversion is intensified. [*See* Appendix F, Radiation Transfer.] Thus, a positive feedback may occur wherein inversions concentrate pollution which intensifies inversions. The converse may also occur when an initial vertical distribution of aerosol burden diminishes exponentially with height, as is frequently the case in unstable air. Incoming radiation may then penetrate the upper and more tenuous aerosols without much heat deposition and, instead, heat the air at lower altitudes. In this case, negative feedback may occur and the added heating rate at low altitudes may enhance vertical mixing so as to reduce low level pollution, which then in turn reduces the radiation heat input. Thus, radiation heating by aerosols may operate either to intensify periods of pollution or to speed their dispersal, depending upon the vertical distribution of the aerosols.

A second interesting consequence of multiple scattering of aerosols is that heating rates by molecular absorptions, as with NO_2, are also enhanced as a result of the lengthened effective optical path traced by the more diffused light. Factors of 2 are common for this enhancement effect. An average daily heating of 4 °C in Los Angeles has been ascribed to NO_2.

Global Effects

Like the weather, the climate of the earth fluctuates with time, but on a longer time scale. Such fluctuations can have a profound effect on man and his activities, as well as on animals and plants. Prior to the industrial revolution, changes in climate were almost certainly unrelated to human activity. However, in recent years the question has arisen whether the activities of man might be changing world climate.

The atmospheric constituent most often mentioned in this regard is carbon dioxide (CO_2). The concentration of CO_2 in the air has increased by about 10 percent since the beginning of the Industrial Revolution. This increase is attributed to the consumption of fossil fuels. Simple theoretical models predict that increases in the concentration of CO_2 in the air should result in increases in temperature at ground level due to the "greenhouse" effect. Climatological data indicate that the earth's average annual surface temperature did, in fact, increase by about 0.6 °C from 1880 to 1940. Since 1940, however, this temperature has been decreasing, and is now about 0.3 °C lower than in 1940.

The changes in temperature in recent years raise the question of possible climatic effects attributable to increased particulate loading. There are indications that there is an upward trend in the concentrations of particles in the air in the northern hemisphere, and in the southern hemisphere at some locations that are close to large cities or industrial areas. The meteorological effects of airborne particles depend on their optical and chemical characteristics, as well as on their sizes. Most important are the optical absorption and scattering properties of particles, about which very little is known.

At the present time, it is not possible to predict with certainty even the sign of the ground-level temperature change that would accompany an increase in the concentration of atmospheric particles. The first possibility that comes to mind is that increases in particulate loading would increase the amount of solar energy reflected back into space and the atmosphere would be cooled. This might be the reason for the observed decreasing temperatures in recent years. However, if the particles had an absorption to backscattering ratio greater than a critical value, the lower atmosphere would be warmed by an increase in particulate loading. Also, the sign of the effect depends on the distribution of the particles between and above cloud layers. The weight of arguments at this time favors a cooling, rather than a warming effect, due to increased particulate loading. It is the opinion of the panel, however, that coupled effects between particles and clouds, mentioned above, are likely to outweigh direct albedo effects from the particles themselves.

The earth's stratosphere, which is situated between 10 and 50 km above the earth's surface, is particularly sensitive to pollutant impact. Particle residence times are longer than in the troposphere (e.g., the residence time of micrometer-sized particles or smaller is 1–3 years, compared to 1 or 2 weeks in the troposphere). Photochemical processes occur in the stratosphere, especially ozone-forming reactions, and the dominant heating results from absorption of solar energy by ozone. Moreover, ozone absorbs solar radiation at wavelengths shorter than about 3000 Å, providing a shield for protoplasm in the troposphere, which is damaged by these wavelengths.

These considerations have stimulated concern over possible modifications to stratospheric chemistry which might be caused by supersonic aircraft. In particular, it appears that nitrogen oxides released in the stratosphere by such aircraft could lead to a significant reduction in the ozone content if the mixing ratio of the natural nitrogen oxides in the stratosphere is significantly less than 10^{-8}. Unfortunately, good measurements of the concentrations of nitrogen oxides in the stratosphere are not yet available. The destruction of atmospheric ozone through "wet photolysis" might also be important. [*See* Appendix F, Global Effects of Pollutants on Climate.]

CRITERIA FOR THE CLASSIFICATION OF ATMOSPHERIC POLLUTANTS

In this section some basic principles upon which a preliminary classification of pollutants might be made are outlined, according to their likely effects on the atmosphere.

Physical Properties

Molecular Weights and Vapor Pressures   For a chemical to affect the atmosphere significantly, it must have a physical state compatible with residence in the atmosphere. In principle any chemical with a finite vapor pressure can become airborne and exist in the atmosphere at concentrations up to an equilibrium value. For example, a chemial compound with a vapor pressure of only 10^{-6} torr can reach its equilibrium concentration of approximately 1 ppb in the air (1 ppb = 2.46×10^{10} molecules/cm^3 at 25 °C and 760 torr). Similarly, a chemical with a vapor pressure higher than the ambient pressure boils in the atmosphere and may be present at any concentration level.

For species which are molecularly dispersed, the requirement for appreciable vapor pressure immediately sets upper limits upon molecular weights and dipole moments. For nonpolar molecules (e.g., alkanes) vapor pressures at 20 °C correspond approximately to mixing fractions of 1 ppm of $H_2(CH_2)_{16}$, and to 1 ppb of $H_2(CH_2)_{22}$, which have molecular weights of 230 and 310 gram-atoms, respectively. For increasingly polar molecules, the lower the molecular weight the less the volatility. Thus, nitrobenzene ($C_6H_5NO_2$) has a mixing fraction at room temperature near 10 ppm, despite its molecular weight of only 123. Therefore, for chemical species with molecular weights substantially higher than

2–300, molecular residence in the atmosphere is incompatible with appreciable mixing fractions; nevertheless, many of these heavy species can and do significantly affect the atmosphere—but as aerosols rather than as dispersed molecules.

Dipole Moments, Ionicities, and Solubilities   Molecular dipole moments affect not only vapor pressures but act also to enhance solubility in polar fluids, such as water. Similarly, strongly ionic crystals dissolve more readily than covalent or metallic substances. Consequently, polar and ionic species which may enter the atmosphere are preferentially absorbed, dissolved, and concentrated in aqueous clouds. This process facilitates both heterogeneous and aqueous chemistry, which may transform the chemical nature of the original tracer species, and precipitation washout, which may remove these species from the atmosphere entirely.

Surface Activity and Nucleation   One of the most profound potential effects of extraneous material added to the atmosphere is its possible action as cloud condensation nuclei for cloud droplets or as ice nuclei for ice crystals. This subject was treated earlier and is discussed in detail in Appendix F, Clouds and Precipitation. For three reasons, however, it is appropriate to mention nucleation here: (1) to emphasize that the effectiveness of any particular nucleating agent is related largely to its physical properties (e.g., crystal structure and the surface heats of absorptivity; (2) to emphasize that these physical properties are therefore cardinal flags for cautionary action; and (3) to avoid an impression of misordered priorities which may possibly be drawn by our discussions of other, perhaps less profound, effects of trace species on the atmosphere.

Optical Scattering and Absorption   Other sections of this chapter deal more fully with interactions between radiation and atmospheric trace species. Appendix F deals with the active interactions of photochemical change. Together, these may appreciably affect the distribution of heat in the atmosphere and therefore change temperatures and winds. Here again, relevant physical properties of the candidate species could be assessed before licensing a major discharge into the air.

Energy States and Spectra   The total internal energy of a molecule is composed of electronic, vibrational, and rotational degrees of freedom; hence, the corresponding energy states and the resulting spectra represent the origin of virtually all the physical and chemical properties of a chemical. These spectra exhibit a high degree of resemblance among chemicals that possess similar physical and chemical properties. Thus, these properties constitute a fundamental basis for the classification of chemicals, and they also serve as an important method for identifying and monitoring chemicals in the atmosphere.

Thermodynamic Properties   While energy states and resulting spectra refer to the individual quantum levels of a molecule, such thermodynamic parameters as enthalpy, entropy, and free energy describe the overall energy content of a molecule with respect to its equilibrium state in a given chemical environment. These thermodynamic properties are a measure of the physical and chemical stability of a system of chemical constituents. They do not explicitly define the time-independent behavior of the physical and chemical transformation of a given chemical compound. Nevertheless, chemical reactivity can be correlated to some extent with these thermodynamic parameters. For example, endothermic reactions require kinetic activation energies comparable to the endothermicity; since activation energies appear exponentially in rate factors, even a few kJ/mol suffice to make many otherwise plausible reactions too slow to affect air chemistry. Similarly, at equilibrium, considerations of detailed balancing require the ratios of forward to reverse rate coefficients to equal the thermodynamically derived equilibrium constant.

Chemical Properties

The distinction between chemical and physical properties is arbitrary because all of the former derive ultimately from the latter. However, it is conventional and probably useful to distinguish as chemical those interactions that result in rearrangements between more or less tightly associated atoms. These rearrangements in turn affect those exterior physical properties which may influence the atmosphere.

Among many others, the following kinds of molecules are likely in various ways to interact strongly with photochemical oxidation sequences in the air:

1.   photo-active molecules that may form O, OH, H, or halogen atoms in ultraviolet or visible radiation (especially active if any mechanism exists for a regenerating chain);

2.   free-radical scavenging molecules (especially active if any mechanism exists for a regenerating chain);

3.   molecules with double bonds, $-C=C-$ (especially conjugated double bonds, $-C=C-C=C-$);

4.   molecules with aromatic and heterocyclic rings (especially adjacent to vinyls, nitrates, sulfates, and amines);

5. molecules that form long-lived triplet states by absorption near 3000–4000 Å (substituted napthalenes and anthracenes, etc.); and

6. strained, that is 3, 4, 7 membered, rings.

From this list, and from the host of other complexities not discussed, it is evident that the list of chemical alarm criteria can easily get too long to be useful. It is tautological, but still informative, to say that every "reactive" molecule added to the air will interact in some way with the atmosphere.

CONTROL CRITERIA AND MONITORING

Wise control implies a sense of direction toward a desired goal; however, in the case of weather and climate modification, there is no consensus on the nature of that goal. Many, perhaps most, citizens yearn for a return to pristine nature: The fact remains that weather and climate are frequently hostile to man and that a desire for control over the elements is deep-seated in human psyche. Theoretical studies based on modeling and careful experimentation in certain aspects of deliberate weather modification (Appendix F, Clouds and Precipitation) offer hopes for some control over weather phenomena and, also, throwing light on inadvertent weather modification. Until such time as the principal effects of air pollution on weather and climate can be predicted with some certainty, however, certain controls and monitoring programs need to be established. Some principles on which to base these controls and monitoring efforts are given below.

Control Criteria

The most elementary precautionary criterion to signal possible disturbance to the atmosphere of a chemical discharge is that of amount. For each possible chemical constituent, a concentration exists below which the effect of a chemical on the atmosphere will either not be measurable or be of less significance to some measurable property of the atmosphere than natural atmospheric constituents. However, the difficulties of defining any acceptably "negligible" background of radioactive wastes must be taken as a warning that similar difficulties are likely to affect future control levels for many other chemical discharges into the atmosphere. Ultimately, "significant," "acceptable," and "negligible" are subjective terms. Nevertheless, certain levels of chemical contamination can be suggested below which it is increasingly improbable that "significant" atmospheric effects can be expected by looking at present minor atmospheric species and noticing the concentrations at which atmospheric phenomena begin to be attributed to these species.

Table 12 illustrates some of these species and their associated thresholds for affecting particular processes. The direct influences of certain trace gases upon state variables, such as temperature and wind velocity, can be expected at concentrations as low as 10^{-2} kg/km^3 of air. Owing to the great variety and complexity of measurable effects in the atmosphere, the panel judges it likely that most chemicals will measurably affect one process or another when their concentrations approach or exceed 10^3 kg/km^3 of air, or mixing fractions near 1 ppm; it is unlikely that any added chemicals will appreciably affect the atmospheric state of concentrations near to or below 1 g/km^3 of air (or 10^{-3} ppb), except those that act as ice nuclei or cloud condensation nuclei and modify the structure of clouds.

Since the concentration of a tracer chemical on any scale, from microclimate (tens of meters or less) up to global systems ($\sim 10^4$ km), results from the time-dependent interplay of sources, transport, and sinks, the rates of discharge for each of these processes must be considered in estimating both the levels of concentration and the spatial distributions that may be attained by atmospheric chemicals. The transport and dispersion of atmospheric materials and their sources and sinks have been discussed above; only the obvious point that upper limits in acceptable concentrations also imply upper limits in acceptable input rates is emphasized here.

Since the transport of chemicals in the atmosphere and their sinks are not constant, an acceptable source rate may be difficult to specify. As an example of what is probably an excessive rate, a single source of SO_2 at 5 kg/s, which has the effect of reducing the mean pH of rainfall, is measured at 70 km downwind, one pH unit below its normally CO_2-buffered value of 5.6. This illustrates a condition where both sources and sinks are rather rapid, yet concentrations of ambient SO_2 and sulfate aerosols remain fairly low (5–20 ppb) by comparison with other localities that enjoy comparable input, but less active transport and washout. For this circumstance a control limit on input flux of chemicals to the atmosphere would probably be more sensible than a limit on ambient concentrations. Which of these alternate control criteria will best suit any particular chemical depends principally upon the nature of the sink, since transport is not likely to be affected by the chemical nature of the tracer species. In general, rapid sinks mean relatively intense local deposition and make more sensible a flux criterion, while slow sinks permit remote and more dilute deposition and suggest a concentration criterion. To guess beforehand which should apply requires knowledge of the physics and chemistry of the chemical.

TABLE 12   Approximate Minimum Concentration Thresholds for Atmospheric Effects due to Minor Constituents

Species	Effect	Threshold Species Volume per Unit Volume of Air	Concentration in Air, kg/km^3
Ice nuclei	Cloud structure and precipitation	10^{-18}	10^{-6}
Cloud condensation nuclei	Cloud structure and precipitation	10^{-15}	10^{-3}
Aerosols	Visibility and heating rates (pH of rain)	10^{-12} (10^{-10})	10^{0}
Hydrochloric and sulfuric acids	pH of rain	10^{-11}	10^{-2}
Ammonia	pH of rain	10^{-10}	10^{-1}
Sulfur dioxide	pH of rain	10^{-8}	10^{1}
Nitrogen dioxide	Visibility and heating rates	10^{-7}	10^{2}
Ozone	Heating rates	10^{-6}	10^{3}

Several specific suggestions on control criteria follow:

• First, the panel believes the influences of chemical wastes on weather and climate to be greatly amplifed when they affect clouds. The presence or absence of clouds and their nature can have dramatic effects, as can small changes in their frequency or placement; therefore, changes in clouds produced by aerosols generate enormous relative differences per unit of aerosol mass. Consequently, control attention should be directed especially to a chemical's prospective effects on cloud modification and aerosol dynamics.

• Second, regenerating chains of chemical interactions—for example, those involving OH and NO_x (*see* Appendix F, Photochemical Reactions in the Atmosphere)—are especially sensitive to modification by additional chemicals which may compete for the chain-carrying radicals. The panel particularly emphasizes the importance of OH and the need to develop and deploy analytical apparatus to measure its role in photochemical smogs.

• Third, the panel believes present control criteria for many constituents based on ambient concentration levels might profitably be re-examined based upon area-flux levels, or throughput. Variable emission licensing, adjusted to the local dispersive capacity of the air, might be explored. However, care must be taken that acute local problems are not converted into chronic regional or global problems.

• Finally, the panel suggests that air pollution modeling activity, which has been restricted largely to cloud-free dispersion models, be expanded to include cloud processes. Economic factors should also be included in theoretical models.

Measurements and Monitoring

Although dispersion models can be used to estimate the possible impact of a specific pollutant emission, measurement and monitoring programs should also be employed. The size of the monitoring program should reflect the estimated magnitude of the problem, including such factors as probable emission rate, probable source location, and possible severity of any toxic impact. Although it is not feasible here to discuss monitoring programs in detail, it is possible to establish the guidelines or program design that a toxic substance monitoring program should include.

Schedule The monitoring program should begin before the introduction of the toxic compound into the region, so that background or blank levels can be obtained. These observed levels may be fictitious, as a result of analytical problems such as a lack of sensitivity or specificity, or real because of actual but unanticipated emissions. Monitoring should continue after the material has been introduced and the emission rate has stabilized. When any possible hazard can be completely evaluated and shown to be negligible, the monitoring program can be terminated.

Monitoring System   Much thought should be given to designing a monitoring system appropriate to each toxic compound. There will be a strong temptation to use some or all of an existing system; however, the compromises required in order to use sampling sites and devices already in service may often adversely affect success. In the monitoring of toxic substances, very low concentrations of materials have to be considered; therefore, sample handling and subtle intrumental effects can be significant. In a specific system, these can be checked and controlled; for a toxic compound monitoring program, the selected analytical methods must be specifically designed for ambient air samples and must include methods to eliminate the effects of interferences that would be present in the atmosphere, either as gases or particles. The averaging time selected for the instrumentation should be compatible with the nature of the postulated toxic impact: Expensive real-time concentration monitoring should only be undertaken when short period exposures are of concern for the toxic compound under study. The design of the monitoring system must include access to meteorological data with sufficient resolution to establish the effects of the weather on concentrations to an accuracy compatible with the resolution required of the concentration pattern.

Locations of Monitoring Stations   The purpose of toxic compound assessment is to determine the maximum likely impact from the emission; therefore, the location of the sampling stations should facilitate maximum detection of disturbances. To meet this need, the monitoring network might not have to be extensive over any given test area. However, as a result, the data will not be interpretable as indicative of "average concentrations" since, by design, areas with maximum levels will often be singled out for monitoring.

Monitoring Schedules and Risk Functions   In conventional monitoring for toxic materials, the risk function is usually assumed as an increasing function of concentration times exposure. With monitoring for meteorological disturbances, similar risk functions may, or may not, be appropriate. Often, risks may maximize during periods that do not coincide with exposure levels (e.g., clouds might be particularly susceptible to modification during periods of high humidity and moderate supercooling). In this case, a monitoring program geared to peak concentration episodes may be seriously misleading. In general, each postulated contaminant has to be considered in the light of a likely contaminating mechanism or impact, and control schedules and risk functions redefined, case by case.

CONCLUSIONS

A summary of the panel's conclusions on the principles of protocols for evaluating the effects of chemicals on the atmosphere is contained in Table 13.

TABLE 13   Some Questions and Comments on Atmospheric Pollutants

Question	Comments
1. What atmospheric process is the discharge likely to affect?	Controls should be based on known or postulated effects of the pollutants (Table 12).
2. Is the discharge large or small compared to the same or other agents in the atmosphere that act similarly?	A discharge must cause an appreciable change in the concentration of similar agents in order to affect an atmospheric process.
3. Are all the constituents of the effluent known?	Tract substances might have more impact on the atmosphere than the primary constituents.
4. Will any of the chemicals in the discharge react with atmospheric constituents?	Beware of regenerating chemical chains, especially those known to take place with OH and NO. Small influences on these two species may have large secondary effects (e.g., photochemical reactions leading to smog).
5. Can chemicals in the discharge interact in the atmosphere to amplify their effects?	If so, beware! (The reaction of SO_2 and NH_3 in the gaseous phase is slow, but in the presence of cloud droplets it is accelerated enormously to produce sulfates.)
6. Is the discharge concentrated (a point source) or diffuse (an area source)?	The first may stimulate more complaints, but the latter more damage.
7. What concentrations are to be expected downwind from sources of pollutants?	Simple model calculations can be used to estimate these concentrations, but not conclusively.

Table 13   (continued)

Question	Comments
8. Is the weather stagnant or dispersive?	Controlled emissions are generally best vented in dispersive conditions; however, in some cases discharges in dispersive conditions might produce more damage.
9. What are the lifetimes and sinks of the pollutants?	Rapid sinks depress concentrations but the throughput may remain high and the deposition concentrated.
10. Are the pollutants water soluble or hygroscopic?	If so, they will concentrate in clouds, are potentially active in modifying warm clouds, and will experience relatively short residence times in the atmosphere with possibly large local deposition.
11. Are the pollutants surface active?	Surface active molecules may coat cloud droplets and affect cloud and aerosol evaporation and coagulation.
12. Do the solid pollutants have crystal structures and dimensions similar to ice (i.e., hexagonal) and are they insoluble?	If so, they may nucleate ice in cold clouds and affect precipitation processes, even at very low concentrations.
13. Do the chemicals interact with visible light? If so, (a) do they photodissociate? (b) do they form reactive fragments such as free radicals and metastable atoms? (c) do they sensitize other chemicals?	If so, they may contribute to atmospheric heating. In addition, affirmative answers to questions a, b, or c imply activity in photochemical processes affecting smog.
14. Do the chemicals interact with infrared radiation?	If so, they will affect radiation transfer, especially if they absorb between the strong lines of H_2O and CO_2. Absorption at these wavelengths will cause warming near the earth's surface but cooling in the stratosphere.
15. Most critical of all, do the pollutants affect aerosols or clouds?	If so, the structure of clouds may be changed by the pollutants, thereby causing changes in precipitation and optical scattering. Research priority should be given to this area.

SUGGESTED READINGS

Junge, C.E. 1963. *Air Chemistry and Radioactivity*. Academic Press, New York. 382 pp.

Leighton, P.A. 1961. *Photochemistry of Air Pollution*. Academic Press, New York. 300 pp.

National Research Council. Committee on Atmospheric Sciences. 1966. *Weather and Climate Modification: Problems and Prospects*. 2 Vols. National Academy of Sciences, Washington, D.C.

National Research Council. Committee on Atmospheric Sciences. 1973. *Weather and Climate Modification: Problems and Progress*. National Academy of Sciences, Washington, D.C. 258 pp.

Wilson, C.L., and W.H. Matthews, eds. 1970. *Man's Impact on the Global Environment: Assessment and Recommendations for Action*. M.I.T. Press, Cambridge. 319 pp.

Wilson, C.L., and W.H. Matthews, eds. 1971. *Inadvertent Climate Modification*. M.I.T. Press, Cambridge. 308 pp.

XIX

Inanimate
Materials

INTRODUCTION

The damaging effects that certain types of chemicals have had on inanimate materials are well recognized (e.g., deicing salts on roadways and automobiles; sulfur gases on lead based house paints; sulfur acids on concrete, masonry, and stone; and ozone on rubber products). It is not the intent of this report to review each and every one of these instances where chemicals released to the atmosphere have had deleterious effects on materials but instead to discuss the need for testing to screen a chemical substance for its environmental effects to prevent future problems.

The field of inanimate materials is extremely broad, and it is obviously impossible to include every inanimate object in a study of this type. However, it is also obvious that a limited list of categories of materials can be chosen that will encompass the majority of those inanimate objects whose preservation is of principal concern to mankind. The following list has been chosen as the domain of this study.

- Ferrous metals
- Nonferrous metals
- Glass
- Wood, paper, natural fibers

- Concrete, mortar, stone
- Plastics and synthetic fibers

Each of these categories is further subdivided in Appendix G.

Although natural formations and deposits of rock and soil are not specifically considered, the discussion of concrete mortar and stone would be generally applicable. Similarly, water is also not specifically considered here, but pollutants dispersed in water may change some of its physical characteristics, such as surface energy. However, the effects of such changes on materials will probably be minimal.

The screening of a chemical substance for its effects on inanimate materials would logically begin with certain information supplied by the producer of the substance. Table 14 shows a recommended list of information, which should be supplied as a condition for acceptance of the chemical in the screening program.

NECESSITY FOR TESTING

By comparison with the toxicological interactions of chemicals and the environment, the interactions of chemicals with inanimate materials are relatively uncomplicated. Furthermore, practical experience with the production and use of chemicals has led to the accumulation of an enormous volume of detailed quantitative information on the behavior of materials in a wide variety of chemical environments (Appendix G). It is therefore probable, that for many existing chemical substances, it will not be necessary to conduct any experimental tests because enough information may already be available in published form. Even for *new*

TABLE 14 Information to be Supplied by Chemical Producer

1. Structural formula of the chemical substance. If uncertain or unknown, the elemental analysis, stability, functionality, and other known chemical and physical data.

2. Proposed uses for the substance.

3. Annual production of the substance.

4. Existing information on the effects of the substance during normal usage on inanimate objects.

5. Anticipated method of disposal, biodegradability, safety of sewer or landfill disposal, gaseous products produced on incineration.

chemical substances, it will often be possible to make an adequate pre-diction, based on experience and established chemical principles, of ef-fects on materials without testing.

In cases where the published data are insufficient, it will often be pos-sible to limit the required testing to those specific classes of materials that are potentially susceptible to the substance in question and are likely to come in contact with the chemical in the course of normal usage. Ex-isting methods for testing inanimate materials with regard to the deteriora-tion by chemicals are listed in Appendix G for guidance purposes; the purpose of the section, "Performance of Materials" is to provide the in-formation necessary for the choice of susceptible classes of materials.

There is little need for testing those chemicals that are not released in-to the environment in their normal processes of production, usage, and disposal. Nitric acid, for example, is used almost exclusively for the pro-duction of other chemicals and is handled within the confines of the chem-ical industry in equipment that is adequate for safe handling.

Concentration and exposure time are important variables. Most inani-mate materials are relatively resistant to small concentrations of chemi-cals that are aggressive at higher concentration, particularly if the exposure time is short. Consequently, tests would be warranted only if the pro-jected conditions of usage indicate that the chemical may be brought into frequent contact with inanimate materials at high concentrations or pro-longed contact at low levels of concentration. A familiar example of the former is the use of deicing chemicals on highways and bridges.

Tests designed to simulate a "spill" should be of reasonably short dura-, tion, representative of the time required to clean up the spill. It should also be recognized that the consequences of a spill will frequently and foreseeably be limited to replacement of the materials directly involved within an isolated area. Extensive testing and evaluation of such exposures will rarely be necessary.

SUMMARY

The problem of determining the effects of chemicals on inanimate materials is relatively uncomplicated because of the existence of stan-dardized testing procedures and because of the accumulation of a con-siderable body of knowledge on the effects of existing chemicals. [*See* Appendix G.] For many new chemicals, the kinds of information listed in Table 14 will provide an adequate basis for predicting effects. In other cases, the anticipated production, use, and method of disposal will be such as to limit the extent of testing required.

SUGGESTED READINGS

American Concrete Institute Committee 201. 1962. Durability of concrete in service. *J. Am. Concr. Inst.* 59:1771–1820.

American Concrete Institute Committee 515. 1966. Guide for the protection of concrete against chemical attack by means of coatings and other corrosion-resistant materials. *J. Am. Concr. Inst.* 63:1305–1392.

American Society for Testing and Materials. 1968. *Metal Corrosion in the Atmosphere.* STP 435. ASTM, Philadelphia. 396 pp.

Bacon, F.R. 1968. The chemical durability of silicate glass. *Glass Ind.* 49:438–439, 442–446; 494–499, 554–559.

Bolam, F., ed. 1958. *Transactions of the Symposium on Fundamentals of Paper Making Fibers.* British Paper and Board Makers' Association, Kenley, Surrey, England. 487 pp.

Brydson, J.A. 1966. *Plastics Materials.* D. VanNostrand Co., Princeton, N.J. 576 pp.

Casey, J.P. 1960. *Pulp and Paper: Chemistry and Chemical Technology,* 2nd ed., rev. 3 Vols. John Wiley and Sons, Inc., New York.

Cook, J.G. 1968. *Handbook of Textile Fibres,* 4th Ed. 2 Vols. Merrow Pub. Co., Ltd., England.

Ernsberger, F.M. 1972. Properties of Glass Surfaces. In Huggins, R.A., ed., *Annual Review of Materials Science.* Vol. 2. Annual Reviews, Inc., Palo Alto, Calif. pp. 529–572.

Fenner, O.H. 1968. Plastic materials of construction. *Chem. Eng.* 75:126–138.

Fontana, M.G. 1957. *Corrosion: A Compilation.* Hollenback Press, Columbus, Ohio. 240 pp.

Fontana, M.G., and N.D. Green. 1967. *Corrosion Engineering.* McGraw-Hill Book Co., New York. 391 pp.

Hall, A.J. 1969. *The Standard Handbook of Textiles,* 7th ed. Heywood Books, London. 369 pp.

Harris, M., ed. 1954. *Handbook of Textile Fibers.* Harris Research Labs., Washington, D.C. 356 pp.

Holland, L. 1964. *The Properties of Glass Surfaces.* John Wiley and Sons, Inc., New York. 546 pp.

Koch, P. 1972. *Utilization of the Southern Pines.* 2 vols. Agric. Handb. No. 420. U.S. Government Printing Office, Washington, D.C.

Kuenning, W.H. 1966. Resistance of Portland cement mortar to chemical attack—a progress report. *Highw. Res. Rec.* 113:43–87.

La Que, F.L., and H.R. Copson, eds. 1963. *Corrosion Resistance of Metals and Alloys,* 2nd ed. Monogr. Ser. No. 158. Reinhold Publ. Corp., New York. 712 pp.

Lever, A.E., and J. Rhys. 1957. *Properties and Testing of Plastics Materials.* Chemical Publ. Co., Inc., New York. 197 pp.

Mauersberger, H.R., ed. 1947. *Matthews' Textile Fibers,* 5th ed. John Wiley and Sons, Inc., New York. 1133 pp.

McKay, R.J., and R. Worthington. 1936. *Corrosion Resistance of Metals and Alloys.* ACS Monogr. Ser. No. 71. Reinhold Publ. Corp., New York. 492 pp.

Miner, D.F., and J. Seastone, eds. 1955. *Handbook of Engineering Materials.* John Wiley and Sons, Inc., New York, 1380 pp.

Modern Plastics Encyclopedia. 1971–1972. Vol. 48. No. 10A. Hightstown, N.J.

Peters, R.H. 1967. *Textile Chemistry*. 3 Vols. American Elsevier Publ. Co., New York.

Rydholm, S.A. 1965. *Pulping Processes*. John Wiley and Sons, Inc., New York. 1269 pp

Seymour, R.B., and R.H. Steiner. 1955. *Plastics for Corrosion-Resistant Applications*. Reinhold Publ. Corp., New York. 423 pp.

Simonds, H.R., and J.M. Church. 1963. *A Concise Guide to Plastics*, 2nd ed. Reinhold Publ. Corp., New York. 392 pp.

Speller, F.N. 1951. *Corrosion: Causes and Prevention*, 3rd ed. McGraw-Hill Book Co., New York. 686 pp.

Stamm, A.J. 1964. *Wood and Cellulose Science*. Ronald Press, New York. 549 pp.

Stamm, A.J., and E.E. Harris. 1953. *Chemical Processing of Wood*. Chemical Publ. Co., New York. 595 pp.

Sutermeister, E. 1941. *Chemistry of Pulp and Papermaking*, 3rd ed. John Wiley and Sons, Inc., New York. 529 pp.

Technical Data on Plastics. 1957. Manufacturing Chemists' Association, Inc., Washington, D.C. 213 pp.

Uhlig, H.H. 1963. *Corrosion and Corrosion Control: An Introduction to Corrosion Science and Engineering*. John Wiley and Sons, Inc., New York. 371 pp.

U.S. Department of Agriculture. 1955. *Wood Handbook*. Agric. Handb. No. 72. U.S. Government Printing Office, Washington, D.C. 528 pp.

Wise, L.E., and E.C. Jahn, eds. 1952. *Wood Chemistry*. 2nd ed. 2 Vols. ACS Mongr. Ser. No. 97. Reinhold Publ. Corp., New York.

Woods, H. 1968. *Durability in Concrete Construction*. ACI Monogr. No. 4. American Concrete Institute, Detroit. 190 pp.

Part Six

ANALYSIS
AND
MONITORING

XX

Analysis and
Monitoring

The need to know what chemicals may escape to the environment and at what levels they may be harmful leads rather quickly to a realization that until one can identify these compounds with certainty and measure their presence in selected compartments of the environment, effective control of these chemicals is essentially impossible. This chapter presents a discussion of principles underlying the sound use of chemical analysis and monitoring in the evaluation and continued assessment of the safety of chemicals to man and his environment.

Analysis consists of the identification of chemical entities and the quantitative measurement of amounts present. For purposes of toxicological evaluation, it is important to know whether the toxic effects of a commerical product are due to the major component or to contaminants that may be present as isomers, by-products, or unreacted intermediates. Knowledge of secondary products formed in the environment may be extremely helpful. While compositional, or assay, analysis to establish purity is essential in establishing a standard of identity for a chemical, the determination of amounts in the environment lies at the other end of the measuring scale. The detection of concentrations over the range of 0.01–100 ppm is not unusual in a modern, adequately staffed laboratory equipped with readily available instruments. This sensitivity is due largely to the immense reservoir of skill, knowledge, and techniques that have emerged from several decades of experience following the complex trails of pesticide chemicals in the environment.

Monitoring is the process of following a specified chemical through the environment. The selection of the most effective means is not necessarily simple. It requires a wide range of considerations, including, for example, the toxicity of the chemical which determines the limit of detection desired of the analytical method, its behavior in the environment as often predictable by chemodynamics, and statistical planning.

The ultimate decisions to monitor, what to monitor, how to monitor, when to monitor, and when to stop monitoring, involve the allocation of considerable resources. The quality of planning in a monitoring program will control the utility of information produced and thereby the success of monitoring. The principles that should guide that planning follow.

BASIC INFORMATION

It would hardly seem necessary to point out the need for basic chemical information about a compound for purposes of analysis and monitoring, including assessment of whether the chemical is likely to be found in the environment; yet this is a much underexploited area of information. Physical and chemical data on the compounds, easily and quickly obtainable from laboratory studies, provide a valuable basis for the development of analytical methods and monitoring strategy, and for devising toxicological studies of the compound (Freed, 1969). How the interpretation and application of data from some rather simple laboratory measurements provide a basis for analyses and monitoring is discussed below.

Structure and Reactions

Such basic knowledge as elemental composition, structure, and formula weight are required in identifying any compound. In many instances, this information is sufficient to indicate to the chemist making the analysis the more common reactions that the chemical may undergo. However, general knowledge of the chemistry of new structures or new classes of compounds may be restricted, so that another chemist would not necessarily be in a position to predict characteristic reactions of the group: This necessary information must be provided. There are certain reactions commonly encountered, particularly in biological systems, that should be evaluated for each new chemical: Among these are oxidation, reduction, hydrolysis, alkylation and dealkylation of oxygen, nitrogen, or certain metallic atoms of molecules, esterification, isomerization, and conjugation with naturally occurring plant and animal metabolites—such as amino acids, polypeptides, or saccharides (Menzies, 1969). Many of these reactions are readily explored in the laboratory and should be investigated for chemicals likely to have wide distribution in the environment.

It is not sufficient, however, to know just what reactions may occur, but in certain instances knowledge of the rates and extents of those reactions is highly desirable: for example, in analyses of environmental samples for persistent organochlorine compounds, that DDT and lindane will dehydrohalogenate with base, while the PCB's will not. The relative rates of hydrolysis between certain organophosphate esters and carbamic acid esters in an analytical procedure is also useful information. Beyond the utility of kinetic data in development of analytical procedures, this same information is useful in assessing the probable persistence of a compound in certain compartments of the environment. [*See* Chapter IV, Estimation of Exposure Levels.]

Physical Properties

Physical data are equally important in devising analytical procedures, assessing behavior and flow through the environment, and devising protocols for toxicological studies. Elementary physical constants, such as melting point, boiling point, decomposition temperature, flash point, physical state, vapor tension, and crystalline form are useful, not only for secondary characterization of the substance, but also for a preliminary assessment of purity and mobility. A number of other physical measurements have considerable utility in one or more aspects of the problem being considered: For example, absorption spectra (ultraviolet, visible, and infrared) are useful in developing analytical and confirmatory methods for micro- and semimicro quantities of the chemical. Mass spectral data, where appropriate, may be invaluable for confirmation of identity.

In the development of analytical methods, solubility in solvents of various polarities and solvent–solvent partitioning data comprise an initial basis of separation and purification for final analysis. Differential solubilities on a microscale (*p*-values) may also be useful for analytical segregation and characterization of isolates (Beroza *et al.*, 1969).

Contaminants of Commercial Products

Impurities in commercial products must be considered in an evaluation of environmental effects. These impurities include foreign matter, residues of reactants, residual solvents, and congeners, the products of side reactions. Some commercial products are deliberate mixtures of more than one major ingredient.

Very few known chemical reactions yield but a single product. Because of energy distributions between the molecules and within the atoms of the molecules, there is a finite probability that one or more side reactions will occur. Congeners may differ from the principal product only slightly as with 2,4,6-trichlorophenoxyacetic acid in 2,4,5-T, or the product of the side reaction may be vastly different from the compound of interest.

Problems of contaminants are, of course, not new to the chemist and chemical engineer who must deal with them daily in the laboratory and the manufacturing plant. The toxicologist should recognize that contaminants may be significantly more toxic than the principal constituents of commercial products.

There have been some recent notable examples of contaminants in chemicals widely distributed in the environment. One of these is the tetrachloro-p-dibenzodioxin found in 2,4,5-T (Wilson, 1971). Dioxin arises, not in the synthesis of 2,4,5-T, but in the preparation of the trichlorophenol used in its manufacture. This contaminant is highly toxic (LD_{50} for guinea pigs is 1 μg/kg) but, fortunately, modification of the manufacturing process has permitted very substantial reductions of the level of the material. Another example of a contaminant in a widely distributed chemical is the toxic chlorodibenzofuran found in some preparations of PCB's (Vos, 1972).

Reaction conditions—such as temperature, pressure, concentration of reactants, and the presence or absence of catalysts or foreign materials—will cause both the kind and amount of contaminant to vary. If the contaminants are likely to present environmental problems, it becomes important to know the variability of the contaminants with changes in the manufacturing process. It should be observed that frequently the chemist can predict by inspection the probable contaminants resulting from a reaction.

As part of the toxicological assessment, it will often be desirable for purposes of comparison to study highly purified samples of a compound in parallel with samples of the technical product. If these studies indicate that contaminants are a problem, and if fluctuations in the level of contaminants from one batch to the next are significant, it would be necessary to determine the quality of each batch or to standardize the product. The toxicity of contaminants should also be considered in any change of process technology that could affect the composition of the product.

ANALYSIS AND ANALYTICAL PROCEDURES

Action directed toward environmental protection must ultimately be grounded on analytical data. The quality of the data will directly influence the logical choice of control measures and their effectiveness. Different analytical methods may be needed to determine the purity of a technical product, to establish the assay of a mixture, and to characterize and measure residues in environmental samples. Which types of analytical methods, if any, should be provided by the manufacturer will depend largely upon the hazard to be associated with its use and the need for monitoring as discussed later in this chapter.

The expense of developing and validating sophisticated procedures for residue analysis should be weighed carefully against the advantages to be gained from them.

The various operations involved in the measurement of low concentrations of foreign chemicals in environmental samples have evolved over nearly 40 years of experience with the analysis of pesticide residues; such references as Gunther and Blinn (1955), Zweig (1963–1972), and Zweig and Sherma (1972) should be consulted for a more thorough discussion than is possible here.

Sampling Considerations

The aim of sampling is to provide a miniature reproduction of the larger portion of the environment which is to be examined, but on a scale that will enable the sample to be manipulated in the laboratory. It is essential that the purpose of the desired analysis be thoroughly understood so that an appropriate sampling scheme can be constructed. Materials that are tightly adsorbed on soil and remain near the surface, for example, may not be detectable if excessively deep soil cores are taken. Conversely, materials that are more readily leached may penetrate to considerable depth and may be detected only by taking successive layers to construct a profile of penetration. Huge water samples put through adsorption columns over week-long intervals may provide impressively small numbers as a lower detectability limit, but cannot reveal whether the measurements reflect a steady-state situation or a situation with an average of a few transient peak loads.

If analysis at the time of collection is impossible, the sample must be stored in such a way that it will continue to reflect the original concentrations of the constituents of interest. The stability of stored samples should be verified by the use of suitably fortified samples or extracts stored under the same conditions.

Dry storage, storage in the cold or in the dark, freeze-drying, chemical digestion in acid or base, dissolution or immersion in solvent, sealing to avoid loss or uptake of solvent, and addition of preservatives are among the techniques that can be utilized to ensure the integrity of samples, but suitable verification of the acceptability of the techniques utilized should be exercised.

Although the analyst can be considered to be directly responsible only for the sample presented to him, he should share some responsibility in ensuring that each sample truly reflects the original material and thus merits the cost and effort incident to its analysis.

Contamination of a sample during storage may result from adsorption onto, or leaching of, a constituent of the container; from breakdown due to effects of heat, light, dissolved oxygen, the presence of water; or from biological activity. Adsorption of the desired constituent on the walls of the container can also affect the integrity of a sample.

In the planning of a sampling program it is imperative that adequate consideration be given to the method for storing samples, to minimize chemical alteration of any of the analytes of interest and to prevent contamination.

In general, the fewer number of times a sample is handled, the less chance there is for contamination. Ideally, the sample on which analysis is actually performed should be an aliquot taken from a larger, homogeneous sample. When subsampling is either necessary or desirable, the techniques followed should be those which have been established by long usage or confirmed by statistical methods.

When a sample is stored in the expectation that verification analysis or analysis for other constituents may eventually be required, the whole history of the sample, including every manipulation performed on it, should be recorded as an aid toward assessing the validity of such analysis.

Determinative Step

Extraction and Concentration   Soil, water, air, and biological samples generally cannot be analyzed directly for chemical residues because the level of the desired constituent may be below the limit of detection of the determinative method or may be masked by other constituents. Consequently, it is often necessary to remove the desired constituent from the substrate and concentrate it in a form more suitable for determination. The usual techniques include solvent extraction, centrifugation, filtration, selective adsorption–desorption, impingement, and distillation or codistillation, often in various combinations.

Since extraction and concentration are vital parts of the analytical procedure, the efficiency of recovery must be evaluated. This can be determined by using repeated extractions with a single solvent or with different solvent systems and types of extraction, or by using radiotracer techniques. Once the efficiency of the extraction has been established, the recovery from the concentration step can be determined simply by fortifying the extract prior to concentration. Test samples used in the development and validation of extraction procedures should be representative of the material ultimately to be analyzed.

Cleanup Although the determinative step of an analytical scheme is designed to be suitably selective in its response, certain natural and man-made constituents of environmental samples, and contaminants in reagents and solvents, can interfere with analytical detection systems, including bioassays, either by evoking a positive response or by inhibiting their response to the desired constituent. For this reason, further purification of concentrated extracts by means of partition distribution between immiscible solvents, selective adsorption, distillation, codistillation, crystallization, derivatization, and the like are often necessary. All cleanup procedures should remove as much interfering material as feasible with as little loss of the desired constituent as possible, and must be carefully evaluated for their ability to accomplish these objectives.

Determination Analytical methods required will vary with the intended purpose, i.e., for monitoring in the environment, for quality control in the manufacturing process, or for the assay of formulated products. Similar analytical techniques might be selected for the above purposes, differing from one another only in sample preparation, extraction, and cleanup. This similarity would extend to determinations based on gas–liquid, liquid–liquid or thin-layer chromatography; infrared, ultraviolet or visible range spectrometry; spectrophotofluorometry; polarography; atomic absorption; and mass spectrometry. The last technique is usually interfaced with gas chromatography for maximum utility. Bioassay techniques would be entirely appropriate in certain monitoring situations; however, the relatively nonspecific nature of these techniques would require some prior information on the presence, or likelihood of presence, and the desired measurable response of a specific chemical in the system monitored.

From the standpoint of efficient utilization of manpower, multiresidue screening procedures offer enormous advantages. It is likely, therefore, that comprehensive monitoring schemes would of necessity be based largely on multiresidue methodology. However, it is doubtful that a single screening procedure or even an integrated scheme of multiresidue methods can be devised that would detect all of the substances for which monitoring would be desirable. For this reason, the manufacturer of a specific compound should not be required to develop multiresidue methods of analysis.

Improving the Reliability of Analytical Data

Validation of Method Quantitative data for the accuracy, precision, and lower limit of detection of an analytical method should be available when its use in a monitoring program is contemplated. The sensitivity and reliability required should depend primarily on the hazard associated with the substance in question, but will usually be mediated by analytical interferences in each substrate to be investigated.

In its simplest form, the validation of a method consists of fortifying several replicates of an environmental sample (free of the sought analyte) at three decadal levels and carrying them through the entire analytical procedure. These data and standard curves for absence or presence of substrate extractives in the concentration range expected for unknown samples, provide normally adequate information for reliability, accuracy, precision, sensitivity, and lower limits of detection under both ideal (no substrate) and practical (substrate) conditions. Intralaboratory comparison involving several analysts represents an intermediate degree of validation. Full-scale validation would involve interlaboratory collaborative study of a procedure under the auspices of a professional analytical society, leading to its adoption as an "official" method.

Modern methods of analysis for trace contaminants in biological samples, particularly those designed for multiresidue screening purposes, frequently include alternative extraction procedures, complex cleanup schemes, split detection systems, and optional or required confirmatory steps. The application of these methods requires extreme attention to technique and practical training with the procedures before reproducible results are attainable. It is suggested that adequate interlaboratory programs be initiated to assure reliability of analytical results obtained in most monitoring programs involving significantly toxic analytes.

Repository for Analytical Materials A repository for analytical reference standards should be maintained by the regulatory agency for use in monitoring programs or for examination of materials containing the regulated substance. Purified samples suitable as primary analytical standards should be obtained along with samples of the technical grade product and major congeners and contaminants which occur in the manufacturing process.

The apparent finding of certain chemicals in monitored samples is sometimes attributed to artifacts in the sample substrate that give the same response as the analyte. In addition, the compound or element sought may be endogenous to the specimen (e.g., mercury in fish). A judgment as to whether an industrial use is contributing increments of a toxic substance to the monitored specimen will depend on correction for this background response or "control." The control is usually determined experimentally by carrying an untreated (control) sample through the entire analytical procedure. It cannot be assumed that uncontaminated control specimens can be found after a chemical has had wide usuage; therefore, a repository of important biological and inanimate specimens should be acquired for this purpose and maintained by the regulatory agency.

Confirmatory Methods   It must be recognized that no analytical method is completely specific. With the expectation that serious sanctions can be applied upon the finding of an undesirable contaminant in an ecosystem, it is imperative that the indicting analyses be confirmed by an independent procedure. The degree of assurance required will depend on the seriousness of the occurrence of the toxicant in the system. A confirmatory analysis by thin-layer chromatography may add a degree of assurance that toxicant X found by gas-liquid chromatography is in fact toxicant X, but does not provide absolute certitude. In the pesticide field, several other useful identification-supporting techniques have been developed that would be applicable to industrial contaminants in the environment. These include use of partition coefficients, infrared spectrometry, preparation of derivatives, and, most important, mass spectrometry interfaced with gas–liquid chromatography when applicable.

Assembling, Interpreting, and Using Data

After the necessary analytical data have been gathered, the analyst must assemble it in a convenient form, such as annotated tables, for evaluation. Both the raw data and the computed results must be available for ready reference. The analyst must report his interpretation of his data as to reliability (i.e., his certainty that the sample he analyzed contained the toxicant he reported and in the concentrations he is reporting) with an indication of variability encountered. These data must contain only positive concentration values; lower values must be reported in terms of "less than the lower limit of detection," including values often reported as "traces" which might be interpreted from very small responses of the detector. Only the analyst can know how much reliance can be placed on his results, and he has the responsibility for making this known, since the ultimate recipient of the data cannot be expected to know their reliability and might therefore misinterpret their biological significance.

MONITORING

The term *monitoring* as used here carries the operational meaning of measurements made over time. There are at least four types of monitoring, which differ according to the purpose for which the observations may be gathered: They are (1) reconnaissance monitoring, (2) surveillance monitoring, (3) subjective monitoring, or spot-checking, and (4) objective monitoring.

Reconnaissance monitoring involves periodic observations with the objective of determining changes or the trend with time, often with the implication that some, perhaps undefined, corrective action may be taken if trends become alarming. In surveillance monitoring, observations are made periodically to support an enforcement program and to ensure compliance with regulations. Subjective monitoring, or spot-checking, may be undertaken for a variety of purposes, but—broadly speaking—it is monitoring for the purpose of exploring the parameters of a problem, whether it be the investigation of an accidental spill or determination of general levels of hazard. In some such cases, the element of time may enter only in that positive findings will indicate a change since some presumed original zero level in the environment. The purpose of objective monitoring is to provide data primarily for use in developing and confirming quantitative models and simulation. This last definition of *monitoring,* while accepted, has not been considered particularly applicable to the present discussion.

In the present context, monitoring of a hazardous chemical can be considered as a means of determining whether existing controls are adequate and will continue to protect man and his environment. Although it may often be appropriate to start monitoring before the chemical has been released, monitoring information becomes useful only after the chemical has entered the environment. Thus, monitoring serves as a feedback mechanism in the decision-making process.

Although monitoring is expensive, the losses that result from an inadequate monitoring system are considerable. These losses must be calculated, first, as the cost of the monitoring, and, second, as that cost accountable to the delay in detecting a hazardous situation. The costs of monitoring include the direct costs plus those of tying up scientific manpower. Costs of delay in detection might include damage to human health, effects on the environment, and influence on the future well-being of the nation. The last costs, however, are only those due to *delay* in action; they do not include the costs of abatement except as these may become greater by the delay. Serious contamination will eventually be detected, although, without monitoring, detection of the problem may occur only after critical damage has been done. If contamination is *never* to be detected, then by definition the problem does not exist.

Each monitoring program should be justified by the utility of the information sought. With the magnitude of the task and the always-too-limited resources, one of the greatest dangers is the dilution of resources and effective effort by including too many programs on the "nice-to-know" basis. It follows that there is need for some operational definition of the relative utility of monitoring information and for objective methods of optimizing monitoring systems in terms of the utility of combined information from the component programs.

Each monitoring program should ideally be planned according to the characteristics of single materials or single indices of status. Often, however, operational monitoring systems must, for economy, include a number of parallel monitoring programs—each planned for a single chemical or index, but with necessary concessions to allow for their inclusion in a single system.

Measurements Used in Monitoring

Both direct chemical analysis and measurement of biological response may be applicable to monitoring programs. Direct chemical measurement may be made of the material in question, or of its recognizable breakdown products, in the physical substrate or in the biota. Data may be gathered on concentrations in the water, the soil, or the air, and in the tissues of animals, plants, or man, in food substances, or in the products of industry.

Beyond the chemical determination of residues in tissues, monitoring of the biota is useful for determining the nature and the extent of the effects of chemicals on intact organisms (Slack *et al.*, 1973). Chemicals may produce specific physiological responses in individual species: For example, some organochlorine insecticides cause eggshell thinning in certain predator birds, thereby reducing hatching success and threatening reproductive capabilities. Another example is the inhibition of cholinesterase in man and animals following exposure to certain organophosphate chemicals. Appropriate methods for determining the effects of chemicals in the environment are discussed elsewhere in this report.

(See the discussion of epidemiological methods in Chapters VIII, XV, and XVI.)

Once a measurable response of a living organism to a chemical is known, this response can be used in a biological monitoring program as a measure of the concentration of that chemical in the environment. For example, cages of fish placed at intervals in a stream could indicate how rapidly an upstream source of contaminants is being diluted or decontaminated; also, plants grown in a filtered air enclosure in the field could indicate by contrast the degree of certain types of air pollution.

As a first approximation, the species chosen for monitoring would be the one likely to receive the highest exposure to a chemical based on its probable distribution in the environment; however, such other factors must be considered in the selection of a species as its availability, sensitivity, and value to man.

The species should be reasonably available, both currently and in the future, if long-term monitoring is contemplated. The most sensitive species would usually be desired, provided that it is not so uniquely responsive to certain chemicals that erroneous conclusions might result. Conversely, choice of highly resistant species may lead to a false sense of security. Is the species of economic or aesthetic value? Species of direct commercial value to man will, of course, be important, but monitoring should not exclude species of lesser economic value that are good indicators of environmental change. Ease of studying and the availability of monitoring methods for a particular species must also be considered.

Storage and Retrieval of Monitoring Data

The value of monitoring information is in making comparisons over time; therefore, the information must be stored in some way for use in the future. Questions of systematic storage and access systems arise when series of data are accumulated by numbers of agencies over time. Aside from the practical questions of whether the storage will be by computer, or what agency will support and service the system, and the operating safeguards to prevent the perversion of the system to other ends, there are more general questions. There may be a legal question of whether data gathered and made available voluntarily by an agency can properly be used in action against the interests of the same agency. Further, there are important difficulties in the future interpretation of data gathered and stored in the past. Considerations here emphasize the importance of also recording the qualitative characteristics of the data, the precise methods used in sampling and analysis and their reliability, and the character of the sample material.

Strategy of Monitoring

The precise character of a monitoring program must be determined by what is known of the properties of the chemicals in question and by the specific objectives of the program. Together, these determine whether monitoring should be done, where, with what materials, how often, with what statistical precision, and how the monitoring effort may best be divided among the several programs of a monitoring system, or among the parts of one monitoring program.

While the objectives of monitoring programs all come within the range of protecting man and the environment, the immediate objectives of specific programs vary over a broad range. Where concern is whether the discharge of a single industrial plant into a river stays within defined tolerance, the objectives are relatively narrow and well-defined. Where the concern is whether a chemical is reaching man, the scope is much greater and the selection of the materials to be sampled becomes complex. Where concern covers a whole ecosystem, the objectives become very broad and the selection of sample materials tends to become increasingly arbitrary.

Expected Flow Models   Models developed to predict the flow of chemicals through the environment (Chapter IV) will also be helpful in determining whether monitoring is necessary and in the planning of monitoring programs. Although expected flow models may often be qualitative, they should be sufficiently detailed to serve as a basis for determining where and what to sample. They should, therefore, indicate which parts of the environment are exposed to the chemical in question, and should identify the major pathways and sinks. Where uncertainties exist, it may be necessary to obtain additional information through means such as preliminary surveys.

It can be argued that one of the ultimate goals of monitoring should be the development of a quantitative model of the flow of a chemical through the environment with accompanying predictions of exposure levels at critical points in time and space along the route. Development of such models proceeds iteratively, from theoretical considerations to empirical observations to revised theory, until reasonable agreement is reached between prediction and observation over a wide range of conditions. At this point, a model becomes a useful tool in predicting the environmental impact of new but adequately closely related chemicals.

Where feasible, the planning of a monitoring program should include consideration of supplementary data requirements such as might be specified for model validation. The data gathered will be of maximum benefit to the evaluation program as a whole if field collections can be so designed as to satisfy more than the immediate objectives of the monitoring program.

When to Monitor   The decision to initiate, continue, or terminate a monitoring program is essentially one of balancing the cost of monitoring against the cost of damage to man and the environment if contamination exists and continues undetected. Typically, it will not be made by the persons who will carry out the monitoring. It must be an advised policy decision based on the best available technical knowledge, which may often be limited, and the best technical advice. Its elements are almost as complex and varied as those involved in the decision to restrict the production or use of a chemical.

Adequate consideration must be given to the consequences of serious exposure and to the likelihood that the chemical will be encountered in the environment at levels requiring corrective action. Therefore, the decision to monitor will rely heavily on the estimate of exposure levels and on the results of tests for effects, both on man and on the living and nonliving components of his environment. The estimate of exposure levels should be revised periodically to account for changes in the volume of production, pattern of use, and method of disposal.

The intensity of the monitoring effort should be no greater than that required to detect important changes in the level of contamination in time to permit effective reaction. Some materials of low volume and low toxicity may require only infrequent determination because rapid changes in hazard are unlikely. Other materials of high volume or great toxic potential may require more frequent determination. Because of limited resources it is often necessary to weigh the cost of more frequent monitoring against the possible losses due to failure to detect a change in the level of some other hazardous material. When important changes are not anticipated for some extended period, monitoring can be stopped without loss of essential information.

The elements entering into the decision of when to monitor are complex and varied. The details could be overwhelming if some criteria were not available to order the problem. It is evident, however, that certain identifiable factors are pivotal in considering the amount of study required on a chemical and whether or not to monitor for it. Among the factors to consider in the decision are: the physical and chemical properties of the substance, the toxicity and spectrum of biological activity, the use pattern including volume, and, finally, disposal of the material after use.

Physical and Chemical Properties   As outlined earlier, application of information on physical and chemical properties of chemicals gives an indication of the probable fate and other behavior of the chemical in the environment. It may be used to predict the compartment of the environment in which the chemical may be found. Thus, on the basis of their known properties, one would predict that PCB's would accumulate in lipids of biota, magnify in concentration as they move through food chains, and be strongly adsorbed by soil. These same types of data are essential in modeling the flow of the chemical through the environment (Chapter IV).

Toxicity and Biological Activity   Obviously the greater the biological activity (toxicity) the greater the need to monitor in order to take corrective procedures as needed. [*See* Chapters VII-XVI.]

Effect on Inanimate Materials   Should a substance have a material deleterious effect on metals, ceramics, textiles, etc., its concentration in the environment should be monitored and controlled to minimize damage to buildings, clothing, and other objects. [*See* Chapter XIX.]

Use and Discharge into the Environment   The pattern, volume, and nature of use are considerations in whether or not to monitor. This factor may be subdivided as follows:

1. Volume of use (total tonnage)—Volume must be subject to surveillance because changes are normally not predictable.

2. Spatial character of use—The spatial aspect may be characterized as (1) point, i.e., only at a manufacturing plant; (2) limited, i.e., at several scattered but defined points; and (3) dispersed.

3. Temporal character of discharge—The temporal aspect may be characterized as (1) intermittent or infrequent; (2) pulsating, i.e., variable; and (3) continuous.

4. Systems of use—Systems may be either closed, restricted, or open.

Disposal and Its Possible Impact   How will disposal be accomplished, under what controls, will there be any probable environmental contamination, and how important can this be?

It is believed that the foregoing represent most of the important elements needed in a decision tree. Though no attempt has been made to give quantitative limits, it is felt that reasonable and useful estimates could be made even at this time for many chemicals.

Precision Required in Monitoring   The objectives of planning a sampling program, in monitoring as elsewhere, may be stated either as obtaining the maximum best quality information for the budget, or as obtaining maximum information of some stated quality at a minimim cost; these statements are equivalent. As used here, *quality* means statistical precision, even though it is recognized that a broader meaning of the term must include the quality of the chemical analysis. The two methods of increasing statistical quality are by improving the sampling designs or, sometimes, by increasing the sample size. For a given sampling design, an increase in statistical quality translates directly into an increase in dollar cost of the program.

For any one monitoring program, therefore, the precision required must be just adequate to detect changes reliably of an order judged to be important. Precision beyond this level may be wasteful and inhibit other parts of a multiple program monitoring system. With less than this level of precision, a monitoring program will fall short of achieving its objectives.

Sampling in Monitoring Studies

There are two different ways of selecting sample materials for analysis. The first method may be termed selection of an *index*. This is by far the more common procedure and perhaps always used from some points of view. Here materials are selected because they are judged to be representative of the universe of interest, with judgment and availability predominating in the selection. In the second method of selection, an attempt is made to obtain an unbiased estimate of an average or total value by using methods of probability sampling, or procedures as close as practical to this ideal. The emphasis here is on the avoidance of the well-known bias inherent in judgment sampling. Both kinds of methods of selection may be employed at different levels of the same monitoring program.

Index material is selected because it is practical to obtain, ordinarily at relatively low cost, and may be obtained reliably on a continuing basis. A common criterion is that it must be *representative,* or correspond in some usually undefined way to the broader population or universe of interest. In the context of monitoring chemicals in the environment, the use of index material rests upon an implicit assumption: that the universe can be described by a multicompartment model with ready exchange among all compartments—either directly or through other compartments—with the transfer functions being such that the direction of change in one compartment will reveal the direction of change in the whole system. Under these conditions the arbitrary choice of any compartment may be justified solely on the basis of convenience of access. Use of several compartments as samples of the environment reduces the bias introduced when the applicability of the model is assumed. Examples of use of index material are the selection of a single species of fish to represent all fish, or perhaps all aquatic biota, or the use of established stations for the sampling of air.

The establishment of unbiased estimates based upon anything reasonably close to probability sampling procedures is practical in only a limited set of monitoring problems. The basis requirements that the probability of selection be known for each item of the sample seems impractical, if not impossible, in most monitoring programs. There are, however, some problems where approximations to this method have been used and others where they could be used more extensively. An example of present use is in the determination of the average pesticide content of various foods in the human diet. An example of potential use is in the determination of average concentration of a chemical in soil, where land could be sampled by area methods.

The exact details of the best sampling system for a particular monitoring program cannot be specified in this general discussion. Each program will present its own problems and require a separate design for greatest efficiency. Sound sampling procedures—such as stratification, systematic sampling, subsampling, compositing, and related procedures—should guide the selection of units to be included.

In studying trends, the use of repeated measurements on the identical primary sampling units will often increase precision. In some cases, the methods of statistical quality control may be adapted for use in monitoring, especially where some defined action is to be taken locally when a trend reaches a certain point. Methods of sequential sampling may increase efficiency of effort in special cases.

Samples taken in monitoring often fall into the form of a nest sampling design. There are three commonly identifiable levels of sampling with their corresponding types of variability: the field variability between sampling stations, the biological or local variability among samples taken at a particular station, and the analytical variability introduced in the process of chemical or biological analysis. The existing, well-established theory and practice of sampling can be used to guide the optimal allocation of effort in such designs, provided that the variability is estimated at the several levels and that the corresponding costs of sampling can also be stated (Cochran, 1963). The technique of compositing samples may allow increased precision without seriously affecting the cost of monitoring because often a single chemical analysis is so much more expensive than an additional local sample at a station.

SUMMARY

A considerable array of information—such as chemical structure, reactivity, and basic physical and chemical properties—is needed for the development both of analytical methods and of predictive models that serve as a basis for monitoring strategy.

Various methods of chemical analysis may be employed to determine the composition of commercial products and to measure residues of these materials and their alteration products in environmental samples. In some cases, minor constituents or alteration products may be as hazardous as the principal ingredient and may require special methods of analysis.

The generation of reliable analytical data demands that care be taken in each of the five unit operations of residue analysis—sampling, extraction, cleanup, determination, and analytical interpretation—and that the method be adequately validated. Many of the principles and techniques that have evolved from pesticide research during the past 40 years are applicable to the study of other chemicals.

Monitoring is designed to measure the success of existing controls in preventing contaminants in the environment from reaching harmful or otherwise undesirable levels. Decisions relating to the need for monitoring and to the intensity of the monitoring effort must consider the cost of monitoring weighed against the cost of damage to human health and the environment if significant contamination exists and continues undetected.

In selecting a strategy for monitoring, some kind of expected flow model based on the physical and chemical properties of a chemical and on its anticipated production, use, and method of disposal (Chapter IV) is essential, for it indicates where the chemical is likely to accumulate and at what concentrations. In addition, there is a special need for statistical planning to ensure full utility of the information gained. Access to the monitoring information must be provided by carefully planned storage and retrieval methods.

REFERENCES

Beroza, M., M.N. Inscoe, and M.C. Bowman. 1969. Distribution of pesticides in immiscible binary solvent systems for cleanup and identification and its application in the extraction of pesticides from milk. Residue Rev. 30:1–61.

Cochran, W.G. 1963. *Sampling Techniques,* 2nd ed. John Wiley and Sons, Inc., New York. 413 pp.

Freed, V.H. 1969. Chemodynamics—Transport and Behavior of Chemicals in the Environment. Task Force on Research Planning in Environmental Health Science. Background Document FW-7:1 for *Man's Health and the Environment—Some Research Needs.* Deposited at National Library of Medicine, Bethesda, Md.

Gunther, F.A., and R.C. Blinn. 1955. *Analysis of Insecticides and Acaricides.* John Wiley and Sons, Inc., New York. 696 pp.

Menzies, C.M. 1969. *Metabolism of Pesticides.* Spec. Sci. Rep.–Wildl. No. 127. Bureau of Sport Fisheries and Wildlife, U.S. Department of the Interior, Washington, D.C. 487 pp.

Slack, K.V., R.C. Averett, P.E. Greeson, and R.G. Lipscomb. 1973. Methods for collection and analysis of aquatic biological and microbiological samples. In *Techniques of Water Resources Investigations: Book 5, Laboratory Analysis.* Chapter A4. U.S. Government Printing Office, Washington, D.C.

Vos, J.G. 1972. Toxicology of PCB's for mammals and birds. *Environ. Health Perspect.* (Experimental Issue) 1:105–117.

Wilson, J.G. 1971. *Report of the Advisory Committee on 2,4,5-T to the Administrator of the Environmental Protection Agency.* Office of Pesticides, Environmental Protection Agency, Washington, D.C. 76 pp.

Zweig, G. 1963–1972. *Analytical Methods for Pesticides, Plant Growth Regulators and Food Additives.* Vol. 1–5. Academic Press, New York.

Zweig, G., and J. Sherma. 1972. *Analytical Methods for Pesticides, Plant Growth Regulators and Food Additives.* Vol. 6. Academic Press, New York.

SUGGESTED READINGS

American Society for Testing and Materials. 1973. Water, atmospheric analysis. In *Annual Book of ASTM Standards,* Part 23. ASTM, Philadelphia.

Bryan, R.J. 1968. Air Quality Monitoring. In A. C. Stern, ed., *Air Pollution. Vol. II: Analysis, Monitoring, Surveying,* 2nd ed. Academic Press, New York. pp. 425–463.

Carver, T.C. 1971. Estuarine monitoring program. *Pestic. Monit. J.* 5:53.

Chou, W.T. 1964. Statistical and probability analysis of hydrologic data. In W. T. Chou, ed., *Handbook of Applied Hydrology,* Section 8. McGraw-Hill Book Co., New York.

Cliath, M.M., and W.F. Spencer. 1972. Dissipation of pesticides from soil by volatilization of degradation products: I. Lindane and DDT. *Environ. Sci. Technol.* 6:910–914.

Coulston, F., and F. Korte, eds. 1972. *Environmental Quality: Global Aspects of Chemistry, Toxicology and Technology as Applied to the Environment.* Vol. 1. Academic Press, New York. 267 pp.

Federal Interagency Work Group on Designation of Standards for Water Data Acquisition. 1972. *Recommended Methods for Water Data Acquisition—Preliminary Report.* Office of Water Data Coordination, U.S. Geological Survey, Washington, D.C. 415 pp.

Freed, V.H., R. Haque, and D. Schmedding. 1972. Vaporization and environmental contamination by DDT. *Chemosphere* 1:61–66.

Freed, V.H., and R. Haque. 1973. Adsorption, Movement, and Distribution of

Pesticides in Soils. In W. Van Valkenburg, ed., *Pesticide Formulations.* Marcel Dekker, Inc., New York. pp. 441–459.

Hartley, G.S. 1969. Evaporation of pesticides. *Advan. Chem. Ser.* 86:115–134.

Kenaga, E.E. 1972. Guidelines for environmental study of pesticides: Determination of bioconcentration potential. *Residue Rev.* 44:73–113.

Lambert, S.M., P.E. Porter, and R.H. Schieferstein. 1965. Movement and sorption of chemicals applied to the soil. *Weeds* 13:185–190.

Lambert, S.M. 1968. Omega (Ω), a useful index of soil sorption equilibria. *J. Agric. Food Chem.* 16:340–343.

Murray, W.S. 1971. Criteria for defining pesticide levels to be considered an alert to potential problems. *Pestic. Monit. J.* 5:36.

Plimmer, J.R. 1971. Photochemistry of pesticides: A discussion of the influence of some environmental factors. In A. S. Tahori, ed., *Proceedings of the Second International IUPAC Congress on Pesticide Chemistry.* Vol. 6. Gordon Breach Science Publ., New York. pp. 47–76.

Wilson, C.L. and W.H. Matthews, eds. 1970. *Man's Impact on the Global Environment: Assessment and Recommendations for Action.* M.I.T. Press, Cambridge, Mass. pp. 121, 172.

World Meteorological Organization. 1970. *Guide to Hydrometeorological Practices,* 2nd ed. Publ. No. 168 (also TP #82). World Meteorological Organization, Geneva, Switzerland. 294 pp.

World Meteorological Organization. 1973. *Casebook on Hydrological Network Design Practice,* Chapters I-1.2, I-5.3, I-10.2, II-2.1, III-1.2, III-3.3. Publ. No. 324. World Meteorological Organization, Geneva, Switzerland.

APPENDIXES

A

Short Term
Toxicity Tests

Supplementary Material to Chapter VII

The state of knowledge of the application of nonmammalian animals
and of isolated mammalian organs or cells to questions in cell biology,
genetics, mutagenesis, teratogenesis, and carcinogenesis is sufficiently
promising to recommend that such systems be further examined for
possible use in evaluating toxic effects of environmental chemicals.
These systems are most likely to be useful in *in vitro* short-term screening studies. They need to be employed in parallel with studies in intact
mammals in order to build a framework of comparative data with which
to judge the relative reliability, sensitivity, cost, and utility.

The test systems identified here may be only a fraction of the
number and variety that can be deployed. The value at this time of
these systems does not depend on their replacing animal and human
exposure models unless they prove suitable as substitutes; rather, their
value lies in serving as adjunctive probes of the biologic action of
environmental chemicals.

MOLECULAR PHARMACOLOGY

The field that has come to be known as molecular pharmacology is
as advanced in technology as molecular biology and genetics. This
field will expand if it is supported and financed in the way that is

appropriate to a national pursuit of means to understand and protect human health in a complex environment. Methods in this field are contributing to the capacity to define biochemical functions and lesions in small numbers of cells or small amounts of tissue. Skilled manpower is available for applying those tests to *in vitro* systems in pursuit of the rationale described above.

CELL CULTURE

Cell culture methods have been applied to a large range of critical biological questions; they comprise the basic technology for studies of neoplastic transformation by viruses and chemical carcinogens. Conditions for isolating, maintaining, and growing cells have become highly developed and some characteristics of cells as individuals and as populations are being elucidated. A major gap in this development is in the isolation and maintenance in cell culture of epithelial cells as compared to connective tissue (fibroblastic) cells. Epithelial cells are the first cell types to be hit upon exposure to the environment and are the major cell types that metabolize, detoxify, and excrete environmental chemicals. Development of culture methods for epithelial cells is a high priority objective in research in cancer, lung diseases, and cell biology.

Preparation

Dispersed cells of appropriate organs provide a cell population representative of cells able to survive dispersing methods. With appropriate methods a portion of these cells will be epithelial, and may emerge as a majority cell type. Epithelial cells for toxicologic studies specific to an organ should be used within 1 or 2 days of setting up cultures and only after establishing that they are the predominant cell type in a culture.

Types of Observations

Test chemicals can be added to media in vehicles which have proven not to be toxic for cultured cells. Cells or media can be recovered for biochemical measurement of the chemical under test or for measurement of tracers for macromolecular syntheses and nutrients. Localization of radioactive, fluorescent, or colored compounds in selected parts of cells is aided by their flattened aspect on the surface of a culture vessel. Cell population size and cell characteristics can be scored and normality of the appearance of cells recorded by microscopy in living cultures.

Applications

Applications of cell cultures are listed below:

1. metabolic characterization of representative cells cultured from an organ;
2. metabolism of an environmental chemical by such cells;
3. effect of an environmental chemical on the metabolic activity of the cultured cells; and
4. comparison of the metabolic characteristics and of the response to an environmental chemical of cultured cells taken (1) from several different organs of a single species, and (2) from the same organ taken from two or more species.

ORGAN CULTURE

This technique maintains an organ segment in which all cells of the organ are present in their normal relationships. The method aims at retaining cells in the functioning state representative of the living animal. Organ pieces can be maintained in a reasonably intact state for several weeks. This period is long enough for some toxicologic observations.

Preparation

Organ fragments can be maintained submerged or on the surface of nutrient media. A high oxygen content in the atmosphere tends to preserve the initial state of differentiation of cells on the surface. Deep cells in solid organs die in 3–5 days despite high oxygen content.

Types of Observations

Modes of observation are as described for cell culture except that histologic preparations take the place of direct examination of living cells by microscopy. Cell population size cannot be counted directly; hence indirect measures of cell number such as DNA content are used.

Applications

These are the same as those described for cell culture. Observations made in 1–3 days may not reveal histologic changes caused by test chemicals, but, by 5 or more days, histologically identifiable cell and tissue alterations may appear.

TISSUE SLICE METHODS

This technology depends on the survival for several hours of meta-bolically active cells. Time is too short for enzyme induction *in vitro,* and tissues must be "primed" *in vivo* if induction is needed. This feature constrains the use of the method with human tissue. Modification of this method to permit 1–3 days survival is not a known development but may be feasible.

VALIDATION AND INTERPRETATION OF *IN VITRO* DATA

At this time no decision about toxicity or safety for man can be made from *in vitro* tests described in this section. The component technolo-gies are now adequate for identifying mechanisms of cell–chemical interaction. These technologies are also at a stage ready for assembly into a program of expanded studies to probe the effects of environ-mental chemicals on animals and man. As such studies are done *in vitro,* parallel *in vivo* studies are required to validate the culture find-ings. This means that the *in vitro* data will be regarded as meaningful only if they yield data similar to those obtainable from the same organs in intact animals exposed to the same chemicals. Sensitivities of *in vivo* and *in vitro* measurements would be compared to correct for extreme differences as a guide to future deployment of *in vitro* methods as a predictive screening method.

NONMAMMALIAN SYSTEMS

Some of these systems are reviewed briefly as examples of available methods deserving consideration.

Drosophila have been used for mutagenesis testing and for evaluation of genetic effects on behavior. This fly has a rapid reproductive rate, genetic mapping of it is highly advanced, and mutations are readily scored. Its suitability in probes of some mutagenic and toxic chemi-cals is limited by its range of metabolic capability as compared to mammals. Applications to the study of environmental chemicals warrants review.

Embryonated avian eggs represent a closed system in which nutrients and chemicals are delivered from one repository (yolk sac) and metabolites are delivered to another (allantois). The embryonated egg can be manipulated by the injection of material into the yolk sac for alimentary incorporation, into the amniotic sac for access to both alimentary and respiratory systems, and into the chorio-allantois vein for systemic dissemination. Neuromuscular activity and cardiac rates are readily recorded electrically.

Embryonated avian eggs were used extensively for viral infection and tumor virus assays, as well as for virus production, before the development of cell cultures; another use has been in limited teratologic and toxicologic work.

POTENTIAL ADVANTAGES OF SHORT-TERM TESTS

There are four major reasons to expand research and development of short-term systems.

Utilization of Human Materials

Human organ pieces or representative cells can be exposed to chemicals that could not safely be given to living human subjects. Human tissues can be examined for ability to metabolize chemicals or undergo functional, chromosomal, or morphologic alterations.

As a corollary, comparative *in vivo–in vitro* tests in animal tissues have confirmed the validity of *in vitro* observations in sufficient instances to warrant application of cell and organ culture systems for study of tissues from rare or expensive animals. Samples may be obtained by biopsy, or multiple samples may be obtained at autopsy, to extend observations beyond those made during life.

Flexibility with Regard to Quantity

Smaller quantities of material can be tested than would be required in animal trials. This consideration can be important when only small quantities of material can be collected from airborne or other effluents released by commercial or consumer processes. In this context, the whole effluent may be too complex to be analyzed for specific components. The crude product may be tested in a few animals and/or in a variety of *in vitro* systems to broaden the range of information obtainable from small amounts of material in order to provide leads for more detailed investigations.

Favorable Cost Factors

Costs may be lower for short-term methods. Many *in vitro* systems are inexpensive in labor, materials, space, and equipment. Replicate samples are readily taken; dynamic events, such as changes in population or in precursor utilization, can be recorded by sequential sampling; and quantitative dose–effect and rate estimates can be made with statistically suitable numbers of determinations, but without great cost or expenditure of time. Such tests may be helpful in setting priorities.

Sensitivity

Systems can be chosen that are selective in sensitivity to environmental chemicals. Some single components of environmental effluent mixtures are so toxic for whole animals that the remaining potentially important materials cannot be used at high enough concentrations to test for toxicity in intact animals. *In vitro* systems can be chosen that are responsive to some, but not all, components of a complex environmental material.

B

Target
Organ
Study

Supplementary Material to Chapter VII

Subchronic toxicity studies concepts are discussed in general terms in Chapter VII. Their main purpose is to lay a base for the design and conduction of chronic studies and to predict the kinds of effects to be observed in the chronic tests. Since the effects to be observed are likely to be of small magnitude, it is important to know where to look and what to look for. The target organ study is designed for that purpose.

It is not a purpose of this presentation to define specific protocols, but certain principles will be suggested for the design of target organ or target system studies with the following goals:

- To determine the system most susceptible to the effects of the agent.
- To determine the rate of development of the effect as related to dose level.
- To determine reversibility of effect upon withdrawal of the agent.
- To determine the relation of blood or tissue levels of the agent or its metabolites to the appearance and development or persistence of an effect.
- To determine possible equilibration of degree of effect at a fixed dose level; i.e., to determine whether there is a progressive cumulation of effect with time at a fixed dose level or whether each dose level is characterized by a plateau effect.

It is recognized that such studies would require thoughtful and individualized consideration of each material investigated; the use of sufficient numbers of animals to permit evaluation of all parameters considered to be toxicologically significant, including histopathologic changes, at all prescribed intervals during the study; and continual exercise of judgment with regard to progressive adjustment of dosage. Having completed one such study, however, one would be in a position to design more meaningful chronic studies or perhaps even to eliminate the necessity for conducting certain traditional chronic studies (*e.g.,* long-term cholinesterase inhibition studies at fixed dose levels). The results of a well-designed target organ study would alert investigators to specific anatomical, physiological, and biochemical parameters requiring special attention and would contribute much toward elimination of the number of sensational episodes such as have occurred with hexachlorophene and other substances.

The target organ study requires the following information from the acute toxicity tests in addition to LD_{50} data: (1) species variability; (2) sex differences; and (3) signs of intoxication—including the relationship of signs to the activity of primary interest and the dose–response curve.

SPECIES SELECTION

Studies should be conducted in two species, usually rats and dogs, unless there is some reason to avoid these species or to select others. In general, it would be preferable to employ species whose metabolic pathways are most similar to those of man, but it is unlikely, in most instances, that metabolic information will be acquired prior to the time that a compound will have passed the test of a subacute or target system study. Some guidance is available from the accumulated knowledge of comparative metabolism. The monkey would be unsuitable for evaluation of a uricosuric agent since uric acid is not an end product of nitrogen metabolism in the monkey. The rabbit would probably be unsuitable for studies of compounds that are detoxified to a major extent by glycoside formation since the rabbit is extraordinary in the ability to conjugate.

NUMBER OF ANIMALS

If rats and dogs are employed, at least 60 rats (30 males and 30 females) and 12 dogs (6 males and 6 females) should be used. This would permit sacrifice of 5/5 rats and 1/1 dogs after each of four intervals on test and after each of two periods of recovery.

DOSE LEVELS

In a typical 90-day study, it is a common practice to select a high dose level equivalent to 0.2–0.25 times the acute LD_{50}. If the dose–response curve is unusually steep, a higher fraction of the LD_{50} might be chosen; if the dose response curve is flat, a smaller fraction would be advisable. If, for a target study, one starts at one-fourth the acute LD_{50} and increases the dose level by 0.2 log increments at selected intervals, sequential dose levels would be 25, 40, 63 and 100 percent of the acute LD_{50} during four consecutive intervals of testing.

INTERVAL SELECTION

It is suggested that the interval for evaluation be 3 weeks, increasing the dose level at the end of each 3-week period, except for a provision to continue any dose level for an additional 3-week period in the event of a questionable effect. This would permit continuation of the study for a period of time comparable to that usually employed for traditional subacute studies. Cumulative toxicity (as with reserpine) or tolerance (as with a narcotic analgesic) might be evidenced by the early or delayed appearance of evidence of toxicity.

PARAMETERS

Food consumption, growth, and behavioral effects should be noted and standard hematologic and clinical determinations should be made at the end of each 3-week period. Special studies that might be suggested by the known pharmacodynamics of the compound or by knowledge of the activity of structurally related compounds should be conducted. Blood levels of the agent, and of its metabolites, if known, should be determined in an effort to relate blood levels to the appearance of signs of toxicity. All data should be evaluated before making a decision to continue a dose level or proceed to the next higher level. If the decision is made to increase the dose level, an appropriate number of randomly selected animals would be sacrificed for gross and histopathologic examination, using special staining techniques when indicated. Because of the time involved in preparing specimens for examination, histopathologic data would be delayed and could not be conveniently used as a basis for continuing or increasing the treatment level. Any animal that might die would be subjected to gross and histopathologic study.

DURATION OF STUDY

The study would continue until clear signs of toxicity developed, after which time treatment would be terminated and the remaining animals maintained for a period of recovery. During the recovery period, special attention would be directed toward the organs or systems judged to be affected for evidence of disappearance or diminution of effects.

COMMENTS

Having defined the systems affected by the test material and having knowledge of the time of appearance of effects as related to dose levels and blood levels, one would be prepared to design chronic studies on a rational basis. In instances in which the effect plateaus in a short time at a given dose level, the need for long-term studies directed toward this effect might be obviated, but long-terms studies would still be required to determine the effects of extended low-level exposure, nonplateau toxicologic effects, and, particularly, carcinogenic and genetic effects.

If a compound continues to be of interest after completion of the target study, it is suggested that metabolic studies in animals and in man should precede the design of the chronic studies. This is of importance for proper selection of animal species for the chronic investigations and to provide comparative data to assist in the extrapolation of results in animals to expectations in man.

Special Risks
due to
Inborn Errors
of Metabolism

Supplementary Material to Chapter VIII

In 1923, Garrod published his book, *Inborn Errors of Metabolism*, based on his observations on alcaptonuria begun in 1899 and followed by similar studies on cystinuria, pentosuria, and albinism. Garrod developed the concept that certain diseases of lifelong duration occur because an enzyme governing a single metabolic step possesses reduced activity or is missing altogether. A half century later, LaDu *et al.* (1958) proved Garrod's hypothesis by demonstrating the absence of homogentisic acid oxidase activity in the liver of a patient with alcaptonuria. Beadle (1945) had already enunicated his one gene–one enzyme principle, which stated the following:

- All biochemical processes in all organisms are under genic control.
- These biochemical processes are resolvable into series of individual stepwise reactions.
- Each biochemical reaction is under the ultimate control of a different single gene.
- Mutation of a single gene results only in an alteration in the ability of the cell to carry out a single primary chemical reaction.

By 1971, at least 1,500 distinguishable human diseases were known to be genetically determined (McKusick, 1971), and new examples are being reported annually. Although the molecular basis for most of these diseases is not known, McKusick (1970) has listed 92 human disorders for which a genetically determined, specific enzyme deficiency has been identified. The disorders and the causative enzymes are listed in Table C-3. The third edition of *The Metabolic Basis of Inherited Disease* identifies more than 150 diseases of genetic origin (Stanburg, 1972).

CATEGORIES OF GENETIC ERRORS OF METABOLISM

The 92 presently known human disorders identified by a variation in a specific enzyme can be grouped into five general categories, Table C-1. These five types in turn may be accounted for by a general schema. Figure C-1 shows, in a hypothetic and greatly oversimplified metabolic pathway, how defective enzyme systems derived from mutant genes can lead to the various abnormal conditions given in Table C-1. A mutant gene 3 (in Figure C-1, for Category 1 of Table C-1) may result in either complete or partial inhibition in the conversion of metabolite C, so that the conversion to D does not proceed, or is deficient in amount, resulting in absence or deficiency of an essential substance.

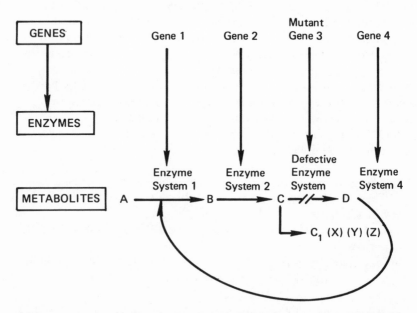

FIGURE C-1   General schema showing how defective genes cause altered metabolism that leads to hypersusceptible reactions.

For Category 2, gene 3 is missing, or so altered that no enzyme 3 is produced or is produced in subnormal amount, leading to a deficiency or absence of an enzyme. For Category 3, defective enzyme 3 is unable to perform metabolic conversion to D at a normal rate, and so alters the rate of cellular transport of metabolite. In Category 4, a mutant gene 3 would appear to offer a rational mechanism for the development of abnormal protein (Category 5): either a double mutation in gene 3, an intracistronic recombination that results in a slightly modified protein denoted by C_1 (as in hemoglobin S with amino acid substitutions), or more profound changes represented by products (X) (Y) or (Z).

The importance for research protocols is that genetic errors of metabolism, with the few exceptions noted later, give rise to exaggerated toxic responses, so-called hypersusceptible or hypersensitivity reactions, which should be identified in any overall toxicologic evaluation of a new substance.

Figure C-2 gives some indication from the more than twofold levels of phenylalanine, what the degree of hyperactivity might be in a phenylketonuric individual further subjected to a substance whose metabolism involves phenylalanine hydroxylase.

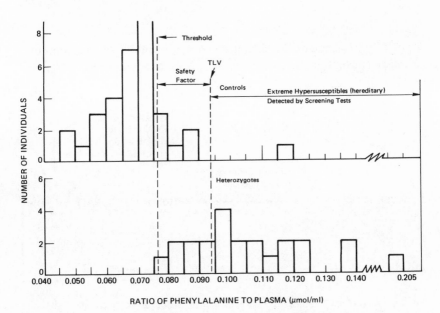

FIGURE C-2   Distribution of plasma phenylalanine level in 33 controls and 23 heterozygous individuals.

GENETIC DEFECTS AFFECTING BROAD CATEGORIES OF CHEMICAL SUBSTANCES

Although the foregoing example concerned a rather restricted group of chemical structures, there are several genetic defects that comprehend a broad spectrum of chemical substances, notably glucose-6-phosphate dehydrogenase (G-6-PD) deficiency, serum antitrypsin (SAT) deficiency, and allergic sensitivity to certain chemicals of commerce. These particular three defects are of more than ordinary importance because of one common characteristic: a high prevalence in either the general population, or among certain ethnic groups. From a survey of a worldwide prevalence of G-6-PD deficiency, Beutler (Beaconsfield, 1965) concluded it to be the most widespread prevalence of a clinically significant human genetic abnormality. Allergic sensitivity (of the ragweed pollen type) is comparable in prevalence to that of G-6-PD deficiency; the prevalence of SAT deficiency, heterozygous form, may occur as high as 5 percent in certain population groups.

CATEGORIES OF CHEMICAL SUBSTANCES SHOWING EXAGGERATED TOXICITY

G-6-PD Deficiency

Table C-2 lists some of the chemical substances and types of groups of chemical substances that can result in hyperactive responses, hemolytic

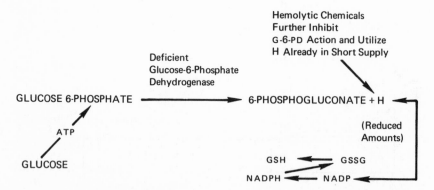

FIGURE C-3   G-6-PD Defective red cell enzyme system. Genetically modified, chemically sensitive, red blood cells with defective G-6-PD cannot maintain NADP and GSSG in reduced form at a rate necessary to maintain red cell integrity in the face of extra demands for H by hemolytic chemicals and drugs. Methemoglobin forms by direct action of chemical metabolites or because inactive catalase allows H_2O_2 to accumulate.

crises, in those individuals with G-6-PD deficient red-cell enzyme system according to the mechanism diagrammed in Figure C-3.

SAT Deficiency

Respiratory irritants, gases, dusts, mists, fumes, and smokes, comprise those substances that can result in an exaggerated response, familial pulmonary emphysema, in those individuals with serum antitrypsin deficiency according to the mechanism outlined below.

Basis of Test for Detecting Serum α_1-Antitrypsin (SAT) Deficiency.

1. The antitrypsin factor, a glycoprotein, is 90 percent in the α_1-globulin fraction of serum.

2. Normally, antitrypsin prevents proteinases (trypsins) from attacking pulmonary alveolar walls.

3. Persons deficient in SAT factors and exposed to respiratory irritants increase risk of inability to counteract trypsin activity and thus increase risk of pulmonary emphysema.

A Simple Test—The capacity of the patient's serum to prevent known amounts of trypsin from digesting gelatin is a measure of the amount of serum antitrypsin and, hence, a measure of the defect.

Allergic Sensitization

The substances capable of allergic sensitization in hypersensitive reactors comprise those with antigenic or haptenic structures, foreign proteins—simple or complex—or chemicals with strong haptenic structures, such as the industrial organic isocyanates represented in Figure C-4 along with their mode of action.

ADVANTAGEOUS EFFECTS OF INBORN METABOLIC ERRORS

It is of interest to note that not all of the physiologic consequences of defective enzyme systems are deleterious. It is recognized, for example, that G-6-PD deficiency, which is related to a low reduced glutathione in the red-blood cell, acts favorably to prevent the development of falciparum malaria, which has high metabolic requirements for the reduced form of glutathione, GSH.

This same enzyme defect has been correlated with a marked decrease in carcinoma rates for selected sites for Israeli Jews among certain racial subgroups of whom the G-6-PD deficiency incidence may be as high as 60 percent; carcinoma rates for stomach, colon, pancreas, and kidney were markedly lower among oriental Jews as compared to occidental

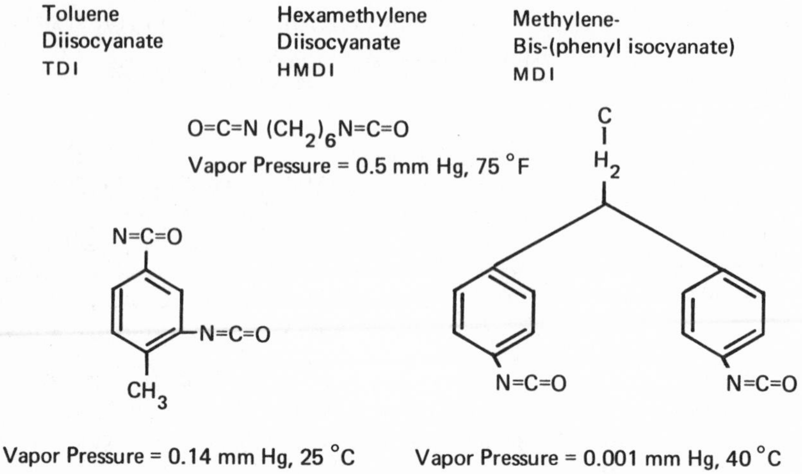

Toluene	Hexamethylene	Methylene-
Diisocyanate	Diisocyanate	Bis-(phenyl isocyanate)
TDI	HMDI	MDI

$$O=C=N \ (CH_2)_6 N=C=O$$

Vapor Pressure = 0.5 mm Hg, 75 °F

Vapor Pressure = 0.14 mm Hg, 25 °C   Vapor Pressure = 0.001 mm Hg, 40 °C

FIGURE C-4 Industrially important isocyanates in plastic coating of foaming operations (polyurethane foam). Nitrogen–carbon–oxygen groups of the isocyanates combine with protein to form a ureido linkage with proteins (antigens), which gives rise to antigenically distinct antibodies. Hapten-specific antigens have been made in the laboratory and can be used (1) to identify past exposure to isocyanates and (2) to determine hypersensitivity to these isocyanates.

Jews (e.g., stomach, 120 versus 258; colon, 22 versus 70; pancreas, 24 versus 48; kidney, 10 versus 36 respectively) (Beaconsfield, 1965).

It is apparent that, of the 92 defects with recognized specific enzyme deficiencies, the 3 noted above alone embrace a wide and varied range of inciting substances for those harboring these defects. It now remains to consider the required protocol for identifying those substances newly introduced into the environment that can pose additional health problems for certain of the genetically defective members of the population.

PROTOCOL FOR IDENTIFYING SUBSTANCES WHOSE TOXICITY MAY BE MODIFIED BY INBORN ERRORS OF METABOLISM

The indicated protocol for identifying substances posing additional health problems among genetically defective groups can be a simple consideration of

1. The chemical structural relationships of the substance under investigation with that of substances known to act unfavorably in a defective system (e.g., substances bearing the primaquin-type structure or the sulfonamide structure, or which can be metabolized to these structures), and

2. The metabolic enzyme relationships to those given in Table C-3 (e.g., substances with structures affecting cholinesterases, such as organophosphate insecticide-like structures, Item 11, Table C-3).

No simple screening procedure is available; however, some interesting advancements are being made in special inbred strains of animal carrying genetic defects. This field of research has not yet advanced to practical laboratory procedures that could be used to predict special toxic responses in people with inborn errors of metabolism.

REFERENCES

Beaconsfield, P., R. Rainsbury, and G. Kalton. 1965. Glucose-6-phosphate dehydrogenase deficiency and the incidence of cancer. *Oncologia* 19:11.

Beadle, G.W. 1945. Biochemical genetics. *Chem. Rev.* 37:15.

LaDu et al. 1958. The nature of the defect in tyrosine metabolism in alcaptonuria. *J. Biol. Chem.* 230:251.

McKusick, V.A. 1970. Human genetics. *Ann. Rev. Genet.* 4:1.

McKusick, V.A. 1971. *Mendelian Inheritance in Man*, 3rd ed. Johns Hopkins Press, Baltimore.

Stanbury, J.B. *et al.*, eds. 1972. *The Metabolic Basis of Inherited Disease,* 3rd ed., McGraw-Hill Book Co., New York City.

Stokinger, H.E., and J.T. Mountain. 1963. Test for hypersusceptibility to hemolytic chemicals. *Arch. Environ. Health* 6:495–502.

TABLE C-1   Categories of Genetic Variation in Man

Category	Example
1. Essential substance missing or deficient	α_1 Antitrypsin deficiency
2. Enzyme system missing or deficient	Glucose-6-phosphate dehydrogenase
3. Alteration in cellular transport of metabolite	CS_2 Sensitivity
4. Abnormal antibody production	Reaginic antibodies to allergenic pollen antigens in "hayfever" cross-reacting to certain industrial chemicals
5. Presence of abnormal protein	Hemoglobin S in sickle-cell anemia

TABLE C-2   Some Hemolytic Industrial Chemicals

Acetanilid	Cresol	o-Nitrochlorobenzenes
		Oxygen (Hyperbaric)
Amyl nitrite	Dinitrobenzenes	p-Phenylenediamine
Aniline	Dinitrotoluenes	Phenylhydrazine
Arsine	Guaiacol	Phosphorus
Benzene	Hydroxylamine	Selenium dioxide
Benzidine	Lead	Stibine
Carbon tetrachloride	Methylcellosolve	Tetrachloroethane
Chlorate	Naphthalene	Toluidine
Chloronitrobenzenes	Nitric oxide	Toluylenediamine
Chloroprene monomer	Nitrites	Trinitrotoluene
	Nitrosamines	
Antimalarial and numerous N-containing drugs		

SOURCE: Stokinger and Mountain (1963).

TABLE C-3   Disorders in which a Deficient Activity of a specific Enzyme has been demonstrated in Man

Condition	Enzyme with Deficient Activity
Acatalasia	Catalase
Acid phosphatase deficiency	Lysosomal acid phosphatase
Adrenal hyperplasia I	21-hydroxylase[a]
Adrenal hyperplasia II	11-beta-hydroxylase[a]
Adrenal hyperplasia III	3-beta-hydroxysteroid dehydrogenase[a]
Adrenal hyperplasia V	17-hydroxylase[a]
Albinism	Tyrosinase
Aldosterone synthesis, defect in	18-hydroxylase[a]
Alkaptonuria	Homogentisic acid oxidase
Angiokeratoma, diffuse (Fabry)	Ceramidetrihexosidase
Apnea, drug-induced	Pseudocholinesterase
Argininemia	Arginase
Argininosuccinic aciduria	Argininosuccinase
Aspartylglycosaminuria	Specific hydrolase (AADC-ase)
Carnosinemia	Carnosinase
Cholesterol ester deficiency (Norum's disease)	Lecithin cholesterol acetyltransferase (LCAT)
Citrullinemia	Arginosuccinic acid synthetase
Crigler–Najiar syndrome	Glucuronyl transferase
Cystathioninuria	Cystathionase
Formiminotransferase deficiency	Formiminotransferase
Fructose intolerance	Fructose-1-phosphate aldolase
Fructosuria	Hepatic fructokinase[a]
Fucosidosis	Fucosidase
Galactokinase deficiency	Galactokinase
Galactosemia	Galactose-1-phosphate uridyl transferase
Gangliosidosis, generalized	β-galactosidase
Gaucher's disease	Glucocerebrosidase

TABLE C-3   (continued)

Condition	Enzyme with Deficient Activity
G-6-PD deficiency (favism, primaquine sensitivity, nonspherocytic hemolytic anemia)	Glucose-6-phosphate dehydrogenase
Glycogen storage disease I	Glucose-6-phosphatase
Glycogen storage disease II	Alpha-1-4-glucosidase
Glycogen storage disease III	Amylo-1-6-glucosidase
Glycogen storage disease IV	Amylo (1-4 to 1-6) transglucosidase
Glycogen storage disease V	Muscle phosphorylase
Glycogen storage disease VI	Liver phosphorylase[a]
Glycogen storage disease VII	Muscle phosphofructokinase
Glycogen storage disease VIII	Liver phosphorylase kinase
Gout, primary (one form)	Hypoxanthine guanine phosphoribosyl-transferase
Hemolytic anemia	Diphosphoglycerate mutase
Hemolytic anemia	Glutathione peroxidase
Hemolytic anemia	Glutathione reductase
Hemolytic anemia	Hexokinase
Hemolytic anemia	Hexosephosphate isomerase
Hemolytic anemia	Phosphoglycerate kinase
Hemolytic anemia	Pyruvate kinase
Hemolytic anemia	Triosephosphate isomerase
Histidinemia	Histidase
Homocystinuria	Cystathione synthetase
Hydroxyprolinemia	Hydroxyproline oxidase
Hyperammonemia I	Ornithine transcarbamylase
Hyperammonemia II	Carbamyl phosphate synthetase
Hyperglycinemia, ketotic form	Propionate carboxylase[a]
Hyperlysinemia	Lysine-ketoglutarate reductase
Hyperoxaluria I Glycolic aciduria	2-oxo-glutarate-glyoxylate carboligase
II Glyceric aciduria	D-glyceric dehydrogenase
Hyperprolinemia I	Proline oxidase deficiency
Hyperprolinemia II	δ-1-pyrroline-5-carboxylate dehydrogenase[a]
Hypophosphatasia	Alkaline phosphatase
Isovalericacidemia	Isovaleric acid CoA dehydrogenase
Lactase deficiency, adult, intestinal	Lactase
Lactose intolerance of infancy	Lactase
Leigh's necrotizing encephalomyelopathy	Pyruvate carboxylase
Lesch–Nyhan syndrome	Hypoxanthine-guanine phosphoribosyl-transferase
Lipase deficiency, congenital	Lipase (pancreatic)
Lysine intolerance	L-lysine:NAD-oxido-reductase
Mannosidosis	α-mannosidase
Maple sugar urine disease	Keto acid decarboxylase
Metachromatic leukodystrophy	Arylsulfatase A (sulfatide sulfatase)
Methemoglobinemia	NADH-methemoglobin reductase
Methylmalonicaciduria	Methylmalonyl-CoA carboxymutase

TABLE C-3 (continued)

Condition	Enzyme with Deficient Activity
Myeloperoxidase deficiency with disseminated candidiasis	Myeloperoxidase
Niemann-Pick disease	Sphingomyelinase
Oroticaciduria	Orotidylic pyrophosphorylase orotidylic decarboxylase
Phenylketonuria	Phenylalanine hydroxylase
Porphyria, congenital erythropoietic	Uroporphyrinogen III cosynthetase
Pulmonary emphysema	α_1-antitrypsin
Pyridoxine-dependent	Glutamic acid decarboxylase[a]
Pyridoxine-responsive anemia	δ-aminolevulinic acid synthetase[a]
Refsum's disease	Phytanic acid α-oxidase
Sarcosinemia	Sarcosine dehydrogenase[a]
Sucrose intolerance	Sucrose, isomaltase
Sulfite oxidase deficiency	Sulfite oxidase
Tay-Sachs disease	Hexosaminidase A
Testicular feminization	Δ^4-5α-reductase[a]
Thyroid hormonogenesis, defect in	Iodothyrosine dehalogenase (deiodinase)
Trypsinogen deficiency disease	Trypsinogen
Tyrosinemia I	Para-hydroxyphenylpyruvate oxidase
Tyrosinemia II	Tyrosine transaminase
Valinemia	Valine transaminase
Vitamin D resistant rickets	Cholecalciferase[a]
Wolman's disease	Acid lipase
Xanthinuria	Xanthine oxidase
Xanthurenic aciduria	Kynureninase
Xeroderma pigmentosa	Ultraviolet specific endonuclease[a]

SOURCE: Adapted from McKusick (1970).

[a] In some conditions marked in this way (as well as some that are not listed) deficiency of a particular enzyme is suspected but has not been proved by direct study of enzyme activity.

D

Environmental Toxicology

Supplementary Material to Chapter XIII

TERRESTRIAL TEST SPECIES

Considerably less work has been done on terrestrial species (exclusive of crop plants) than on aquatic. Because there is a paucity of literature on certain terrestrial groups, the reasons for selection of test species are considered at some length. Selection of test species will depend on usages and geographic areas, i.e., mink and fish-eating birds for stable, lipid, soluble material that escapes into Lake Michigan.

Microorganisms

Experience indicates that most of the soil microorganisms are highly resistant to effects of environmental chemicals at the concentrations usually found in the field, the principal exception being the nitrifying bacteria. (An exception is the fungicidal class, members of which are highly antimicrobial.) Thus, it is comparatively unlikely that the balance of these organisms will be directly affected. However, chemicals could readily alter availability of oxygen and nitrogen, etc., which could have profound effects on the microflora and fauna. A main thrust for the use of these organisms would be to study the conversion of the original toxicants to metabolites.

Vegetation

The choice of vegetation types depends upon the problem under investigation. No specific test species have been developed for these toxicological type studies, although many are commonly used in laboratories. In specific studies the use of lichens and/or mosses might be advantageous. However, in most cases, angiosperms should be used—gymnosperms in a few study areas. Due to the many choices available, recommendations have been broken down into use types with two or three examples. It must be borne in mind that with certain pollutants, considerable variation in response exists between cultivars within a species as well as between species. Experience to date suggests that generalities in terms of family or genera susceptibilities are impossible.

1. Gymnosperms—pine, larch
2. Angiosperms (species of economic value; selection of "noneconomic" species should be from those characteristic of the region)

> cereals—oat, rye, corn
> field crop—soybean, peanut, tobacco
> fiber—cotton
> vegetable (leaf)—lettuce, spinach
> vegetable (fruit)—bean, tomato
> vegetable (storage)—potato, radish
> floricultural—rose, petunia
> fruit—strawberry, apple, cherry
> forage—alfalfa, grass, clover
> native—trees, perennial herbaceous, annual

Invertebrates

Earthworms and honeybee would be suggested species for initial tests.

Vertebrates

Reptiles The garter snake (*Thamnophis sirtalis*) has a wide distribution throughout the United States. It can be maintained in captivity and will reproduce in captivity; it is viviparous. Its food includes fish, tadpoles, small mammals, and insects. It is suggested as the primary test species for reptiles. The rat snake (*Elaphe obsoleta*), with closely related species of *Elaphe*, can be found in most parts of the United States. It can be maintained in captivity and reproduces well in captivity; it is oviparous. Its food includes small mammals, young birds, and lizards. It is suggested as a secondary test species. The fence lizard (*Sceloporus*

undulatus) is found in most of the United States except the extreme
northern belt. It can be maintained in captivity but does not reproduce
readily under these conditions. Its food includes insects, spiders, and
snails. It is suggested as secondary test species. The range of the painted
turtle (*Chrysemys picta*) includes much of the eastern, central, and northwestern United States. This species can be maintained in captivity but
does not reproduce well in captivity; it requires several years to mature.
Its food includes fish, frogs, tadpoles, insects, and aquatic plants. It is
suggested as a secondary test species.

Amphibians   Experience with persistent pesticides suggests that amphibians are somewhat more sensitive than reptiles. This difference may be
due to the character of the skin: Reptiles have a heavily keratinized skin,
and respiration is solely through the lungs. Amphibians have a highly
vascularized skin and carry out some dermal respiration. Species tied to
shallow waters are likely to be at greater risk due to lack of dilution and
from oily compounds that are likely to concentrate at the air–water
interface

The leopard frog is widely distributed throughout the United States,
except the Pacific coast. Artificial reproduction can be readily carried
out in the laboratory.

The tiger salamander is distributed throughout the United States, except mountainous areas and the Pacific coast. It is largely a terrestrial
species, which does not reproduce easily in captivity.

The spotted newt is found throughout the eastern half of the United
States. It is largely an aquatic species (the eft stage is terrestrial). It does
not reproduce readily in captivity.*

Birds   The mallard is widely distributed throughout the United States. It
can be maintained and bred in captivity readily and has been widely used
for toxicological studies.

The robin is widely distributed throughout the United States. The
Organisation for European Co-operation and Development (OECD)
species for a worm-eating bird is the woodcock (*Philohela minor*), but
this is a very difficult bird to keep in captivity (W.H. Stickel, private communication, 1972). The robin would be easier, although no earthworm-
eater is easy. The supply of food alone can be a considerable difficulty.

The bird-eating birds that have been shown to be most affected by
persistent pesticides, i.e., peregrine (*Falco peregrinus*), European sparrow

* We would like to thank Dr. Harvey Pough, Section of Ecology and Systematics, Cornell
University, for his assistance with Amphibian and Reptiles.

hawk (*Accipiter nisus*), and Cooper's hawk (*A. Cooperii*) (Hickey, 1969; Ratcliffe, 1970) are not readily bread in captivity. The American kestrel (*Falco sparverius*), although not primarily a bird-eater, will eat birds and is in the same genera as the peregrine. This species has been shown to be sensitive, in the case of persistent pesticides, to contaminants of the environment (Porter and Wiemeyer, 1972; Peakall *et al.*, in press) and can be bred in captivity (Willoughby and Cade, 1964). The chemical levels would be expected to be considerably lower for a field monitoring species, at least for persistent lipid soluble materials, than for the species listed above, which are at a higher trophic level.

The night heron breeds throughout the United States except in mountainous areas and has been bred successfully in captivity (Temperley, 1954). Further, since it is a colonial species, it would be possible (indeed, probably necessary) to have many birds in a single cage. This would make for good experimental groups. Kolar (1966) gives an account of a breeding group of 14 cattle egrets (*Bubulcus ibis*) in a cage 15 × 8 × 5 m. Food consists of fish, crustaceans, frogs, and aquatic insects.

The chicken is included as a test species because of its commercial value.

Mammals Domestic species, if feeding on untreated forage, could be used as herbivorous mammals. The rat is included because of its wide-scale use in toxicological work and its ready availability.

Seals are the OECD species and have been shown to have very high levels of organochlorines in some areas (LeBoeuf and Bonnell, 1971; Gaskin *et al.*, 1971). The seal is a difficult and costly animal for laboratory studies. A preferable species would be the mink, which is widely distributed along streams and lakes throughout the United States, except in the arid southwest. Its food includes fish, small mammals, birds, and frogs. Studies with organochlorines suggest that this is a sensitive species (Gilbert, 1969) and can be bred in captivity. This species could be used as both fish-eater and predatory mammal. Another possibility would be to use the red fox as the predatory mammal, but this would be a more difficult experimental animal.

ILLUSTRATIVE SERIES OF TOXICITY TESTS FOR TERRESTRIAL SPECIES

The following suggests a graded series of tests. Once a suitable species has been chosen, a sequence of tests of progressively greater depth can be made.

Minimum Initial Testing (1A–1C)

   1A. Acute toxicity (LD_{50}), two mammals, one bird

   1B. Acute toxicity with invertebrates (two species of different phyla)

   1C. Acute toxicity with plants (three species from different vegetation groupings). Seed germination and seedling growth determination for chemicals with materials added directly to the soil in the course of normal usage (e.g., pesticides, herbicides, fertilizers) and via irrigation water (e.g., industrial materials and sewage effluents). Gross damage photosynthesis and transpiration loss from exposure of 2–4-week-old seedlings in chambers, for chemicals involved in aerial fallout (e.g., around large industrial areas, along highways, from agricultural operations) or in gaseous pollutants (e.g., industrial materials, including products of photochemical reactions).

   If initial testing indicates that the compound is unlikely to accumulate and is not stable, and tests 1A–1C show low toxicity and low damage, then further testing would generally not be required.

   Chronic testing for stable materials (accumulative or not) to include metabolites and products of transformation.

Minimum Testing (2A–2F)

   2A. Chronic feeding studies (90-day on two species of each of the mammals and birds); for one species each, studies to be continued for one year. Reproductive studies on one mammal (observation of such parameters as gestation period, size of litter, number of corpora lutea) and one bird (parameters such as eggs for female, number embryonated, hatching rate, percent raised to given age).

   2B. Acute toxicity to reptiles and amphibians

   2C. Thirty-day tests on soil invertebrates with standard soil (two species, different phyla).

   2D. Tests on nitrifying bacteria

   2E. Thirty-day closed ecosystem tests with radiolabeled compound involving terrestrial degradation, uptake in food chain organisms, determination of nature and amount of degradation products, ecological magnification biodegradability index, and biotransformation in soil

   2F. Chronic studies on vegetation using primarily annual plants. To include continuous and intermittent exposure or growth in both natural and artificial soils to varying toxicant concentrations. Effects on growth, yield, competitive abilities, and reproductive processes to be considered

If these tests do not show serious effects and partition coefficient data do not indicate accumulation, then no further tests would be required. If accumulation or series effects occur, proceed to 3A–3B. Additionally, field studies on seminatural ecosystems (Chapter XVI) would also be required.

Field Studies

3A. Chronic feeding studies on sensitive species at the top trophic levels, i.e., fish-eating mammals and birds, worm-eating birds, and predatory mammals. The feeding should be done in such a manner as to be equivalent to exposure in the natural environment. Reproductive studies with these species would be conducted.

Similar studies on one or more reptiles and amphibia. Pre-adult stages of amphibians may be a sensitive index, i.e., tail resorption and metamorphosis. In this case, environmental stress is superimposed on normal stress. Growth rate of tadpole stage has been shown to be directly correlated with pollutant levels.

3B. Competition studies between two or more plant species over several generations (annual) or for 2–3 years for perennial plants. These test systems could incorporate animals for food chain studies.

ILLUSTRATIVE SERIES OF TOXICITY TESTS FOR AQUATIC SPECIES

1. Exploratory 48-hour static toxicity test with a duplicate to which the test organisms are added 24 hours after the test begins. (For the compounds that are slowly transformed, one week and one month should be considered.) This will demonstrate significant changes in toxicity should they occur. (One marine and freshwater species each, representing fish, invertebrates, and algal groups.)

2. Continuous-flow acute lethality tests should be conducted until a constant proportion of test organisms die. Analytical procedures for the toxic substance and its degradation products in the test water are necessary to specify the quantitative dose–response relationship. (One marine and freshwater species each, representing fish, invertebrates, and algal groups.)

3. Same tests as above, but with three fish, three invertebrate, and three algal (e.g., green and blue-green algae and diatoms) marine and freshwater species to determine range of biological variation within groups of organisms.

4. Continuous-flow toxicity tests up to 30-day duration:

   a. Using the most sensitive marine and freshwater fish species, determine egg, larvae, and juvenile growth and survival, avoidance or attraction of the toxic substance, organoleptic property of toxic substance, and determination of tissue residue with subsequent feeding studies, using a fish-eating species. Fish food organisms, exposed to the toxic substance, should be fed to fish during a 30-day exposure to determine effects of food chain accumulation by fish. Tissue residue analysis of the food and fish are necessary.

    b. Using two invertebrate species with short life cycles from both marine and freshwater environments, determine chronic effects including effects on reproduction, through one generation.

    c. Using two algal species from both marine and freshwater environments, determine effects on growth during a 30-day exposure.

    5. If fish are most sensitive, continue testing with steps 6 and 7; if invertebrates are most sensitive, continue testing with step 8; if algae are most sensitive, additional 30-day tests for population growth (4c) for two additional species are needed; if predator feeding study is most sensitive, continue testing with step 9. When more than one group are generally similar in sensitivity, testing should continue for each of these similar groups.

    6. Continuous-flow, one generation chronic tests, including effects on reproduction, with one marine and freshwater fish species having a short life cycle (6 months or less). The toxic substance and its degradation products will be measured in the test water and tissue residue determinations will be made during and at the end of the chronic test. The loss rate of these residues will be determined also.

    7. Continuous-flow, one-generation chronic tests, including effects on reproduction, with additional fish species having longer life cycles, and a two-generation study with the fish species used in step 6. Water and tissue concentrations of the toxic substance will be measured as in step 6.

    8. Continuous-flow, one- or more-generation (when species has short life cycle), chronic tests including effects on reproduction with four marine and four freshwater invertebrate species.

    9. Chronic feeding studies with representative fish-eating mammal and avian species.

REFERENCES

Gaskin, D.E., M. Holdrinet, and R. Frank. 1971. Organochloride pesticide residues in harbour porpoises from the Bay of Fundy region. *Nature* 233:499–500.

Gilbert, F.F. 1969. Physiological effects of natural DDT residues and metabolites on ranch mink. *J. Wildl. Manage.* 33:933–943.

Hickey, J.J., ed. 1969. *Peregrine Falcon Populations: Their Biology and Decline.* University of Wisconsin Press, Madison. 596 pp.

Kolar, K. 1966. Breeding the cattle egret (*Bubulcus ibis*). *Avic. Mag.* 72:45–46.

LeBoeuf, B.J., and M.L. Bonnell. 1971. DDT in California sea lions. *Nature* 234:108–110.

Peakall, D.B., J.L. Lincer, R.W. Risebrough, J.B. Pritchard, and W.B. Kinter. (In press.) DDE-induced eggshell thinning: Structural and physiological effects in three species. *Comp. Gen. Pharmacol.*

Porter, R.D., and S.N. Wiemeyer. 1972. DDE at low dietary levels kills captive American kestrels. *Bull. Environ. Contam. Toxicol.* 8:193–199.

Ratcliffe, D.A. 1970. Changes attributable to pesticides in egg breakage frequency and eggshell thickness in some British birds. *J. Appl. Ecol.* 7:67–115.

Temperley, G.W. 1954. Night heron in Northumberland. *Br. Birds* 47:351.

Willoughby, E.J., and T.J. Cade. 1964. The breeding behavior of the American kestrel (sparrow hawk). *Living Bird* 3:75–96.

SUGGESTED READINGS

Bloom, S.E., G. Povar, and D.B. Peakall. 1972. Chromosome preparations from the avian allantoic sac. *Stain Technol.* 47:123–127.

Cooke, A.S. 1970. The effect of p,p'-DDT on tadpoles of the common frog (*Rana temporaria*). *Environ. Pollut.* 1:57–71.

Cooke, A.S. 1972. The effects of DDT, dieldrin, and 2,4-D on amphibian spawn and tadpoles. *Environ. Pollut.* 3:51–68.

Heath, R.G., J.W. Spann, and J.F. Kreitzer. 1969. Marked DDT impairment of mallard reproduction in controlled studies. *Nature* 224:47–48.

Mathematical Simulation of Ecosystems, An Example

Supplementary Material to Chapter XIV

An example of one of the more elaborate models designed for dynamic simulation is that of Chen and Orlob (1972) in which 23 variables were utilized. Their model is a mathematical translation of Figure E-1.

The variables in this model are temperature, total dissolved solids, biochemical oxygen demand, pH, carbon, nitrogen (NH_3, NO_2, and NO_3), phosphorus, etc. Biological variables are biomasses of algae (classified into two types according to growth characteristics), zooplankton, cold-water and warm-water fish, and benthos feeders. The physical space considered in the model is dissected into interconnected cells, allowing transfer of mass between cells. Mass balance equations are written to account for changes due to processes such as advection, diffusion, settling, inflow, outflow, decay, chemical transformation, biological uptake, respiration, growth, mortality, and grazing. For each cell there are 23 differential equations, one for each environmental variable.

Very little can be said analytically about such complex systems, so the equations are solved by numerical simulation on a computer. The equations are solved step-by-step to follow the changes in each variable over space and time, with provision for periodic printout of data.

The advantages of such large-scale numerical simulations are (1) the large number of equations that can be handled simultaneously; (2) the ability to utilize nonlinear rate-coefficients for biological processes, as

349

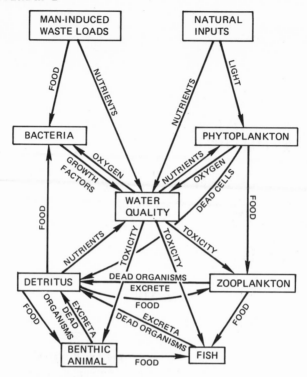

FIGURE E-1   Definition of an Ecosystem (Chen and Orlob, 1972).

derived from experiment; (3) the ability to change rate-coefficients (such as per capita growth rate) at intervals, providing correction mechanisms; and (4) the flexibility in choice of boundary conditions and input values.

The main disadvantage of this kind of computer model is the uncertainty of the "robustness" of the results: that is, their independence of details in the structure of the models, their underlying assumptions, the specific values chosen for the rate constants, and the choice of initial conditions. Other disadvantages include the lack of specific biological information about the behavior of single-species populations and 2-species interactions, and the possible masking of system properties as simple assumptions are made about interactions between components. There are also mathematical difficulties connected with the choice of a finite steplength in proceeding from a differential to a difference equation, even when the rate-coefficients are updated.

REFERENCE

Chen, C.W. and G.T. Orlob. 1972. *Ecologic Simulation for Aquatic Environments.* Report to U.S. Department of the Interior, Office of Water Resources Research. OWRR Report No. C-2044, Washington, D.C.

Atmosphere

Supplementary Material to Chapter XVIII

SOURCES AND DISPERSAL OF ATMOSPHERIC POLLUTION

Short-Range Dispersion

Introduction　The assessment of possible impacts from new toxic air pollutants must include considerations of the meteorological dispersion of these materials. Various types of sources might be involved in the use and dissemination of new compounds. In general it will probably not be possible to have detailed design data on proposed sources; thus the initial assessment of toxic impact will have to depend on basic relationships between meteorological parameters and atmospheric concentrations. The following discussion outlines techniques that can be used to make this initial atmospheric dispersion assessment. This initial assessment should provide indications as to whether atmospheric concentrations might present a toxic or environmental hazard. This described estimation process should provide a conservative estimate of possible atmospheric impacts: If no hazard is indicated, further calculations should not be needed; if some degree of hazard seems to be indicated, measurements and monitoring should be undertaken and the initial evaluation refined on the basis of a more detailed assessment of actual source and meteorological parameters.

Environmental impacts in any initial screening process should be based on an estimate of probable maximum concentrations. These in turn can be calculated using meteorological and topographic parameters that are most conducive to the occurrence of high environmental concentrations, rather than average or mean values. In addition, it has been assumed that these toxic materials will probably be longer term or cumulative hazards rather than acute toxic agents, and thus it has been assumed that the dispersion calculations should estimate likely maximum concentrations for 30-day exposures. If it were useful in a special case, the procedure could be readily modified to estimate either shorter or longer term exposures.

Emission Source Types The downwind dispersion patterns of pollutant emissions are determined to a significant degree by the nature and geometry of the source. Sources may also be classed as instantaneous (e.g., explosions) or continuous. With relatively few exceptions, air pollution sources are   continuous. Also, sources may be classified as point, line, or area. Within each class there can be considereable differences between individual sources; in some cases, there may be some doubt about how a given source should be classed. Thus, some discussion of these three source types may be useful.

The *point source* is typified by the isolated smokestack. In this case, even though the stack may be 30 feet in diameter it is still a "point" insofar as the downwind emission pattern is not affected by the area or dimensions of the source. The height of the emission above the ground is important, but this is not unique to point sources.

A *line source* is defined in mathematical terms as an integrated summation of point sources aligned in a given direction. Probably the most common air pollutant line source is a well-traveled highway where the continual passage of vehicles produces a long ribbon of pollutant that disperses downwind. The line source may be distinguished from the point source not only by geometry but by the fact that crosswind dispersion from a line source is not effective in diluting the emission, whereas crosswind or lateral transport does dilute the emissions from a point source. If a typical highway is taken as an illustration of a line source, it is easy to recognize the fact that crosswinds are ineffective because there is no uncontaminated air available for dilution with the pollutant along a line parallel to the source. In the case of the continuous line source, dilution is brought about only through vertical exchange between polluted and cleaner layers.

The designation of *area source* is most often used as a way of considering the downwind effect of a large number of individually small sources (e.g., automobiles in a downtown commercial area) where it is not possible or at least practical to treat each source individually. By designating the emission source as an area source, one can total all the emissions from the small individual sources and express them on a unit area basis as though the emission occurred uniformly over the area. This is considered reasonable because, outside of the designated area, the pollutant dispersion pattern will not be sensitive to any individual source element but only to the total impact. Once an area source is defined on the basis of the integrated sum of the individual sources, it is often possible to estimate mathematically the downwind impact by postulating this emission to come from an imaginary point or line source.

Briefly, a pollutant emission source can be considered as a point source if both lateral and vertical dispersion processes are important in diluting the emission plume. A source can be classed as a line source if lateral dispersion is relatively ineffective in the dilution process. An area source is a means of treating the summation of a large number of small sources: Mathematically, the downwind dispersion of area source emissions may be treated as either point or line sources, depending on whether lateral dispersion is an important factor in the dilution process.

For the purpose of estimating dispersion in the present discussion, air pollution sources will be related to either of two general configurations—point sources or area sources. Materials that would be used at and possibly released from a limited number of locations (e.g., industrial processes) can be considered as point sources, and the dispersion of the material will be a function of emission factors, distance from the source, and meteorological conditions. The area source type can be used for widely scattered, individually small sources. An automobile or individual home heating system can be considered as a basic component for an area source, while the total emissions from traffic or a residential area would be area source functions.

This classification omits the line source for two reasons: First, the usual line source considered in air pollution problems is the heavily traveled highway; and, for the development of dispersion criteria, it seems sufficient to lump such traffic sources into a community area source along with the traffic from the adjacent roads. Second, to include line source estimates in a preliminary assessment such as this would require more detailed estimates of possible source factors—traffic flow rates, for example—than would normally be available for a preliminary assessment. Aircraft operations offer another possible line source with takeoff and landing patterns. For this initial evaluation, however, this type of source could probably be considered as an area source, when assessing effects close to the airport, and as point source for more distant impacts.

Dispersion Estimates for Point Sources* Point source dispersion estimates can be made using an adaption of Gaussian plume dispersion techniques for long-term average concentrations (Slade, 1968). The following assumptions are made for the estimation of toxic material dispersion:

1. The source emission rate is constant.
2. The wind frequency considered is the maximum 30-day frequency from one of sixteen 22.5 degree sectors.
3. The effluent is uniformly distributed crosswind within the sector.
4. All effluents from the source come from a single stack of effective stack height of 10 meters.
5. The distance to the maximum calculated concentration is 150 meters.

The equation used to estimate the concentration-related impact from a point source is the following:

$$\overline{C} = \frac{2FQ}{\sqrt{2\pi}\sigma_z u \left(\frac{2\pi x}{16}\right)} \exp\left[-\frac{1}{2}\left(\frac{H}{\sigma_z}\right)^2\right], \tag{1}$$

where $\overline{C}$ = 30-day average concentration, g/m^3;
F = frequency of wind in the given sector;
Q = emission rate, g/s;
σ_z = vertical dispersion coefficient (a function of stability and distance), m;
u = average wind speed for the sector being considered, m/s;
x = downwind distance, m; and
H = effective stack height, m.

In order to provide a general guide for a maximum concentration estimate or toxic substance impact, it is necessary to postulate likely values for both the meteorological parameters and the emission parameters. The assumed parameter values are $H = 10$ m, $x = 150$ m, $u = 2$ m/s (4.5 mph), $\sigma_z = 6.6$ m (neutral stability, $x = 150$ m), maximum wind direction frequency $F = 0.40$. Substituting these parameter values in the dispersion equation gives

$$\overline{C} = 3.8 \times 10^{-5} Q. \tag{2}$$

*This procedure follows the methods described in "Background Information—Proposed National Emission Standards for Hazardous Air Pollutants: Asbestos, Beryllium, Mercury", Appendix, EPA, Office of Air Programs, Publ. No. APTD-0753 (Dec., 1971).

Because of the parameter values, this expression gives an estimate of the expected maximum value in an urban area and is obviously dependent on these numerical values. The value for stack height (*H*) of 10 meters is equivalent to a small stack or roof emission point typical of a large fraction of small industrial sources. A taller stack, such as a power plant, would reduce significantly the ground level concentration. The 150-meter distance approximates the point of maximum concentration for the assumed meteorological and stack parameters. The average wind speed of 2 m/s is observed as a long term average in some urban and industrial areas, especially where surrounding topography restricts the general wind flow. Neutral stability is selected because it will generally be characteristic of atmospheric dispersion conditions when maximum concentrations are affecting nearby areas. Slightly unstable conditions could be considered for many well-developed urban areas because of heat island effects and turbulence caused by wind flow over buildings. The choice of stability class and the distance for the calculated concentration determines the value of the diffusion coefficient, σ_z. The maximum monthly wind frequency assumed for a single sector is 0.40, which is indicative of a strongly channelled wind frequency. Wind frequencies of this magnitude may be found in some valleys or in some coastal areas where topography combines with a sea breeze cycle to provide a very restricted wind regime.

It should be emphasized that these parameter values are not necessarily typical values, but they are conditions that could be expected to occur and lead to maximum effluent concentrations. Observed conditions in a community in most situations would be expected to be lower in concentration than calculated from Eq. (2) and the set of parameters we have assumed.

Dispersion Estimates for Area Sources   Area source dispersion estimates can be made using the urban area air pollution potential model as described by Holzworth (1972). This model can provide a concentration averaged over the whole urban area as a function of area emission rate, urban mixing layer depth, wind speed, and city size. Urban-area average concentration, $\overline{C}$, may be obtained from

$$\overline{C} = \overline{Q} \left[3.613 \, D^{0.130} + \frac{S}{2Du} - \frac{0.088uD^{1.260}}{S} \right], \tag{3}$$

where $\overline{Q}$ = average area emission rate, g/m^2 sec^{-1} ;

      D = average depth of urban mixing layer, m;

      S = distance across the urban area, m; and

      u = mixing layer wind speed, m/s.

As in the calculations for point source emissions, it is useful in the case of environmental hazard estimates to select a set of parameter values that are representative of generally restrictive dispersion conditions in major urban areas. For this discussion the parameter values that have been selected are $D = 300$ m, $u = $ m/s, $S = 50$ km. The mixing layer depth of 300 meters is representative of high potential air pollution episodes where, even though strong stability occurs, urban heating and building roughness prevent a lower inversion base from occurring. A wind as low as 3 m/s averaged for 30 days through the mixing or transport layer probably occurs during high pollution potential periods and has been reported as an annual mean mixing layer wind for a limited number of stations by Holzworth. This wind is higher than the wind used in the point source equation because it includes winds through the depth of the 300 meters mixing layer, rather than just surface winds as in the case of the point source calculation. A city size of 50 km is probably equal to or greater than the size of most urban areas, with the possible exception of the Los Angeles basin.

Substituting these values into Holzworth's area source equation gives

$$\overline{C} = 35\overline{Q}, \tag{4}$$

where $\overline{C}$ is the 30-day average concentration (g/m^3) of the material over the urban area and $\overline{Q}$ is the average emission in g/m^2 s^{-1}. This value of 35 for the $\overline{C}/\overline{Q}$ ratio is lower than Holzworth's calculations of the ratio exceeded on 10 percent of the mornings in a number of areas in the United States. It is reasonable in this case that a value intended to apply to a period as long as 30 days would be less than a value for a portion of a day. Thus, the expression given above seems to be a reasonable one to use as an initial estimation procedure for maximum 30-day concentrations of possible toxic emissions from urban area sources.

Transport and Removal of Atmospheric Substances over Large Distances[†]

Introduction In this section a practical procedure is described for estimating long-term ground level air concentrations and deposition of pollutants injected into the atmosphere at or near ground level. The reader should be aware that such estimates prepared at this time are far from perfect; thus, a large uncertainty range should be attached

---

[†]This section is taken from an unpublished report by L. Machta, G. Ferber and J. Heffter of the Air Resources Laboratories, NOAA, prepared under contract to the USAEC Division of Biomedical and Environmental Research.

to predicted values, and continued research and development should be encouraged to improve the estimates.

Transport near the source derives from wind roses; the remaining first traverse around the world is based on a climatology of trajectories in the lower atmosphere; the remaining atmospheric lifetime is based on a zonally uniform pollutant concentration and simple numerical two dimensional (vertical and north–south) model of turbulent mixing. Removal by precipitation is derived from maps of average precipitation amounts and the estimated fraction of scavengeable material deposited per unit area on the earth's surface per unit amount of rainfall. Removal at the ground by impaction or other physical or biological processes is accommodated by the concept of the deposition velocity (the ratio of deposition per unit time to the air concentration near the ground). The composite effect of precipitation scavenging and dry deposition also can be incorporated in the concept of a mean residence time. In general, the settling of large particles occurs near a source (if at or near ground level); hence, no account is taken of the gravitational descent of particles beyond that in the deposition velocity.

The time interval over which the "long-term average" concentration is computed depends on the need of the user. The illustration below treats an annual interval, but the principle is equally applicable to a season or even a month. The annual average might be improved by averaging the contributions derived individually from the 4 seasons or 12 months.

The procedure applies to a single point source; emissions from many widespread sources can be obtained by summing the contributions from each.

Finally, it should be noted that the procedures suggested below can undoubtedly be automated. Computers would be required to cope with widespread sources whose distributions are superimposed on one another during the first circuit around the earth.

Transport and Dilution   In the example used, a site in Illinois is selected and the emission rate is assumed to be one gram per year. For any other case, the predicted concentrations should be multiplied by the actual source strength in grams per year. The worldwide distribution of a continuous source of material emitted at ground level for a period of one year from a point source is considered in the following four successive phases.

Phase 1   Pollutant travel times up to about 6 hours or distances to about 150 km are evidenced. In this earliest phase, a local wind rose is used to determine the horizontal distribution of the average annual concentration at ground level. Material emitted continuously throughout the year is assigned to each sector in proportion to the frequency of time during which the wind direction lies in the sector. The vertical distribution of material is given by a half-Gaussian distribution whose mean is centered at ground level; the standard deviation of the Gaussian curve can be related to the vertical diffusion coefficient as shown below. The formula for the mean concentration at ground level from a continuous point source, $\bar{C}$, is

$$\bar{C} = \left(\frac{2}{\pi}\right)^{1/2} \frac{Qf}{\bar{u}\,\theta\,x\,\sigma_z}, \tag{5}$$

where $\sigma_z = \sqrt{2\,K_z t}$;

K_z = vertical diffusion coefficient = 5 m^2/s;

Q = emission rate (= 1 g/yr = 3.2×10^{-8} g/s;

f = frequency of wind in sector;

$\bar{u}$ = mean wind speed in sector, m/s;

θ = sector width (22½ degrees or $\pi/8$);

x = distance from source, m; and

t = plume travel time, s.

Numerical values for $\bar{u}$ and f for each sector were obtained from a wind rose at the source location, and Eq. (5) was used to calculate concentrations at various distances from the source. Concentrations were plotted on a map and isolines were drawn to produce Figure F-1.

Phase 2 Travel times of several days and distances up to several thousands of kilometers are involved. The correct method for estimating the lateral spread of material at these greater distances would involve a climatology of trajectories. It is entirely feasible to prepare such trajectories, although it may be costly in terms of computer time. In the example, a subjective estimate of the average path of air parcels, starting initially in the direction of the wind rose sectors but then curved when deemed necessary to fit annual average lower atmosphere airflow patterns, has been substituted for a more rigorous trajectory climatology. Every air parcel leaving the source is presumed to remain within one of the curved sectors extending across the eastern United States. For the nonmeteorologist, it may be noted that the prevailing wind blows mainly from west to east. Hence, those air parcels starting toward the West will relatively quickly curve either northward or southward and then move toward the East. The average ground level concentrations in the second phase were obtained from the formula,

$$\bar{C} = \left(\frac{2}{\pi}\right)^{1/2} \frac{Qf}{\bar{u}\,d\,\sigma_z}, \tag{6}$$

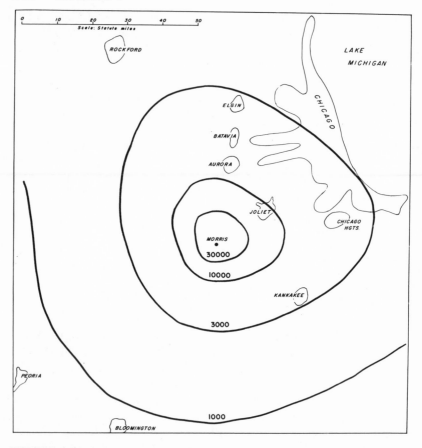

FIGURE F-1   Mean annual surface air concentration (10^{-26} g/cm^3) from the release of 1 g/yr at Morris, Illinois (Phase 1).

where symbols and parameter values are the same as in Eq. (5), except that d is the distance across the extended sector and $\bar{u}$ = 7.5 m/s. Calculated concentrations were plotted on a map and isolines drawn to produce Figure F-2.

Phase 3   This phase deals with transport beyond the Atlantic Ocean until a return to the United States (about 30 days). The average direction of the airflow is from west to east, but the undulations in this flow were obtained from average monthly charts of low level airflow. The typical wind speed for transit through the first few days is taken as 7.5 m/s (15 knots) increasing gradually to 12.5 m/s (25 knots) as the plume of material spreads upward and is transported by stronger winds at higher

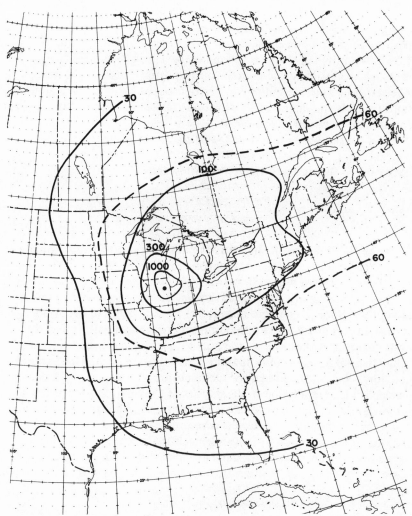

FIGURE F-2 Mean annual surface air concentration (10^{-26} g/cm³) from the release of 1 g/yr at Morris, Illinois (Phase 2).

altitudes. The horizontal spread at the distance of Europe is based on an assumed linear increase in the lateral standard deviation of a Gaussian distribution with travel time; σ_y (nautical miles) $= 2t$, where t is travel time in hours. Actually available tracer information suggests that $\sigma_y = t$ for individual clouds of material (instantaneous releases). This rate of lateral spread has been somewhat arbitrarily doubled here to account for the effects of long-term meander of a continuous plume as well as the spread around the center of mass of the instantaneous position of the plume. However, after 15 days of lateral spread, the growth with time of the lateral standard deviation is stopped to prevent an unrealistically wide north–south spread from 15 to 30 days. The vertical diffusion coefficient is here taken as 6 m² /s. The assumed transit speeds and lateral and vertical standard deviations of the Gaussian spread may be found in Table F-1.

For a continuous ground-level point source, the long-term average concentration at a point on the earth's surface at a distance y from the centerline of the mean air trajectory noted above is given by

$$C = \frac{Q}{\pi \, \sigma_y \, \sigma_z \, u} \, \exp \left(-\frac{y^2}{2\sigma_y{}^2} \right). \tag{7}$$

Figure F-3 is derived from the above information. The approximate travel time in days to various distances along the centerline of the average plume motion is shown in the figure.

Phase 4   Range of time elapsed is from the end of the first transit around the globe to the time of uniform concentration in the atmosphere. In this phase, it is assumed that there is zonal uniformity; that is, every location at the same latitude possesses the same concentration. Thus, there is no net transport and further dilution occurs only upward and north–south. The model for such dilution has been programmed on an electronic computer given the physics of the dilution process and an assumed grid spacing. The usual, if not exclusive, dilution mechanism assumes that the flux of a conservative property (e.g., pollutant material) lies in the direction of the gradient of the property (from high towards low concentrations) with the proportionality constant called

TABLE F-1   Transport and Diffusion Parameter Values

Time (d)	Wind Speed (average over trajectory) (knots)	σ_y (10^7 cm)	$4\,\sigma_y$ (° lat.)	σ_z (10^5 cm)
9	17.0	8.0	30	3.0
12	17.5	10.6	40	3.6
15	18.0	13.4	50	4.0
18	18.3	13.4	50	4.4
21	19.0	13.4	50	4.6
24	20.0	13.4	50	5.0
27	20.5	13.4	50	5.2
30	21.0	13.4	50	5.6

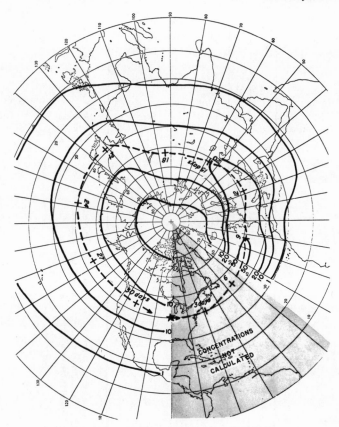

FIGURE F-3 Mean annual surface air concentration (10^{-26} g/cm^3) from the release of 1 g/yr at Morris, Illinois (Phase 3). [*See* Figures F-1 and F-2 for concentrations in shaded area.]

the eddy diffusion coefficient (K_y or K_z). The turbulent diffusive character of the atmosphere in the vertical and north–south direction is incorporated in the choice of the eddy diffusion coefficients. These vary with latitude, altitude, and season. The vertical diffusion coefficient is 5–7 orders of magnitude smaller than the horizontal diffusion coefficient on this global scale. The vertical diffusion intensity is smaller, on the average, in the stratosphere than in the troposphere. Selection of the values for the eddy diffusion coefficients is based on experience in fitting tracers on a global scale.

It must be recognized that the model is rather crude: Not only may the eddy diffusion coefficients be in error by a factor of two (or in some cases even more), but organized meridional circulations, such as

TABLE F-2 Preliminary Estimates of Average Surface-Air Concentration of Pollutants

Concentrations by Latitude, 10^{-26} g/cm³ of air

Year	90–70°N	70–50°N	50–30°N	30–10°N	10°N–10°S	10–30°S	30–50°S	50–70°S	70–90°S
1[a]	42.87	42.57	40.24	32.54	22.71	16.27	13.73	12.08	11.11
2	25.36	25.14	24.87	24.60	24.19	23.83	23.61	23.46	23.38
All Latitudes									
3	24								
4	23								
5	23								
6	23								
7	23								
8[b]	22								

NOTE: There is 1 gram input in a 30–50°N latitude band.
[a] First year values are actually the contributions to the mean annual concentration from the end of month 1 to the end of month 12 (11/12 of the average concentration during this period). To obtain total mean annual concentration, add the value from Figure F-1, F-2 or F-3.
[b] Concentration remains constant at 22×10^{-26} g/cm³ for all subsequent years.

the Hadley cell, have not yet been included in the model. With respect to the omission of the circulations, the eddy diffusion coefficients based on past tracers also ignored the circulation so that the selected values do include the effects of the organized circulation (insofar as the observed distributions of tracers reflect them).

Table F-2 exhibits the mean annual concentrations in 20° latitude bands (the north–south grid spacing) of the dispersed material. The source in this case operates for 1 year and is then shut off permanently. Even in the second year the north–south gradient is very small and, after the second year, the difference is too small to record.

For the first year after a continuous release begins, the mean annual concentration at any location is obtained by adding the value from Figures F-1, F-2 or F-3 to the value in Table F-2. For succeeding years, only Table F-2 is needed.

Effects of Precipitation Scavenging   In the first method of accounting for precipitation scavenging to be discussed here, the initial step in calculating the air concentration and the deposition of material from the atmosphere involves the calculations described in the previous section leading to patterns of air concentration without any scavenging. Engelmann (1970) has collected data from many sources and under diverse meteorological conditions, which yield the ratio of concentration of pollutants in rainwater (or melted snow, which henceforth will be understood when rainwater is stated) to that in air at ground level. If the ratio of the two concentrations is expressed per unit mass (i.e., grams of material per gram water to grams of material per gram air), then most of the observed ratios lie in the range of 100–1000. We somewhat arbitrarily select a ratio of 500. It can be shown that this leads to an annual amount of material deposited per inch of rainfall equal to 10^6 times the ground level annual average air concentration per cubic centimeter (such as g/cm^3). The data that Engelmann used are from cases that had either a uniform concentration of material to the top of the rain-bearing layer (say to about 4 km) or an increasing concentration of material with altitude. However, during the early stages of the plume from a point source, the concentration decreases with altitude and, at first, there is no material present through a substantial layer of the atmosphere above the plume and below the rain-bearing clouds. A correction for this difference between the Engelmann data and that of the present discussion must be made.

The annual deposition can be related to the ground level air concentration to about 30 days through the formula,

$$D = 10^6 \, CPfa,$$

(8)

where D = annual deposition per unit area, (g/cm^2/yr);

C = the mean annual surface air concentration, g/cm^3 as read from Figures F-1, F-2 or F-3;

P = the annual precipitation in inches;

f = a depletion factor which corrects C for the amount of depletion because of prior removal; and

a = a factor which adjusts for the dissimilarity between the vertical distribution of the single source plume and Engelmann's data (converts surface air concentration to average concentration in layer from the ground up to 4 km).

The depletion factor, f, is obtained by successive applications of the formula, and typical values will be given later for the case of the hypothetical source in Illinois.

The adjustment factor, a, is given in Table F-3. The lower (relative to surface air concentration) amounts of deposition occur when the material is more concentrated near the ground than throughout the layer below the raining clouds. There are two modes of scavenging of material by falling precipitation: The first, *rainout,* occurs during the formation of the liquid or ice particles and the second, *washout,* during the descent of the raindrops or ice crystals. Rainout depends largely on the content of the pollutant material at the level of water cloud formation. Definitive data on the relative importance of the two modes of scavenging are not now available.

The deposition formula for precipitation scavenging has been applied to Figures F-1, F-2 and F-3. For the immediate area (Figure F-1) one need only change the labels on the lines, as indicated in Table F-4, since the fraction removed during transit through this nearby area is small

TABLE F-3 Adjustment Factor, a, for Scavenging of a Nonuniform Vertical Distribution Concentration During the Early Phases of a Pollutant Cloud

Travel Time, h	Adjustment Factor, a
0–4	0.08
6	0.14
11	0.20
22	0.28
37	0.38
55	0.45
72	0.50
72–96	0.57
96–120	0.62
120–144	0.67

NOTE: Assume a = 1 after the first week of plume travel.

TABLE F-4 Precipitation Scavenging in the Vicinity of Morris, Illinois

Surface-Air Concentration, 10^{-26} g/cm^3	Annual Wet Deposition, 10^{-18} g/cm^2
30,000	820
10,000	270
3,000	82
1,000	27

(about 6% out to 6 h of travel), a uniform rainfall of 34 inches per year may be assumed constant (0.08).

The mean annual rainfall pattern (Figure F-4) was used with the surface air concentrations in Figure F-2 to obtain the total annual deposition pattern over the eastern United States (Figure F-5) from Eq. (8). Integrations of the material deposited were calculated at various distances from the source to determine the rate of depletion of the plume. The mean annual surface air concentration, taking into account depletion due to precipitation removal is shown in Figure F-6. This may be compared with Figure F-2 where precipitation scavenging was not considered.

The approximate fraction of material deposited as a function of travel time from the source is given in Table F-5. Analysis was extended over the Atlantic using Figure F-3 to obtain removal rates to 6 days (72–144 h).

The plume of pollutant material from a point source in Illinois, in this example, has not reached Europe in 6 days, but about 80 percent of the material has been scavenged by precipitation. These results are regarded as tentative since they depend critically on the assumptions—for example, the depth of the rain-bearing layer and the Engelmann ratio.

An alternative method for modeling the depletion of plume material with time is simply to assume an exponential depletion rate. The cumulative fraction removed at any time t, is then

$$f_r = 1 - \exp(-t/t_r),\qquad(9)$$

where f_r = fraction removed, and
t_r = the mean residence time.

A mean residence time for a ground level source of approximately 3.3 days has been inferred from the use of radon daughters as an atmospheric tracer. The cumulative fraction removed at various times, assuming a 3.3 day mean residence is shown in the last column of Table F-5. The agreement with values obtained using the Engelmann ratio method

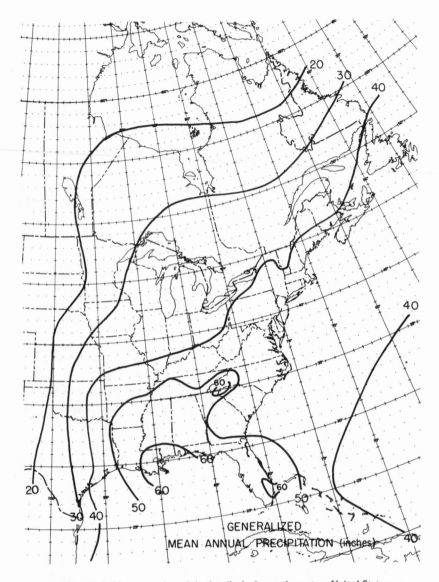

FIGURE F-4   Mean annual precipitation (inches) over the eastern United States.

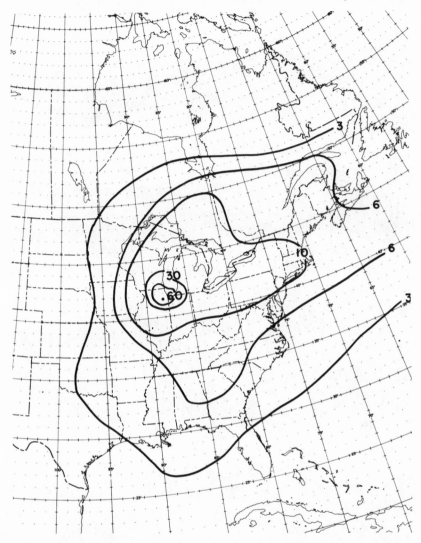

FIGURE F-5 Annual deposition by precipitation scavenging (10^{-18} g/cm^2).

is quite good. It must be stressed that the appropriate residence time is also uncertain, and the agreement may be coincidental. A calculation scheme using exponential removal would be simpler than the scheme employing Engelmann ratios, and the simpler scheme may be adequate for a gross picture of removal by precipitation scavenging. However, it does not take into account the variations in rainfall over the world and cannot

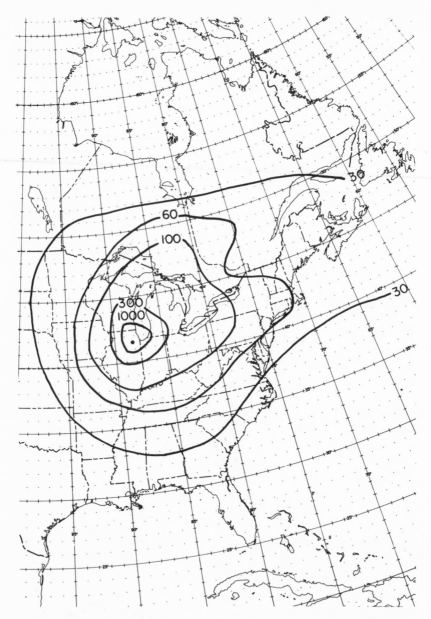

FIGURE F-6 Mean annual surface air concentration (10^{-26} g/cm^3) with depletion by precipitation.

TABLE F-5 Fraction of Pollutant Removed by Precipitation

Travel Period, h	Fraction Removed	Cumulative Removal	
		using ratio of 500	using 3.3-day residence time
0–6	0.06	0.06	0.07
6–12	0.06	0.12	0.14
12–24	0.12	0.24	0.26
24–36	0.15	0.39	0.37
36–55	0.12	0.51	0.50
55–72	0.08	0.59	0.60
72–96	0.10	0.69	0.70
96–120	0.07	0.76	0.78
120–144	0.05	0.81	0.84

reflect local differences due to this factor. Of course, a scheme might be devised to adjust results to some extent with regard to rainfall.

The calculation of precipitation scavenging in the global model (beyond 30 days) is treated differently from that described above. The global mixing model contains many boxes with contaminants and redistributes the latter according to the direction of the gradients of concentration and the coefficients of eddy diffusion. To this is added a fractional removal per unit of time of the contaimant in the box, the effect of precipitation removal. In the lower level temperate latitudes about 20 percent of the box content is removed per day, on the average, and except for the tropics, $10°N–10°S$, very little removal occurs above 5 km.

The results show that ground level concentrations with precipitation scavenging after 1 month, from an instantaneous source at ground level in the $30–50°N$ box, are about 1 percent of the value without removal and, after 6 months, about 0.001 percent of the nonremoval case. After 1 month the peak concentration is above the main rain-bearing layers, rather than at the ground. The accumulated deposition from an instantaneous point source after 1 month is about 96 percent of the input while, after 6 months, almost 99.9 percent of the initial input has left the atmosphere.

Material emitted near the ground, and subject to scavenging by precipitation, will be nearly completely removed from the atmosphere during phase 3, and little error will be introduced into population exposure calculations by assuming it to be totally removed at 30 days.

Dry Deposition The usual technique for incorporating dry deposition employs the concept of deposition velocity, i.e., the ratio of the deposition per unit area and time to the air concentration per unit volume in contact with the ground. Experimentally determined values of deposition velocity generally range from about 0.1 cm/s to several centimeters per second. In general, values greater than 1 cm/s are observed with chemically active materials (^{131}I, SO_2, for example) depositing on surfaces covered with vegetation (grass, sagebrush, etc.) while inert materials or bare soil produce lower values.

Application of the deposition velocity to the patterns in Figures F-1, F-2 or F-3 will provide the deposition of a pollutant and consequent decrease in downwind air concentration. However, a velocity of 1 cm/s removes the pollutant material at a rate equal to (at great distances) or over 10 times faster (near the source) than that from either the application of Engelmann's concept or the mean residence time of 3.3 days. This contradicts existing concepts which ascribe most deposition to precipitation rather than dry weather scavenging.

It is likely that the above inconsistency (i.e., faster dry than wet deposition) results from incorrect treatment of dry deposition. The dry removal occurs at the earth's surface rather than throughout a column as is the case with precipitation scavenging. The vertical profile of concentration is probably affected by the sink at ground level. This means that the concentration at ground level will decrease very rapidly with time or travel distance, faster than the decrease of the average column concentration. This lower ground level concentration reduces the dry weather removal rate over that which might occur if the whole vertical column of pollutants responded to ground level removal. To properly incorporate these qualitative ideas into estimates of air concentration and deposition requires the correct vertical mixing intensities especially near the earth's surface. The response of the vertical profile of pollutant air concentration to vertical mixing in the presence of a ground level sink is beyond the scope of the present report.

Despite this problem, the use of a deposition velocity of 0.1 cm/s appears to give reasonable results, so a preliminary assessment of dry deposition will be provided here.

The annual amounts of dry, wet, and total deposition for each air concentration contour shown in Figure F-1, are given in Table F-6 for the first phase of plume travel. With a deposition velocity of 0.1 cm/s, dry deposition is slightly greater than wet deposition, which is not unreasonably close to the source where most of the plume material is near the ground. Note that the surface air concentrations after depletion due to deposition (last column) are only slightly lower than the initial concentrations (first column), indicating that only a small portion of the source material has been deposited within this region. The lower portion of Table F-6 gives results for a deposition velocity of 1 cm/s. Calculated dry

TABLE F-6 Wet and Dry Deposition in the Vicinity of Morris, Illinois

Surface-Air Concentration (no deposition), 10^{-26} g/cm^3	Annual Dry Deposition, 10^{-18} g/cm^2	Annual Wet Deposition, 10^{-18} g/cm^2	Annual Total Deposition, 10^{-18} g/cm^2	Depleted Surface Air Concentration, 10^{-26} g/cm^3
Deposition Velocity = 0.1 cm/s				
30,000	925	820	1,745	29,700
10,000	306	265	570	9,740
3,000	90	80	170	2,860
1,000	29	26	55	920
Deposition Velocity = 1.0 cm/s				
30,000	8,800	770	9,570	28,200
10,000	2,700	235	2,935	8,560
3,000	710	60	770	2,230
1,000	170	15	185	520

NOTE: Results for a deposition velocity of 1 cm/s are considered unrealistic (*see* text).

deposition is more than a factor of 10 higher than wet deposition and nearly half of the total source material has been deposited within the 1000 contour (air concentration at the 1000 contour has been reduced to 520×10^{-26} g/cm^3).

The annual dry deposition pattern over the eastern United States (phase 2) is shown in Figure F-7 for a deposition velocity of 0.1 cm/s. Deposition amounts were calculated from surface air concentrations in Figure F-2, adjusting the concentration at each point for prior depletion when applying the deposition velocity formula,

$$D_d = (Cf_d)V_g t \qquad (10)$$

where D_d = annual dry deposition, g/cm^2;
$\quad C$ = air concentration before deposition, g/cm^3;
$\quad f_d$ = fraction of source material previously deposited;
$\quad V_g$ = deposition velocity, 0.1 cm/s; and
$\quad t = 3.1 \times 10^7$ s/yr.

The depletion factor, f_d, is obtained by determining the area integral of all material deposited during each time step in the calculation. Note that dry deposition over this region (Figure F-7) is less than wet deposition (Figure F-5).

Mean annual surface air concentration over the eastern United States,

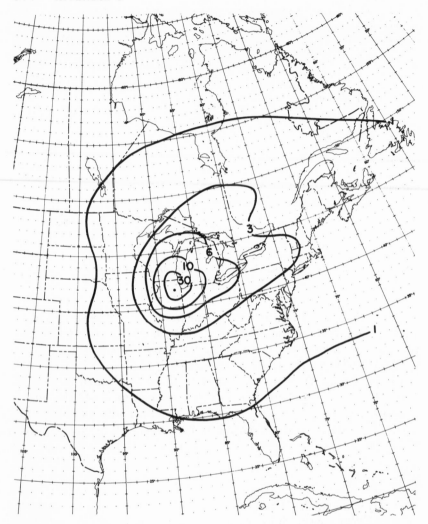

FIGURE F-7   Annual dry deposition (10^{-18} g/cm^2) with deposition velocity of 0.1 cm/s.

taking into account depletion due to both wet and dry deposition, is shown in Figure F-8.

The cumulative fractions of material removed by wet and dry deposition during various plume travel periods up to 6 days are shown in Table F-7. Results for precipitation only (no dry deposition) are repeated from Table F-5. Dry removal rates (assuming no precipitation) are shown for deposition velocities (V_g) of 0.1 and 1.0 cm/s. Even with the lower rate

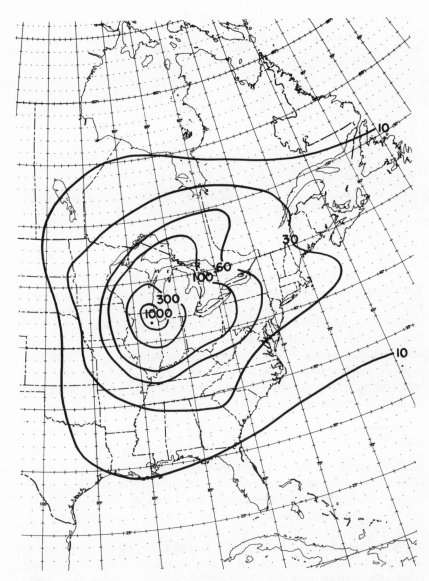

FIGURE F-8 Mean annual surface air concentration (10^{-26} g/cm³) including wet and dry depletion.

TABLE F-7   Cumulative Fractions of Pollutant Removed by Wet and Dry Deposition

Travel Period, h	Precipitation Only	Fraction Removed			
		Dry Deposition Only		Wet and Dry Deposition	
		$V_g = 0.1$	$V_g = 1.0^a$	$V_g = 0.1$	$V_g = 1.0^a$
6	0.06	0.05	0.44	0.11	0.50
12	0.12	0.09	0.66	0.20	0.73
24	0.24	0.14	0.84	0.35	0.94
36	0.39	0.19	0.94	0.53	≈ 1.0
55	0.51	0.22	0.96	0.65	
72	0.59	0.24	0.97	0.72	
96	0.69	0.26	0.98	0.80	
120	0.76	0.29	0.986	0.86	
144	0.81	0.30	0.990	0.90	

[a] Removal rates obtained with a deposition velocity of 1 cm/s are unrealistically high and are shown here only as an illustration (*see* text).

about the same fraction is removed by dry deposition as by precipitation during the first 6 hours, but wet deposition predominates thereafter. Thirty percent of the material is removed in 6 days (144 h) by dry deposition acting alone. With a deposition velocity of 1 cm/s, 44 percent is removed within 6 hours by dry deposition acting alone (and about 99% in 6 days). The probable reasons for this unrealistic removal rate have already been discussed. Finally, removal rates are shown for wet and dry deposition acting together. A deposition velocity of 0.1 cm/s combined with wet removal results in 90 percent removal in 6 days compared to 81 percent for wet removal alone.

GAS-TO-PARTICLE CONVERSIONS

Aerosol particles interact strongly with one another, with water and ice clouds, and with dispersed atmospheric chemicals. From these interactions a complicated and time-varying distribution of aerosol sizes that extend over many decades results—from ionic clusters containing as few as $10-10^4$ molecules and having radii of $10-100$ Å ($10^{-3} - 10^{-2}$ μm), to soil particles and droplets only briefly suspended in the air by violent winds. As no single technique can be used to measure sizes over the whole range, the results from methods special to particular size intervals must be patched together as best one can. When this is done, a spectrum of sizes emerges, which so far shows still increasing number concentrations at the smallest sizes measured reliably (about 10^{-2} μm). A useful empirical expression to summarize the number distribution of measured aerosol sizes is a power law (Junge, 1963):

$$dn/dr \sim C\,r^{-(\nu+1)}$$

or

$$dn/d\ln r \sim C\,r^{-\nu}$$

In the size range of maximum interaction with light (0.1–1 μm) ν usually lies in the interval $2 < \nu < 4$.

Steady-state arguments suggest that aerosols for which $\nu = 3$ may be kinetically self-preserving, and, indeed, values near to this are frequently observed in "well-aged" air (Whitby *et al.*, 1972). For such an aerosol the volume distribution ($r^3\,dn/d\ln r$) is approximately a constant; that is, each logarithmic decade of size interval contains about the same volume, or mass. Whitby *et al.* (1972) has found, however, that superimposed upon this relative uniformity are two recognizable subpopulations—one of sizes greater than 1 μm, which he identifies to be photochemically inactive and likely composed of conventional smoke and soil scour, the other of radii near to 0.1–0.2 μm, which he identifies by its rapid growth in sunlight as photochemically active. A further rearrangement of the aerosol distribution into an area moment $r^2\,dn/d\ln r$, which varies as $r^{-(\nu-2)} \sim r^{-1}$ shows that most of the aerosol's surface area is concentrated at the very small particle end of the size spectrum. (Indeed, the last expression is infinite at $r = 0$, unless ν ultimately declines to 2 or less, as it obviously must.)

Since primary gas-to-particle conversion must be preceded by surface-area limited absorption processes, it follows that the very smallest end of the particle size spectrum—at radii much less than those which best interact with light and clouds—dominates the primary conversion processes. The important potential effects of aerosols on climate—by their interactions with clouds and the radiation flux—are therefore phenomena of secondary aerosol particles, formed in a cascading chain of coagulation by particle-to-particle collisions. This is an important point, because the kinetics of the accretion—and of the primary gas-to-particle conversion—is very sensitive to the chemical type and physical properties of the condensing trace chemicals and their photochemical conversion products. Hence, the final aerosol effects are sensitive to interruptions and modifications induced by relatively minor changes in the type and quantity of chemicals that might enter the atmosphere. It is appropriate, therefore, that questions of influence upon aerosol kinetics be asked as part of a general protocol for alarm on possible deleterious effects of projected chemical influences upon the atmosphere.

PHOTOCHEMICAL REACTIONS IN THE ATMOSPHERE

Photochemical reactions occur as a result of the absorption of solar radiation by a molecule that then produces chemical and physical changes. Knowledge of the spectral features of solar radiation and absorption characteristics of the molecules is prerequisite to the consideration of the chemical fates of compounds in the atmosphere. Photochemical changes that follow molecular excitation by light absorption can be conveniently categorized into primary and secondary processes: The primary process is the act of light absorption i.e., the excited molecule may form highly reactive species such as atoms and radicals; subsequent reactions of these species may be defined as secondary photochemical reactions. It is important to note that photochemical reactions occur in the natural atmosphere and that a number of natural atmospheric constituents can produce a variety of reactive species. These reactive species present in the natural atmosphere can be responsible, in part, for the chemical fate of compounds introduced into the atmosphere. In this appendix the general features of solar radiation, light absorption, and primary photochemical processes will be discussed first. This is followed by a brief discussion of photochemistry in polluted air.

Solar Radiation in the Troposphere

The lower atmosphere near the earth's surface receives visible and ultraviolet radiation, not only directly from the sun, but also from the sky and by reflection from the surface of the earth. The quantity of radiation received is dependent on the solar spectral irradiance outside the atmosphere; the solar zenith angle; the nature and amount of scattering, diffusion, and absorption of radiation by the atmosphere; and the albedo of the surface. The incident solar intensity I_0 in the visible-near ultraviolet region is essentially that of a black body radiator at about 6000 K, crossed by several thousand Fraunhofer absorption lines. The irradiation J_λ, to which air near the ground surface is exposed is given approximately by

$$J_\lambda = I_{0\lambda} T_{a\lambda} \ [T_{s\lambda} + 2g(1 - T_{s\lambda})\cos(z)]$$

where $I_{o\lambda}$ = incident solar intensity at wavelenth λ;

$T_{a\lambda}$ = overall transmissivity (fraction transmitted) in absorption in the atmosphere at λ;

$T_{s\lambda}$ = transmissivity due to molecular scattering and particulate diffusion at λ;

g = value determined by directional distribution of the scattered radiation and by the amount of multiple scattering; and

z = zenith angle.

The most notable feature of J_λ is marked deviation from the incident solar radiation I_0 at wavelengths shorter than 4000 Å (i.e., the sharp cut off at 3000 Å and strong dependence on the zenith angle). This modification is due primarily to the absorption by the ozone layer in the upper atmosphere and to the variations in its column density. This wavelength region is of particular importance to atmospheric photochemistry, since most chemicals with few important exceptions have energy thresholds in the vicinity of 3000 Å for absorption by electronic transitions.

Clearly, no photochemical primary reactions can take place at night or under heavy cloud coverage in the day time. The photochemical lifetime of a given compound is highly dependent on solar irradiation as well as on its inherent molecular properties. Thus, characterization of solar diurnal and seasonal spectral distribution and corresponding flux should be firmly established on a regional basis for photochemical considerations.

Light Absorption

The logical next step in the discussion of photochemical primary processes is to identify the light absorbers and nonabsorbers. In the troposphere these will be the species that absorb in the photochemically active region of the solar spectrum (i.e., in the region of 3000–7000 Å), which roughly corresponds to 1.68–4.2 kJ/mole of the excitation energies. Once a specific chemical is chosen for photochemical consideration, its adsorption characteristics—especially its absorption coefficient—should be determined over the entire wavelengths of interest. To illustrate, ozone absorbs strongly in the region of 2000–3500 Å (Huggins bands), and weekly in the region 4500–7000 Å (Chappius bands). Absorption coefficients of ozone near the short wavelength limit of solar radiation are shown in Figure F-9.

It can be seen from Figure F-9 that the absorption of solar radiation by ozone is extremely sensitive to the wavelength; thus, accurate determination of the absorption coefficients, as well as solar radiation, is crucial for the photochemical consideration of light absorbing chemicals.

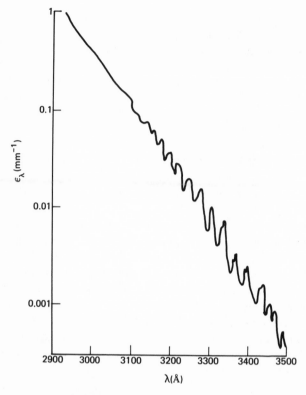

FIGURE F-9   Absorption coefficients of ozone, 2900-3500 Å.
(From Inn and Tanaka, 1953).

In general, there are three types of absorption spectra—line, band, and continuous. Line spectra consist of single, sharp lines even with small dispersion, and originate from the electronic transition between two discrete energy levels of atomic species. Band spectra appear over more or less broad wavelength regions, and range from well-defined, sharp lines to a rather diffuse band even with high resolution. These originate from electronic absorption by diatomic and polyatomic molecules that possess vibrational and rotational sublevels in their electronic states. Continuous spectra occur over extended continuous regions. Both diffuse and continuous spectra result from transitions between two electronic states, the upper one of which can assume a continuous range for energy values by splitting the molecule into atomic components. In view of the great importance of these dissociation processes in photochemistry, treatises on the subject such as the comprehensive work by Herzberg (1950) should be consulted for more detailed discussion.

Photochemical Processes

Following excitation of the molecules, various physical and chemical processes take place depending on the occurrence of bond scission. Among physical processes are re-emission of the absorbed photon by fluorescence or phosphorescence, radiationless transfer of the excitation energy to other chemical bonds within the molecule, collisional transfer of the absorbed energy to an electronic state of another molecule (i.e., photosensitization) and analogous processes without resulting in the electronic excitation of the colliding molecule (i.e., quenching). On the other hand, chemical processes consist of dissociation to atoms and radicals, decomposition into molecules, molecular rearrangement, and reaction with other molecules.

Several of these processes can occur competitively for a given chemical under atmospheric conditions. Notably, only those processes that lead to chemical transformation define the photochemical lifetime for the primary processes. The photochemical lifetime then depends on the absorption rate and the yield of such processes; thus, the assessment of the photochemical fate of a compound requires the determination of the efficiency of each process per photon absorbed (i.e., quantum yield) as a function of wavelength in the presence of air. Although such studies are actively pursued in the field of photochemistry, there is a serious lack of adequate data for most chemicals. Some of the photochemical primary processes in urban air have been estimated by Leighton (1961) and are listed in Table F-8.

Illustrative Case Study: CH_4, CO, and the Oxides of Nitrogen in the Natural Atmosphere

The atmospheric fate of CO deserves special mention. It has previously been assumed (Junge, 1963; Robinson and Robbins, 1968) that combustion is the major source of CO in the atmosphere, and that no atmospheric reactions can remove it significantly. On the basis of this assumption, and an estimated CO tropospheric mixing ratio of 0.1 ppm, Bates and Witherspoon (1952) calculated a CO tropospheric lifetime of up to 4 years. Weinstock (1969) then derived from radiocarbon data a lifetime for CO that was more than 10 times shorter than the earlier estimates. Such a short lifetime requires much larger sources and sinks than had been previously suggested (Bates and Witherspoon, 1952; Robinson and Robbins, 1968; Seiler and Junge, 1970). More recently, Stevens *et al.* (1972) have determined the concentration and the carbon and oxygen isotopic composition of atmospheric CO in the northern hemisphere. The isotopic pattern was found to be different from that for CO from auto-

TABLE F-8   Products of Photochemical Primary Processes in Urban Air

Product (Formula)	Absorber Possibly Forming the Product	Estimated Rate of Formation at $z = 45°$ and Unit Absorber Conc. (pphm h^{-1})
Oxygen atoms (O)	NO_2	~20
	O_2	1.3
Nitric oxide (NO)	NO_2	~20
	Alkyl nitrites	≤5
	Nitroalkanes	≤0.15
Nitrogen dioxide (NO_3)	Nitric acid	≤0.01
	Alkyl nitrates	0.006
Alkyl radicals ($\dot{R}$)	Aldehydes	0.04 to 0.14
	Ketones	0.03
Alkoxyl radicals ($R\dot{O}$)	Alkyl nitrites	≤5
	Alkyl nitrates	0.006
	Nitroalkanes	≤0.15
	Organic peroxides	<0.01
Formyl radicals ($H\dot{C}O$)	Formaldehyde	~0.2
	Aliphatic aldehydes	0.04 to 0.14
Acyl radicals ($R\dot{C}O$)	Diketones	0 to 0.1
	Ketones	~0.03
Hydroxyl radicals ($\dot{O}H$)	Hydrogen peroxide	0.06
	Hydroperoxides	<0.01
	Nitric acid	≤0.01
Hydrogen atoms (H)	Formaldehyde	~0.2
Aldehydes (RCHO)	Alkyl nitrites	≤5.5
	Nitroalkanes	≤0.15
Nitroxyl (HNO)	Alkyl nitrites	≤5.5
	Nitroalkanes	≤0.15
Sulfates (SO_4)	SO_2	<0.5, possibly <0.005

SOURCE: Leighton (1961).

mobile engine combustion, whether compared to combustion in the same region as the air sample or to an estimated world average. These results indicate that there are several natural sources of CO that may be much greater than anthropogenic emissions. Weinstock (1969) suggested that the oxidations of CO by hydroxyl (OH) radicals, first proposed by Bates and Witherspoon (1952), would provide the necessary sink if a sufficient source of radicals could be found. Levy (1972) presented a simple photochemical model of the troposphere that provides both the necessary OH radicals and—by their destruction of methane (CH_4)—a large source of formaldehyde, which subsequently leads to the production of CO.

Calculations by Wofsy *et al.* (1972) and Levy (1972) have shown that the oxidation of CH_4 is a much larger source of CO than is combustion. The major sink would appear to be the oxidation of CO by OH. The calculated sink for this process gives a lifetime in harmony with that predicted from radiocarbon data (Weinstock 1969; Weinstock and Niki, 1972).

A unified model of tropospheric chemistry including various trace gases is shown schematically in Figure F-10. The major features of this scheme can be summarized as follows. The key step is the production of OH by the photolysis of O_3 in the presence of H_2O. The OH is pri-

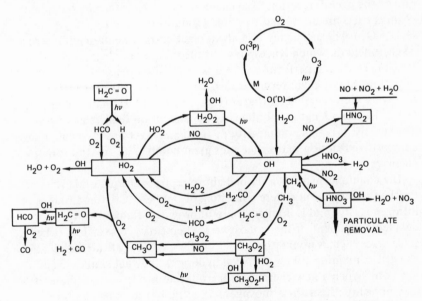

FIGURE F-10 A model of tropospheric photochemistry. (From Levy, 1972.)

marily responsible for the oxidation of CH_4 and CO and H_2, which are the oxidation products of CH_4. In these reaction steps, the OH is transformed to HO_2, which in turn regenerates OH by the reaction with NO (i.e., $HO_2 + NO \rightarrow OH + NO_2$). The resulting NO_2 undergoes rapid photodissociation and regenerates O_3 and NO (not shown in this figure). Thus, the photolysis of O_3 in the presence of H_2O leads to a long series of chain reactions until a certain radical in the chain is converted to a chemically inert form or alternatively removed from the gas phase by some physical processes. It should be noted that formaldehyde, peroxides, nitric acid, and nitrous acid are formed as reaction intermediates in the tropospheric oxidation of CH_4. More formalistically stated, a chain mechanism consists of several functional groups of reaction steps involving chain carriers (i.e., generation, initiation, propagation, and termination steps). For example, in Figure F-10 the OH radicals are formed in the generation step $O('D) + H_2O \rightarrow 2 OH$. If HCHO, HNO_3 and HONO are present as initial reactants, their photolyses also constitute generation steps. The reactions of OH with CH_4, CO, and H_2 are the initiation steps that are the rate controlling steps in the chain. The resulting radicals, such as CH_3O_2 and CH_3O, then propagate the chain until the chain cycle is completed by the regeneration of the OH. Notably, some of the chain propagation steps produce more than one chain carrier (e.g., photolyses of HCHO and H_2O_2) and greatly enhance the rate of the overall reaction. The chain propagation is terminated when chain carriers are converted to stable products (e.g., $OH + HO_2 \rightarrow H_2O + O_2$). The efficiency of a chain reaction may be defined in terms of chain length, which corresponds to the number of chain cycles that a chain carrier can perform before it is terminated (i.e., rate of chain initiation/rate of chain termination). Since a chain carrier reacts competitively with the chain initiator (e.g., CH_4) and terminator (e.g., HO_2) the chain length is nonlinearly dependent on their relative concentrations. It is this nonlinearity of the chain reactions involving many competitive reaction paths that adds great complexity to atmospheric chemistry.

The chain mechanism described above represents a plausible scheme for the "model" atmosphere consisting of only O_3, CH_4, and oxides of nitrogen (NO_x) and is intended here to provide a framework for more detailed assessment of the tropospheric chemistry. Presumably, other trace gases such as nonmethane hydrocarbons, NH_3, sulfides, and halogen-containing compounds can undergo somewhat similar chain reactions. When a new chemical is introduced into the atmosphere, it may not only affect the atmosphere directly, but may also be transformed chemically and alter the residence times of other atmosphere constituents by perturbing the balance of the concentrations of radicals. A quantitative assessment of these effects would require consideration of the spatial and time variances of all the constituents of the atmosphere and the rate parameters for all possible combinations of the relevant species, including radicals. However, it is possible to reduce the size of the reaction matrices by sensitivity tests, thermochemical methods and other basic principles.

The reactions shown in Figure F-10 represent a minimum set of important rate parameters for the O_3-NO_x-CH_4-H_2O system. The majority of these reactions are not known accurately enough for reliable modeling of the atmosphere; they need to be firmly established before reactions involving other trace gases can be incorporated into the model. For example, photochemistry of O_3, H_2O_2, HCHO, nitrates, and nitrites should be determined with better accuracy as a function of photodissociation wavelength. Virtually no direct experimental data are available for the reactions involving triatomic and polyatomic radicals. Activation energies for most of these reactions are still unknown. Concomitantly, reactions of the indicated chain carriers with these trace gases and the subsequent reactions of the resulting products should be determined.

The above-mentioned kinetic studies need to be coordinated with a number of monitoring programs. In view of the important role of OH radicals in the oxidation reactions of nearly all the trace gases, its direct determination will yield the most definitive answers for atmospheric chemistry. At present there are no direct measurements of aldehydes and nitric acid in the natural atmosphere. More extensive monitoring of nonmethane hydrocarbons, NH_3, and sulfur- and halogen-containing compounds is crucial for further development of atmospheric chemistry. These measurements are also of particular importance to pollution chemistry, since many of these gases coincide with man-made chemicals emitted in the atmosphere. The establishment of natural background levels of trace gases would serve as a basis for the determination of the extent of perturbations caused by human activities. Great care and precaution should be taken in these monitoring efforts.

Chemistry of the Polluted Atmosphere

When a man-made chemical is introduced into the natural atmosphere, its chemical fate may be determined by photochemical decomposition or through interactions with reactive species present in the atmosphere. As stated above, O, OH, HO_2 and O_3 are the potential natural reactants for the atmospheric oxidation reactions. Reactions with water and with numerous nitrogenous compounds (NO, NO_2, NH_3, HNO_3, etc.) may also be important in this process.

When high concentrations of man-made chemicals are present in the atmosphere, they may dominate the natural atmospheric chemistry and lead to interactions, which can be characterized phenomenologically as *synergistic effects*: Photochemical smog in urban atmospheres, typical of the Los Angeles basin, serves as such an example.

In the formation of photochemical smog, hydrocarbons and nitric oxide are the two major ingredients. These compounds are, in themselves, generally innocuous at the levels encountered. Their significance lies in the photochemical formation of oxygenated compounds such as ozone, aldehydes, peroxides, and organic and inorganic acids. Atmospheric coloration and visibility reduction are the well-known atmospheric effects of smog.

The chemistry of smog formation resembles that of the natural atmosphere in that both are characterized by photochemical oxidation of hydrocarbons in the presence of nitrogen oxides and ozone. However, smog chemistry exhibits much greater complexity, due primarily to the presence of a multitude of hydrocarbons. For example, in the Los Angeles atmosphere hydrocarbons are present which consist of paraffinic, olefinic, and aromatic hydrocarbons (see Table F-9). These originate from automotive emissions, gasoline and solvent evaporation, and leakage of natural gas and petroleum deposits. The major departure from the natural atmospheric oxidation of methane arises from the chemical reactivity of these hydrocarbons, particularly olefinic compounds toward not only OH but also O and O_3. As a result, the photochemical reactions of the complex $NO-NO_2$ hydrocarbons remove the different classes of hydrocarbons at substantially different rates. Air monitoring data in the Los Angeles basin show significant diurnal variations in hydrocarbon composition. Similar direct observations have been made on the composition of parcels of the polluted air before and after irradiation with ultraviolet lamps in the laboratory.

The chemical fate of hydrocarbons, oxides of nitrogen, and the oxidation products are closely coupled to each other. Basically, there is a fundamental relationship between NO, NO_2, and O_3 concentrations.

$$NO_2 + h\nu \xrightarrow{k_1} NO + O$$

$$O + O_2 + M \xrightarrow{k_2} O_3 + M$$

$$O_3 + NO \xrightarrow{k_3} NO_2 + O_2$$

TABLE F-9 Typical Hydrocarbon Composition of the Atmosphere of the Los Angeles Downtown in 1967

Hydrocarbon	Concentration by Volume, ppb
Methane	2,400
Ethane + ethylene	102
Acetylene + propane	76
Propylene	10.5
n-Butane	46
Isobutane	12
1-Butene + isobutene	5.5
2-Butene	2
1, 3-Butadiene	2
n-Pentane	21
Isopentane	35
1-pentane + 2 methyl-1-butane	3
Nonane + decane	5
Toluene	30
Ethyl benzene	5
p-Xylene	5
o-Xylene	6.5
m-Xylene	12
Propylbenzenes	4.5
Ethyl toluenes	7.5
Other C_9 and C_{10} alkylbenzenes	12

SOURCE: Altshuller *et al.* (1971).

The photostationary relationship is given by

$$[O_3] = \frac{k_1 \left[NO_2 \right]}{k_3 \left[NO \right]},$$

where the square brackets indicate concentrations, and k_1 is a function of light intensity (3000–4000 Å) and the absorption coefficient of NO_2. A typical value of (k_1/k_3) is 100 ppm. It is this relationship that delays the formation of O_3 in the atmosphere until an appreciable fraction of the NO emitted from combustion sources is converted to NO_2. This step of NO-to-NO_2 conversion, and the subsequent formation of O_3, takes place in the atmosphere within a few hours (Figure F-11).

The chemical fate of nitrogen dioxide is presumably due to the formation of organic and inorganic nitrates such as PAN ($CH_3 CO_3 NO_2$) and nitric acid (HNO_3). These highly polar compounds may eventually coagulate as aerosols, or be removed by physical processes, such as washout and adsorption onto other aerosols present in the polluted atmosphere.

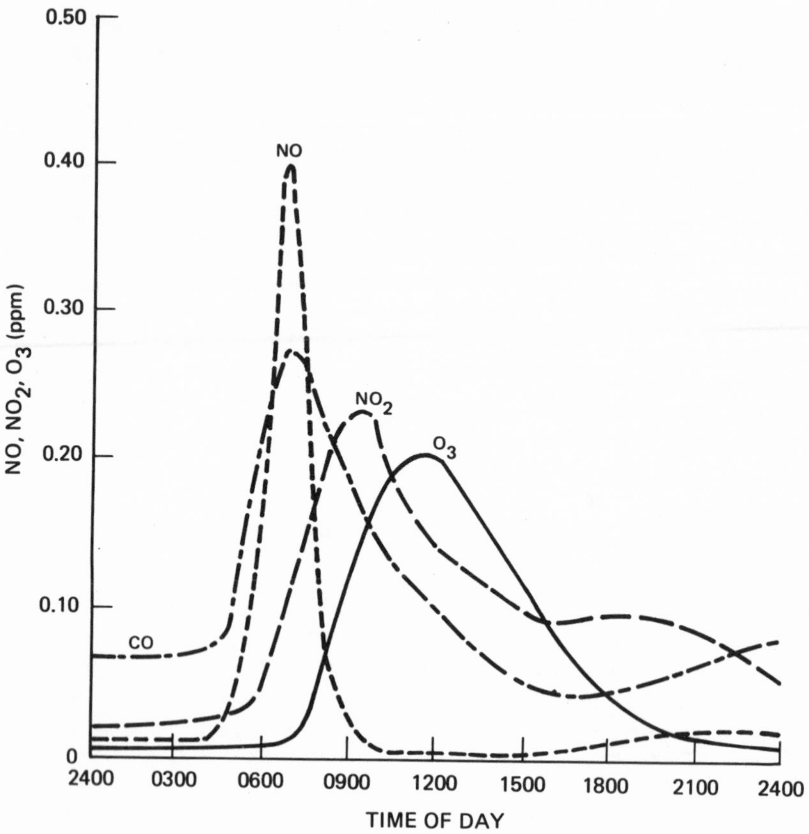

FIGURE F-11   Average daily 1-hour concentrations of selected pollutant in Los Angeles, California, July 19, 1965. [From "Air Quality Criteria for Nitrogen Oxide" (1971) S.C. Air Pollution Control Office Publication No. S.C.-84, Washington D. C.]

CLOUDS AND PRECIPITATION

Field experiments carried out during the past 30 years have shown that, under certain conditions, clouds and precipitation can be modified in a variety of ways by the addition of certain types of particles.* At the present time, deliberate attempts at modifying precipitation and reducing the destructive effects of severe storms by seeding clouds with various chemicals are being carried out in many states of the United States and throughout the world. The application of these techniques can, in many cases, lead to significant societal benefits. However, as with any technol-

* For a detailed review of this topic, the reader is referred to the National Research Council's report entitled *Weather and Climate Modification: Problems and Progress* (NRC, 1973).

ogy, the side effects of the chemicals used in weather modification and also of modifications to the weather on ecosystems, need to be carefully monitored and evaluated.

Apart from deliberate attempts to modify precipitation, evidence is mounting that man is inadvertently affecting cloud and precipitation processes in certain locations. This problem is likely to become increasingly acute in the future due to the growth of metropolitan and suburban areas, the need for increasing supplies of energy, and the extensions of both ground and aerial transportation systems.

Aided by results from deliberate weather modification projects, the increasing amount of data becoming available on the effects of pollutants from cities and specific industrial sources on clouds and precipitation, and the development of numerical models simulating these effects, it seems likely that the major effects of a particular anthropogenic source of chemicals on clouds and precipitation will be predictable in the near future.

In order to understand these effects, the basic physical and chemical processes that take place in clouds and lead to the formation of precipitation are discussed first, followed by an account of deliberate attempts to modify clouds and precipitation, and suggestions for some principles of protocol for evaluating the environmental effects of cloud seeding. Finally, the inadvertent modifications of clouds and precipitation due to man's activities are considered and some principles of protocol for evaluating these effects presented.

A Short Review of Cloud and Precipitation Processes

Cloud Condensation Nuclei   Clouds form when air containing water vapor is forced to rise in the atmosphere. As it does so, the air expands, is cooled, and water vapor is condensed as small cloud droplets or—under appropriate conditions—as ice particles. If the air were completely free of particles and ions, the pressure of the water vapor would have to reach a value 8 times that required to saturate air with respect to a plane surface of water before condensation would occur. This high supersaturation is never reached in the atmosphere because condensation of liquid water takes place on particulates in the air when the supersaturation* reaches

---

* The supersaturation is defined as

$$\left(\frac{e_v}{e_s} - 1\right) 100,$$

where e_v is the actual vapor pressure and e_s the saturated vapor pressure over a plane surface of water at the same temperature.

a value of 1 percent or less. Particles which serve as nuclei for the formation of water droplets in clouds are called cloud condensation nuclei (CCN).

The total concentration of particles in the air is variable in both space and time. However, typical values are of the order of a few hundred per cubic centimeter over the oceans and in the upper atmosphere, to a million or more per cubic centimeter in large cities. These particles, which vary in size from a few angstroms to tens of micrometers, originate from both natural (e.g., windblown dusts, volcanoes) and anthropogenic sources. Of these particles, only about 100 per cubic centimeter serve as CCN. These tend to be the larger (greater than about 0.05 μm in radius) and hygroscopic particles which serve as CCN at supersaturations of a few tenths of 1 percent. The relative humidity, H (in percent), which the air must have to remain in (unstable) equilibrium with a solution drop of radius, r, containing mass, m (in g), of dissolved salt is given by

$$\frac{H}{100} = \exp\left(\frac{2\gamma M}{\rho RTr}\right)\left[1 - \frac{8.6m}{M_1 r^3}\right]$$

where γ, ρ, and M are, respectively, the surface tension, density, and molecular weight of the drop; M_1, the molecular weight of the salt; T, the temperature in K; and R, the universal gas constant. For example, a pure water drop ($m=0$) of radius 1 μm is in (unstable) equilibrium with air of relative humidity 100.12 percent (i.e., air supersaturated by 0.12 percent). However, if the drop contained just 10^{-15} g of dissolved sodium chloride, it could have a radius of about 0.6 μm and still be in (unstable) equilibrium with air of relative humidity 100.12 percent. Furthermore, this same mass of sodium chloride in a drop of radius 0.08 μm could survive evaporation at a relative humidity of 78 percent. It is a consequence of this latter fact that haze droplets can form in the air, causing significant reductions in visibility, even when the air is well below saturation.

Smaller and insoluble particles require much larger supersaturations, not normally attained in the atmosphere, in order to serve as nuclei for condensation.

Growth of Cloud Drops by Condensation and Coalescence   The rate of increase in the radius of a drop due to condensation from the vapor phase varies inversely as the radius of the drop. Consequently, cloud drops initially grow quickly by this process, but their rates of growth decrease with time. Typically, cloud droplets may reach a radius of

20 μm due to growth by condensation in about one hour, but there-after growth by this mechanism is negligibly slow. However, when the droplets reach a size of about 20 μm, their collection efficiencies become significant, and their growth is thereafter dominated by collisions and coalescence. In this process, larger drops (formed, for example, on giant CCN) fall through the cloud with greater velocities than the average, and therefore collect some of the droplets which lie in their path. Once a drop starts to grow by this process, its mass will increase at an accelerating rate, and this can lead to the development of precipitation. The rate of increase in the radius, R, of a drop growing by collisions and coalescences with other drops is given by

$$\frac{dR}{dt} = \frac{Ew}{4\rho}\left(V - v\right),$$

where E is the collection efficiency, w the liquid water content of the cloud, ρ the density of water, and V and v are the fall velocities of the collection drop and the collected drop, respectively. Since both E and V increase with increasing R, growth by this process is an accelerating one.

Stability of Warm Clouds Warm clouds are defined as those which lie completely below the 0° C isotherm in the atmosphere; warm clouds, therefore, cannot contain ice particles. The only way in which precipitation can form in warm clouds is by condensation followed by collection and coalescence as described above.

The stability of a warm cloud is very sensitive to the concentration and size distribution of the cloud droplets and, therefore, to the concentration and nature of CCN in the air. This is clearly demonstrated by comparing warm clouds which form over the ocean with those which form in continental interiors. In the former case, there are comparatively few CCN in the air; consequently, the number concentration of drops in maritime clouds is much less than in continental clouds. Since the liquid water contents of these two cloud types do not differ significantly, the drops in maritime clouds are, on average, larger than those in continental clouds; also, the spread in their sizes is much greater than in continental clouds. For example, a typical maritime cumulus may contain about 50 drops per cubic centimeter, with a median diameter of 30 μm but with some drops up to 150 μm in diameter; whereas a typical continental cumulus contains 200 drops per cubic centimeter, with a median diameter of 10 μm and a maximum diameter of 20 μm. The larger drop sizes and broader spectra in maritime clouds makes a growth by collection and coalescence easier than in continental clouds, which explains the observation that warm maritime clouds rain more easily than do continental clouds.

Nucleation of Ice in Cold Clouds—Natural Ice Nuclei   We turn now to cold clouds, which are defined as clouds that have at least part of their volume above the 0 °C isotherm. In this case, ice particles may be present in the cloud and, as we shall see, another mechanism for producing precipitable particles can operate.

If there were no particles in the air or in cloud droplets, the latter would not freeze until their temperature fell below about −40 °C, which is the homogeneous nucleation temperature for pure water. Water which is in the liquid state below 0 °C is said to be supercooled. Cloud drops are rarely supercooled to −40 °C because they are nucleated heterogeneously at higher temperatures by certain types of particles in the air which are called ice nuclei.

The concentrations of ice nuclei in the air can vary by orders of magnitude from day to day and at different locations. Typically, however, the air contains about one particle per liter, which is effective as an ice nucleus at −20 °C.* Hence, in continental air only about 1 particle in 10^8 is effective as an ice nucleus, even at temperatures as low as −20 °C.

The factors which determine the effectiveness of a material as an ice nucleus are still not completely understood, but the following simple guidelines might be found useful. Most good ice nucleating materials are insoluble in water. (An interesting exception to this general rule is urea, which has a high solubility and a high endothermic heat of solution. As a result, this chemical can cause a drop, which may initially have a temperature as high as 6 °C, to freeze by cooling it well below 0 °C.) They have crystal symmetries similar, but not necessarily identical, to that of ice (which is hexagonal), and their misfit, defined as $a-a_0/a_0$, where a is the lattice parameter of the material and a_0 that of ice. $a_0 = 4.52$ Å for the basal plane, and $a_0 = 7.36$ Å for the prism face with at least one crystallographic plane of ice is often only a few percent. Exceptions to the last two rules are, however, not uncommon.

---

* For temperatures, ΔT (in deg C below 0 °C), in the range $10 < \Delta T < 30$, the average concentration, $n(\Delta T)$, of ice nucleus in the air active at supercoolings ΔT or less is given by

$$n(\Delta T) = n_0 \exp (\beta \Delta T)$$

where $\beta \simeq 0.6$ and $n_0 = 10^{-5}$ liter^{-1}. This expression predicts a concentration of 1 ice nucleus per liter at −20 °C, with the concentration decreasing by a factor of 10 for a rise in temperature of 4 °C.

Several techniques are available for measuring the concentrations of ice nuclei in the air, although none has yet become universally accepted.*

The majority of natural ice nuclei in the air appear to originate from the surface of the earth. Silicate minerals of the clay and mica variety produce ice crystals in supercooled clouds to the extent of about one crystal for every 10,000 particles at -15 °C. Some silicate minerals are active at higher temperatures; for example, covellite (CuS with hexagonal symmetry) can nucleate ice at -5 °C. Common airborne materials, such as sand, are generally ineffective as ice nuclei; this is to be expected in view of the relatively low concentrations of ice nuclei in the air.

From an examination of the particles at the centers of symmetrical snow crystals, it has been deduced that natural ice nuclei have diameters in the range 0.5–8 μm, with a mean diameter of about 3 μm.

Formation of Precipitation in Cold Clouds   Although the growth of cloud droplets by condensation is too slow to form raindrops, the growth of ice particles in a cloud at water saturation is very much faster due to the fact that the equilibrium vapor pressure of ice is much less than that of liquid water at the same temperature.† Therefore, when a few ice particles are nucleated in a cloud consisting primarily of supercooled water droplets, the ice particles increase in size fairly rapidly by condensation, and then by aggregation, to form precipitable particles. (These may, of course, melt to form raindrops before they reach the ground.) We will refer to this mechanism for producing precipitation in cold clouds as the ice crystal mechanism. The ice crystal mechanism is thought to be the main mechanism by which precipitation forms in temperate latitudes.

Deliberate Attempts at Modifying Clouds and Precipitation

The above brief review is sufficient to illustrate that a number of instabilities exist in the chain of events leading to the formation of

---

* Different techniques for measuring the concentration of ice nuclei in a given sample of air can sometimes differ by several orders of magnitude. Moreover, the concentrations of ice particles in some clouds are several orders of magnitude greater than the measured concentrations of ice nuclei. This discrepancy is often attributed to the multiplication of ice particles in clouds without the action of ice nuclei, but it may also be due to shortcomings in the techniques used for measuring ice nuclei.

† An atmosphere at water saturation is 10 percent supersaturated with respect to ice at -10°C and 21 percent supersaturated with respect to ice at -20 °C.

clouds and the development of precipitation that might be conducive to artificial modification. Experiments to test the degrees to which clouds and precipitation can be modified under various conditions have been carried out for the past 25 years, although the subject is probably still in its infancy. A brief review is given of some of the principal types of deliberate cloud modification experiments that are being carried out, with emphasis on the types and concentrations of chemicals used.

Warm Clouds   Comparatively little work has been done on seeding warm clouds. Most of the attempts to modify precipitation from warm clouds are based on the assumption that the introduction of large, hygroscopic particles into the clouds will stimulate the co-alescence process and lead to precipitation. The material most commonly used for this purpose is sodium chloride. A common rule of thumb is to try to introduce about one sodium chloride particle in excess of 3 μm in radius into each liter of cloudy air.

In a recent series of such experiments carried out in India (Biswas *et al.*, 1967), two types of ground generator were used. One type sprayed a water solution of NaCl (about 120 g of salt per liter of water) into the air via power sprayers driven from air compressors, and the other emitted a dry dust through blowers. The sprayers emitted solution drops at a rate of about 200 cm^3 per minute, which, after evaporation, left salt particles about 3–12 μm in radius. The equivalent particle emission rate was about 10^9 per second, which corresponds to an average spray drop-let radius of about 10 μm and a dry-residue radius of about 5 μm. With plausible assumptions as to the rate of turbulent spreading following ejection, a concentration of large salt particles of about 0.2 per liter is estimated at a distance of 20 km downwind of the generator. The dry-dusters used in the Indian trials were fed a mixture of NaCl and soap-stone, in a ratio of 9 to 1, ground to a median particle mass of 10^{-9} g, which corresponds to dry NaCl particles of radius 5 μm. The soapstone was added to prevent caking. At a dispersal rate of 2.5 kg/min, an effective particle emission rate of about 4 $\times$ 10^{10} per second is estimated. The corresponding concentration of large NaCl particles 20 km downwind is estimated at 2 per liter.

The Indian salt-seeding experiments were carried out for eight seasons in Delhi, six in Agra, and four in Jaipur. Statistical comparisons of rainfall were made between target and control areas for seeded and nonseeded days. In 16 out of the total of 18 seasons, an average increase of rain of 41.9 percent occurred in the target area.

Several cloud-seeding efforts involving the dispersal of NaCl are currently being carried out in the United States (e.g., in South Dakota and Oklahoma). In these programs, the salt is dispersed into the bases of the clouds from an aircraft. In a recent case study carried out in South Dakota (Biswas and Dennis, 1971), 350 lb of NaCl was released into a line of stratocumulus clouds. No rain fell from neighboring unseeded clouds, but 280 acre-feet of water were estimated to have precipitated from the seeded cloud.

The apparent successes of the above experiments will probably result in increasing numbers of cloud-seeding experiments involving hygroscopic materials being carried out in the future.

Ninety-five percent of the fogs that occur at airports in the United States are warm fogs (i.e., composed of droplets which are not supercooled). A reliable technique for dissipating these fogs has not yet been developed. However, several techniques have been tried, including seeding with giant ($\cong 10 \, \mu$m radius) hygroscopic particles (generally chlorides and hydroxides, although urea and ammonium nitrate have also been tried), dispersing long-chain alcohols to cover the droplets and inhibit their growth, ion seeding, and using the downdrafts produced by helicopters or the exhaust heat from jet engines.

Finally, it should be noted that it should be possible to stabilize warm clouds by introducing very large numbers of artificial cloud nuclei, which would produce large numbers of relatively small cloud droplets too small to precipitate. Although this technique has not been employed deliberately, there is evidence that it occurs inadvertently (discussed later in this section).

Cold Clouds By far the greatest amount of work in weather modification has been concerned with attempts to increase precipitation from cold clouds by the introduction of artificial ice nuclei. The theoretical basis for this work is that, due to the low concentrations of natural ice nuclei, some cold clouds may be very inefficient in producing precipitation by the ice crystal mechanism. In this case, the introduction of artificial ice nuclei in concentrations of about 1 per liter might initiate the development of precipitations.

The most common artificial ice nucleus used in cloud-seeding experiments is silver iodide (AgI). This material has a very low solubility in ice; it has a hexagonal crystal structure, and a misfit with ice of just a few percent. It can nucleate ice crystals in a supercooled cloud at a temperature of about -5 °C. Moreover, the fact that about 10^{15} submicron-sized particles of AgI can be produced by vaporizing 1 g of AgI, means that only a few grams of this material are required to seed a typical cumulus cloud. The material is often dispersed in larger quantities from ground-based generators, in which a solution of a few percent of AgI in a NaI-acetone base is burned to produce a smoke containing AgI (plus impurities). Dry ice (solid CO_2) is also used for cloud seeding. In this case, ice crystals are produced by homogeneous nucleation in the wake of the very cold air produced behind small pellets of the material dropped into the clouds from an aircraft. Typical seeding rates for dry ice are a few pounds per mile.

When ice is nucleated in a supercooled cloud, the release of latent heat can change the dynamical behavior of the cloud. It is widely believed that careful control of their dynamical behavior through seeding with artificial ice nuclei offers, in the case of convective clouds, the best method for increasing precipitation. Experiments of this kind generally involve releasing an order of 1000 g of AgI into each cumulus cloud.

Many other artificial ice nucleating materials exist. For example— among the inorganics—lead iodide, cupric sulfide, mercuric iodide, silver sulfide, ammonium fluoride, silver oxide, cadmium iodide, vanadium pentoxide, and iodine all nucleate ice at relatively high temperatures. Many organic materials are also good ice nucleators, including phloroglucinol-*l*, 5-dihydroxynaphthalene, and metaldehyde. So far, none of these materials has been used very widely in cloud-seeding experiments. However, as silver becomes more expensive, ice-nucleating materials other than AgI might be sought for cloud-seeding operations.

The seeding of clouds with artificial ice nuclei, in attempts to increase precipitation, are widespread throughout the United States and the rest of the world. Most work of this kind (both experimental and operational) is being carried out on convective and orographic clouds.

If concentrations of artificial ice nuclei much larger than 1 per liter are introduced into a supercooled cloud, many small ice crystals are formed which might evaporate and result in the dissipation of the cloud. This process is referred to as *overseeding*, and is used operationally to dissipate cold fogs at many airports. Dry ice is generally used for this purpose. At the Paris airport, cold fogs are overseeded with liquid propane dispersed from sixty dispensers. In the United States, propane tests have been conducted by the U.S. Army, with a reported success rate of 60 percent at Medford, Oregon.

In addition to seeding clouds to increase precipitation, artificial ice nuclei are also being used in attempts to reduce damage from hurricanes, hailstorms, and thunderstorms and to redistribute snowfall. These experiments generally involve overseeding with relatively large quantities of silver iodide. Major operational programs in hail modification are being carried out in the Soviet Union. In 1969, these extended over an area of 6,000,000 acres of farmland. In these projects, gun shells and rockets are used to disperse several thousands of grams of artificial ice nuclei (AgI or PbI$_2$) into developing hailstorms. Prompted by Soviet reports of success in reducing hail damage by these techniques, the National Hail Research Experiment (NHRE) has been established in the United States. A major goal of NHRE is to develop and test (in Colorado) various techniques for hailstorm modification. Other major experiments in cloud seeding to reduce hail damage are being carried out in the Dakotas, Canada (Alberta), Switzerland, Italy, and Kenya. The U.S. Forest Service has been engaged for many years in a research experiment in Montana to determine whether cloud seeding with AgI reduces the frequency of lightning flashes from thunderstorms. Experimental investigations into the controlled diversion of snowfall are being carried out in the Cascade Mountains of Washington and in the Great Lakes region. In the former experiments, in which a total of about 1 kg of AgI is released over a period of 1 hour, case studies have shown that snowfall can be targeted to designated areas on the ground (Hobbs and Radke, 1973).

Evaluation of Environmental Effects of Deliberate Cloud Seeding

It is clear from the previous discussion that cloud-seeding experiments are widespread, both in the United States and throughout the world. This is a consequence of its potential (and, in some cases, proven) ability to contribute to the solution of many problems, including water shortages, fogs, flooding, and the damages caused by severe storms. However, cloud seeding, in common with most technologies, may have adverse effects on the environment and man that need to be carefully evaluated and weighed against the potential benefits.

Some general principles of protocol for evaluating the environmental effects of cloud seeding are suggested:

1. It should be required as a matter of routine that full information on any attempts to deliberately modify the weather be sent to a designated agency of the federal government.* The information provided should include time and place of the weather modification activity, type of modification activity, type and amount of each modification

---

* Such information is now required by law to be reported to the National Oceanic and Atmospheric Administration (NOAA), except where the modification is being carried out for the federal government; however, most of the research and operational work in weather modification is being carried out under federal grants and contracts.

agent used, and an account of the measurements and observations made before, during, and after the weather modification activity which would aid in evaluating its effects.

2. Chemicals used in weather modification should be carefully evaluated for inadvertent toxic effects on the environment, ecosystems, and man. As an illustration of the type of evaluation that should be carried out, the most widely used chemical for cloud seeding—namely, silver iodide—is evaluated below.

3. The predicted changes in the weather caused by the weather modification activity should be evaluated for both their beneficial and adverse effects on the environment, ecosystems, and man.

4. In carrying out the evaluations referred to in steps 2 and 3 above, a clear distinction should be drawn between long-term, operational weather modification projects carried out in a specific area (e.g., seeding on every possible occasion in order to increase precipitation in a given area year after year), and short-term, or one-shot, weather modification activities (e.g., alleviation of a drought or cloud seeding for research purposes).

In the case of long-term weather modification operations, a careful evaluation should be made of both the toxic effects of the chemicals used and the effects of the long-term changes in the weather (in the direction sought by the weather modification activity) on the ecosystem. Also, in long-term weather modification projects, monitoring of the quantity of seeding agent in and around the target area (in the air, on the ground, and in lakes and rivers) should be mandatory.

In short-term weather modification activities, the main concern should be that the chemicals used are not highly toxic in the amounts in which they will be dispersed.

5. A distinction can often be made also between cold and warm cloud seeding.

Compared to the quantities of chemicals that enter the atmosphere from other sources, those used in the seeding of cold clouds to trigger the ice crystal mechanism of precipitation production are generally minute. In this case, therefore, the main concern is that the substances used are not highly toxic or accumulate somewhere in the ecosystem, and that the changes produced in the weather (e.g., precipitation, cloud cover) will not have dire effects on man, animals, or plants.

The seeding of warm clouds or fogs with hygroscopic materials, on the other hand, generally involve much larger quantities of chemicals than the seeding of cold clouds. For example, about 450 km/h of a hygroscopic material might be required to keep an airport clear of warm fog. Even if the material is only mildly toxic, it might have serious effects when distributed in such large quantities. For example, this amount of NaCl could have adverse effects on vegetation and aquatic life in the waters into which the salt finally drains, let alone on aircraft!

Inadvertent Modification of Clouds and Precipitation Due to Man's Activities

In the light of the above discussions of cloud physical processes and their modification by deliberate cloud seeding, it should come as no surprise that man's activities can and do inadvertently modify the clouds and precipitation in a variety of ways. As cities, suburban areas, industrial activities, and areas under cultivation continue to grow, modifications of this kind are likely to become more pronounced and widespread.

Some of the ways in which clouds, precipitation, and other aspects of the weather may be modified by man's activities are summarized below; then some principles of protocol for evaluating the effects are presented.

Anthropogenic Sources of Ice Nuclei   Man-made particulates that enter the atmosphere and act as ice nuclei at temperatures above about $-20\,^\circ$C have the potential for modifying the ice crystal mechanism for producing precipitation in cold clouds. This mechanism is particularly sensitive to modification since, as we have seen, the concentrations of natural ice nuclei active at $-20\,^\circ$C are only about 1 per liter of air. Anthropogenic sources of particulates give rise to concentrations of ice nuclei in clouds of about this order of magnitude and are likely to enhance the development of precipitation in cold clouds. If, on the other hand, the source is more prolific and produces much higher concentrations of ice nuclei, it may overseed clouds and cause a reduction in the efficiency with which they precipitate.

High ice nucleus counts have been observed by several workers in plumes from steel mills (Langer, 1968). Of greater concern, however, is the recent suggestion (Schaefer, 1966) that lead compounds emitted from automobiles using gasolines containing tetraethyl lead anti-knock agents may combine with trace quantities of iodine in the atmosphere to produce significant concentrations of lead iodine particles that are efficient as ice nuclei at $-6\,^\circ$C. Another suggestion (Langer, 1970) is that the photolytic reaction of lead bromide and related compounds from automobiles may form lead oxides. These processes may explain the abnormally high concentrations of ice nuclei which have been observed in and around some cities. We also note that snow sometimes contains as much as 2 ppm of lead, which is almost 15 times above the safe limit for drinking water set by the U.S. Public Health Service. Much more research is needed in this area in order to establish the principal man-made sources of ice nuclei and the reactions in the atmosphere that may give rise to them.

Anthropogenic Sources of Cloud Condensation Nuclei   The injection of artificial cloud condensation nuclei (CCN) into the atmosphere may modify the microstructure of clouds and the development of precipitation in warm clouds in two different ways: If the concentrations of the artificial CCN in the clouds are not too high and they are very effective (i.e., giant-size hygroscopic particles), they may stimulate the coalescence mechanism and thereby lead to an increase in precipitation. On the other hand, if very large numbers of CCN are emitted, they will tend to increase the concentration of cloud droplets, decrease the average size of the droplets, and increase the stability of warm clouds. In this case, decreases in precipitation are to be expected.

Several industrial sources of CCN have been identified (Hobbs *et al.,* 1970). These include Kraft pulp and paper mills ($10^{14} - 10^{19}$ CCN per second), sulfite pulp and paper mills ($10^{14} - 10^5$ CCN per second), sawmills (10^{18} CCN per second), and aluminum smelters. All of these industries produce sufficient numbers of CCN to cause appreciable changes in the concentrations of CCN in the area over large areas extending up to 100 km or more downwind. The burning of wood products and some other organic materials (e.g., sugarcane) also generate airborne CCN (Hobbs and Locatelli, 1969; Warner, 1968). However, many major sources of general air pollution—such as automobiles, oil refineries, and oil-fired power plants—do not emit appreciable numbers of CCN into the air (Hobbs *et al.,* 1970).

Evidence for Inadvertent Modification of Precipitation   Several studies have been carried out which suggest that precipitation patterns have been modified in some cities and urban–industrial areas. Increases in summer rainfall ranging from 9 to 17 percent, attributable to urban effects, have been observed in or downwind of St. Louis, Chicago, Cleveland, Washington, D.C., Baltimore, Houston, and New Orleans (Huff and Changnon, 1972). Some cities show significantly higher incidences of thunder and hail than the climatic background. An analysis of 50 years of daily precipitation data from 22 stations in the eastern United States (Frederick, 1970) showed that the precipitation during the winter months in urban areas is not randomly distributed but is less on weekends and greater on weekdays. Since there is not a natural

7-day cycle, the implication is that this difference is due to the higher
level of man's activities on weekdays than on weekends.

Due to the variety of pollution sources in large cities, and other
meteorological effects that urban complexes can produce, it is not
possible to ascribe the observed changes in precipitation to specific
causes: They may be due to thermal and dynamical effects as well as
to anthropogenic sources in ice nuclei, cloud condensation nuclei,
gases, and vapor.

More clear-cut, from the physical point of view, have been a few
studies of the effects of specific industries on precipitation: For example, a number of areas downwind of nonurban industrial sources of
cloud condensation nuclei have been observed to have significantly different annual precipitation than neighboring areas unaffected by the
pollutants (Hobbs *et al.*, 1970).

*Some Principles of Protocol for Evaluating Inadvertent Modification
of Clouds and Precipitation*   It should be clear from the above discussion that many factors may play a role in the inadvertent modification of clouds and precipitation, including man-made emissions of
heat, water vapor, particulates, and gases; consequently, it is not
possible, in general, to predict all of the effects of a city or urban complex on clouds and precipitation. Some large cities appear to produce
increases in precipitation, but the effect is variable and probably depends on the predominant natural mechanism for the production of
precipitation, as well as on the nature of the city and its pollutants. It
is unlikely, therefore, that results obtained on inadvertent modification
in any one city can be used to predict the effects of another city. Nevertheless, detailed studies of the effects on clouds and precipitation (and
other aspects of the weather) of a number of large cities are urgently
needed. In addition, it would be of considerable interest to monitor
the increase in pollution and the nature of the changes in all aspects
of the weather resulting through the creation and growth of an entirely
new city.

The effects of a relatively isolated source of pollution on precipitation
are more amenable to evaluation than are the effects of the complex
array of different sources common to most large cities. In the former
case, the following series of questions could be posed:

1. Does the source emit large quantities of heat and water vapor into
the atmosphere to the extent that water clouds are commonly observed
downwind of the source in otherwise cloudless situations? If so, increases
in precipitation are likely to be observed downwind of the source.

2. Does the source emit large numbers of hygroscopic particles greater than a few tenths of a micrometer in size? If so, the source emits cloud condensation nuclei in sufficient numbers to modify the microstructure of clouds for many miles downwind, and it will probably affect precipitation mechanisms. (More direct tests of this can be made by comparing measurements of the concentration and size distributions of cloud droplets upwind and downwind of the source.)

3. Does the source emit particulates in concentrations on the order of 1 per liter of air or greater, which act as ice nuclei at temperatures of $-20\,°C$ or higher? If so, the source is likely to affect precipitation mechanisms. If the concentration of artificial ice nuclei is about 1 per liter, it will probably increase precipitation produced by the ice crystal mechanism; whereas, if the concentration is considerably in excess of this, it may reduce precipitation produced by the ice crystal mechanism due to overseeding.

As an example of the application of the above test questions let us consider the case of large Kraft or sulfite pulp and paper mills. Such mills emit heat and water vapor into the atmosphere as well as hygroscopic particles including Na_2SO_4, NH_4HSO_3, $Ca(HSO_3)_2$, $NaOH$, Na_2SO_3, and H_2SO_4. The particles range in size from submicron to several tens of microns in diameter and should serve as efficient cloud condensation nuclei. Therefore, it could have been predicted that in certain areas clouds and precipitation downwind of Kraft mills would be affected by these paper mills. These have, in fact, been observed (although it was not predicted) in the state of Washington, where a number of areas in the vicinity of large pulp and paper mills have experienced increases in mean annual precipitation during the last 20 years of as much as 30 percent compared to the previous 20 years (Hobbs *et al.*, 1970).

RADIATION TRANSFER

Heating

Parcels of air may absorb radiation through the excitation of electronic, rotational, and vibrational molecular energy and—by subsequent intra-molecular coupling and intermolecular collisions—may redistribute the absorbed energy into heat. The radiation incident upon the air is emitted primarily by the sun, with a spectral peak near 0.5 μm. The absorption may occur both for individually dispersed molecules and for molecular aggregates dispersed as aerosols.

Molecular Absorption A single electron undergoing a semiclassical vibration about a massive charge center displays a total cross section (Q) for interaction with light, averaged over all wavelengths, of about 4×10^{-22} m^2. The upper limit of the resulting heating rate ($\dot{T}$), measured in degree celsius per second, produced by a volume mixing fraction (X) of such electrons in air is

$$\dot{T} = SQX/C_p^m,$$

where, S is the solar constant ($\simeq 1400$ watt/m^2) and C_p^m is the specific heat of a molecule of air at constant pressure ($\simeq 35 \times 10^{-23}$ J/deg). With $X = 1$ ppm, $\dot{T} \simeq 0.02$ °C/s. This heating rate is, of course, about a thousandfold higher than the atmosphere actually experiences from molecular absorption. The purpose of the illustration is to support the corollary observation that few of the earth's electrons behave as semiclassical oscillators. This in turn is another way of asserting that few molecules are intensely colored, and that strong power absorption is a rare—not a common—property of those molecular gases which are present at mixing fractions greater than 1 ppb. However, many molecules do absorb strongly in limited parts of the spectrum, particularly in the infrared: For example, H_2O, CO_2, and O_3 each significantly affect the heat transfer of outgoing thermal radiation from the earth's surface. The infrared is a minor part of the incoming solar power, however, which peaks at wavelengths near 0.5 μm. Around this wavelength only two atmospheric molecules normally occur in concentrations sufficient for their molecular absorptions to affect the atmospheric heating rate significantly, namely, ozone (O_3) and nitrogen dioxide (NO_2). These gases are discussed in turn below.

Ozone absorbs strongly in the ultraviolet, with a maximum cross section of 10^{-21} m^2 in the Hartley Continuum at 0.25 μm. This absorption is responsible for the temperature maximum observed near 30 km in the earth's stratosphere, and for the ultraviolet shield which protects protoplasm at the earth's surface. At longer wavelengths, absorption by ozone is weaker, displaying cross sections near 10^{-23} m^2 at 0.3 μm (the Huggins bands), and—after negligible values between 0.36 μm and 0.4 μm—10^{-24} m^2 at 0.6 μm (the Chappuis bands).

The naturally occurring mixing fraction of tropospheric ozone is about 10 ppb. The absorption by this ozone of the sun's radiation near the earth's surface produces heating rates less than 0.001 °C/d; in dense urban smog, ozone concentrations occasionally approach 1 ppm, with the consequent result that direct heating rates may approach 0.1 °C/d. Even the larger of these rates is negligible compared to advective heat transfer upwards from the hot surface of the earth. Ozone is therefore not a significant direct agent for energy input to the lower atmosphere. However, as discussed under Photochemical Reactions in the Atmosphere, ozone is intimately associated with aerosol formation in photochemical smogs.

Aerosol Absorption We consider first simple scattering in an optically thin atmosphere. It can be shown on the basis of quite general dimensional arguments that for Mie-scattering aerosols of any size distribution, for which $2\pi r/\lambda < 1$,

$$Q^*D/V^* = \frac{9R}{(R^2 + 2)^2};$$

where, Q^* is the absorption cross section per unit volume of aerosol-laden air [dimension:length^{-1}], D is the characteristic absorption length for light in the condensed medium, $[D = \lambda/4I]$, V^* is the total condensed-phase aerosol volume per unit volume of air, and R is the real and I is the imaginary part of the index of refraction of the aerosol. With $R = 1.5$, Q^*D/V^* is about 0.75, and the resulting heating rate of the air is then

$$\dot{T} \simeq \frac{0.75\,SV^*}{C_p^v D},$$

where C_p^v is the specific heat of a unit volume of air at constant pressure.
    The remote troposphere carries an aerosol burden of about 10^{-8} kg/m^3, which corresponds to $V^* \simeq 10^{-11}$; C_p^v is 930 J/m^3/deg; and D is about 10^{-6} meters. Together these parameters correspond to

$$\dot{T} \simeq 10^{-5}\,°C/sec \cong 0.4\,°C/12\text{-h day}.$$

This heating rate for the remote troposphere, which is itself marginally significant, appears more so when parameters are chosen to correspond to urban conditions, where V^* is often greater than 10^{-10} and D may approach 3×10^{-5} meters (for sooty smogs). Then $\dot{T}$ may exceed 1 °C/h. Such a heating rate will profoundly influence the vertical temperature distributions and stabilities above smoggy cities (or in rural sites with dust-bowl or slash-and-burn agriculture, including forest fires). The magnitude and sense of these larger disturbances, however, are influenced by multiple scattering (which, strictly, invalidates the use of the above equations for the urban case) and by the vertical distribution of aerosols. These effects are sufficiently important, and interesting, to require separate discussion. We turn now, therefore, to a discussion of multiple scattering in a thick atmosphere with differing vertical distributions of aerosols.

The expression *multiple scattering* has two different meanings: most commonly it means sequential scattering by several successive events, but occasionally authors use the term to describe simultaneous, or parallel, scattering by several discrete but closely adjacent scattering centers. Both effects become important when the scattering centers are present in high density (two or more particles, on the average, within a volume defined by a cubic wavelength). However, the former effect also obtains with lesser densities, provided only that the columnar optical depth exceeds about 0.3. This criterion is more commonly encountered than the other, and for this reason the first or sequential meaning of multiple scattering is also the more common. It is this meaning which we employ here.

In polluted urban atmospheres, and in dry rural areas where wind lifted soil may generate aerosol burdens occasionally as high as 10^{-6} kg/m^3, optical depths often exceed 0.3. In Los Angeles, for example, measured optical depths range from 0.035 to 0.6 for $\lambda = 0.546$ μm and 0.08–1.1 for $\lambda = 0.365$ μm. In such circumstances a more exact treatment of the radiation-transfer problem becomes necessary. One common higher approximation is the 2-stream model. Conceptually simple, but in practice very expensive of computer time, are Monte Carlo methods. Among the more accurate and economical approximations is a Gauss–Seidel iteration (Herman and Browning, 1965). Try (1972) has investigated the sensitivity of the atmosphere heating to aerosol parameters. Try's calculations give heating rates over 1 °C/h, depending upon many possible variations of the aerosol loading and vertical distribution, the values of the real (R) and imaginary (I) indices of refraction of the aerosol, the particle size distribution (ν), the earth's surface albedo (A_s) and the local optical depth (τ). He finds that the heating rates are more sensitive to both the imaginary part of the index of refraction and the particle size distribution than they are to the other parameters, with the sense of the sensitivity sequence being

$$I > \nu \gg \tau \simeq R > A_s .$$

Cooling

In the troposphere, the dominating manner in which a parcel of air cools is by adiabatic expansion, following lifting. The dominating manner in which a parcel loses energy is by infrared radiation in the numerous molecular bands of water vapor and carbon dioxide, and by grey-body thermal emission from water clouds. In the next section, the "greenhouse" and radiation effects of CO_2 are discussed, and the consequences of rising global CO_2 levels on the radiation balance of the earth.

Again it is convenient to discuss molecular and aerosol cooling under separate headings.

Molecular Cooling   A molecule in a given environment assumes a distribution of internal energy states which may be usefully described by the Boltzmann factors:

$$\frac{n_j}{n_i} = \frac{g_j}{g_i} \exp\left(-\frac{hc}{\lambda_{ji}kT}\right),$$

where n_j/n_i is the relative population between two quantized energy states, j and i, $(j > i \geqslant 1)$; g_j/g_i is a constant ratio of probabilities $\left(\text{for vibration modes } g_j/g_i = 1; \text{ for rotation } g_j/g_i = \frac{j(j+1)}{i(i+1)}\right)$, and λ_{ji} is the wavelength of a possible optical transition between j and i.

Selection rules for permitted radiation or absorption encourage the restriction $j = i \pm 1$. The probability of radiation per unit time for permitted transitions varies with λ^{-3}. The energy per photon varies as λ^{-1}. The power (P_{wr}) radiated per molecule per unit time is therefore given by

$$P_{wr} \sim \lambda^4 \exp\left(-\frac{hc}{\lambda kT}\right)$$

On differentiating with respect to λ, we find that the radiant power of a molecule which should have the greatest chance of affecting the radiation balance of the atmosphere should be centered near the wavelength,

$$\lambda_m = \frac{1}{4}\frac{hc}{kT} \simeq 13 \ \mu\text{m at } T = 283 \text{ K}.$$

However, owing to additional and important terms in their radiation probabilities, molecules may preferentially emit at other wavelengths, even though they also experience transitions near 13 μm. Thus water vapor both absorbs and emits more strongly near 2, 3, and 6 μm and ozone at 9 μm rather than at 13 μm. Other infrared-active minor atmospheric molecules include CO (4.5 μm) CH_4 (3 and 7 μm), N_2O (4 and 7 μm), and HDO (7 μm). The resulting atmosphere is essentially opaque in the center of the infrared region, except for windows between 2–2.5 μm, 3.5–4 μm, 4.5–5 μm, 8–9.5 μm, and 10–12.5 μm. To be effective in cooling, our imaginary molecule should radiate in one of these windows, and especially in the last, which best matches the power maximum we deduced at 13 μm. Molecular transitions most likely to occur near this wavelength are vibrational bending modes engaging a 3-membered sequence of atoms or functional groups, the outer members of which are more massive than hydrogen. (An example is the bending mode of CO_2 at 15 μm.) Molecular transitions most likely to have high transition probabilities will occur when this triad is bent and asymmetrical. (An example is HDO; note that the CO_2 bending mode does not meet this criterion.) An "exact" calculation of the cooling rate of the molecule that we are tailoring to have maximum sensitivity in cooling the atmosphere properly involves a sum or integration of an equation like that given above over a distribution of internal states and radiation probabilities. We may leap at a useful approximation, however, by observing that H_2O effects a net cooling rate of about 1 °C per 12-hour day at mixing fractions near 10^{-2}. We cannot expect our tailored molecule to be much greater than a factor of ten more efficient than is water vapor, and therefore we expect an atmospheric constituent at 1 ppm to effect a differential cooling rate no greater than 10^{-3} °C/d. Since this is a negligible value we conclude that no chemical vent to the atmosphere will significantly affect the cooling rate of the air by direct molecular emission.

Aerosol Cooling Cooling by atmospheric aerosols can operate in two ways: by grey-body radiation and by increasing the albedo (i.e., by reflecting solar energy back into space). We consider these two effects in turn below.

The grey-body radiation from water clouds is a very important term in the heat balance of the atmosphere, which again we neglect here for reasons of space and our emphasis on effects of minor species. We remark, however, that any potential systematic interference of minor species upon the cloud cover (either in horizontal extent or cloud top height) can be expected to have profound effects on the planetary weather. A recent paper by Schneider (1972) discusses some of these effects.

Grey-body emission from noncloud aerosols is not a significant term in the atmospheric heat budget. This follows from the circumstance that very small particles cannot easily radiate at wavelengths greater than their circumference. If, for example, the black-body curve and a Junge power-law aerosol size distribution ($dN \sim r^{-4} \, dr$) are doubly integrated over wavelength from 0 to $2\pi r$ and from R_{min} to R_{max}, then after several approximations the cooling rate for an optically thin aerosol becomes

$$- \dot{T} = \frac{18\ hc^2\ V^*\lambda_0^{-5}}{C_p^v}\ \exp\ \left(\frac{-\lambda_0}{2\pi R_{max}}\right)$$

where $\lambda_0 = hc/kT \sim 53\ \mu m$ and $V^* = 10^{-11}$, $- \dot{T} = 0.001$ °C per 12-hour day. Again, we take this to be negligible even with the more dense aerosol concentrations near cities.

GLOBAL EFFECTS OF POLLUTANTS ON CLIMATE

Like the weather, the climate of the earth fluctuates with time but on a longer time scale. Recorded climate observed by instruments began in the latter part of the seventeenth century, but climatic variations dating back thousands to millions of years have been deduced from in-direct evidence. Prior to the past 50-100 years, changes in the climate were almost certainly unrelated to human activity. But in recent years, man's impact has become progressively more evident in pollution, and the question has arisen whether this might cause changes in world cli-mate. Even relatively small changes in, for example, mean annual air temperatures can have profound effects on the environment and man.

In this section we discuss briefly some aspects of changing air chemis-try due to pollution from human activity which may influence the climate.

Atmospheric Carbon Dioxide

The atmospheric constituent most often mentioned in expressing con-cern that man may be altering the climate is carbon dioxide (CO_2). Its concentration is increasing with time, by perhaps 10 percent since the start of the Industrial Revolution. This increase is attributable to the consumption of fossil fuels. In recent times the only source of atmo-spheric CO_2 comparable in magnitude to the burning of fossil fuels is the decrease in soil humus due to encroachment of cultivation of forests and grassland. The consequences of increasing CO_2 are predicted to be increasing temperatures in the lower atmosphere. This could lead to melting of ice caps, rises in sea level, and the warming of seawater.

The increases of CO_2 in the atmosphere since the early 1960's are sufficiently large that they can be detected with good instrumentation at observatories remote from local sources of pollution. Figure F-12

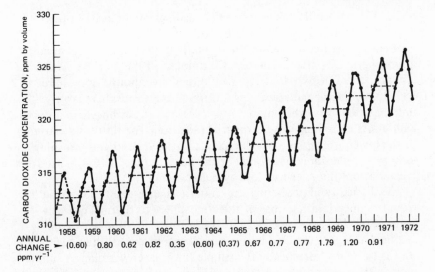

FIGURE F-12 Mean monthly carbon dioxide concentrations at Mauna Loa. Horizontal dashed lines indicate average yearly value. Annual changes in parentheses are based on incomplete record (Keeling *et al.,* in preparation).

shows measurements of the concentration of CO_2 in the air at Mauna Loa (Hawaii) from 1958 to 1972. Two main types of fluctuations are apparent in the record. The first is a seasonal variation with an amplitude of about 6 ppm, having a maximum in April and a minimum in October, due to the excess photosynthetic uptake of CO_2 over decay and respiration during summer in the northern hemisphere. Superimposed on the seasonal variation is a general upward trend with time. From 1958 to 1971, this averaged about 0.80 ppm/yr. If all the CO_2 produced by man's consumption of fossil fuels remained in the atmosphere, this growth would be about 1.44 ppm/yr. This indicates that about 50 percent of man-made CO_2 has remained airborne during this period, while the other 50 percent has gone into the oceans or the biosphere.

Predictions of future atmospheric CO_2 concentrations require knowledge of its fate as well as of fossil fuel inputs. Economists have projected a continued 4 percent annual growth in consumption to 1980 followed by a decrease in growth to 3.5 percent until the year 2000. If the additional fossil fuel from 1972 to 2000 is mixed with the entire mass of the atmosphere, it would increase the atmospheric CO_2 by 93 ppm. However, if we assume that only 50 percent remains airborne, about 47 ppm would add to the 1971 readings of about 323 ppm to suggest a prediction of 370 ppm by the year 2000.

It is more difficult to assess the climatic impact of an increase in atmospheric CO_2 than to predict the amount of the increase. The radiative properties of CO_2 that give rise to the "greenhouse" effect are well known. Solar radiation passes through the atmosphere largely unattenuated; but, when more CO_2 is present, the atmosphere absorbs and remits more long wave terrestrial radiation. The result is a warming of the lower atmosphere which receives both the solar and returning long-wave radiation, but cooling of the upper atmosphere which suffers greater atmospheric energy loss by radiation.

The difficulty in predicting the climatic change due to CO_2 results from the uncertain response of the atmosphere to thermal changes induced by the radiative effects. It is possible that atmospheric circulation, temperature, and moisture patterns might adjust in such a way as to modify drastically the simple lower level warming. A simple model (Manabe and Wetherwald, 1967) predicts that any additional CO_2 would warm the lower atmosphere, which could then hold more moisture. The global average temperature of the lower atmosphere is predicted to warm by about 0.5 °C if the CO_2 concentration is increased to 385 ppm. At altitudes above about 20 km, the temperature decrease exceeds the ground-level increase. A more sophisticated model (S. Manabe, personal communication, 1972) predicts a somewhat larger warming; at high latitudes the warming is about twice as great as the hemispherical average because the higher temperatures force a retreat of the arctic ice and snow.

It should be emphasized that the above predictions, based as they are on incomplete models, are fraught with uncertainties. For example, all models which have been used to predict the effects on the atmosphere of changing CO_2 employ a cloud cover that does not adjust to the increased CO_2. If the warmer lower atmosphere increases lower cloudiness through increased evaporation, the "greenhouse" warming might be negated. For example, an increase of low cloudiness of only 0.6 percent could also decrease the low level temperature by 0.5 °C. Alternatively, the warming of the lower atmosphere may also warm the ocean surface, thereby releasing more CO_2 to the air. This process might have a positive feedback in that the enhanced CO_2 could speed the warming. Despite these uncertainties, the possible effects of increasing CO_2 in the atmosphere due to man's activities are sufficiently profound in their potential impact on the environment and man to warrant very careful attention in the future.

Particles

Particles in the air originate from both natural and man-made sources. Tables F-10 and F-11 list the present estimates in these two categories as well as future predictions for the year 2000 of the man-made contribution. A large fraction of the smaller natural and most of the man-made particles result from indirect production, that is, from gases emitted into the air which are converted mainly in the presence of sunlight, to sulfates and other particles. The subdivision of particles between sizes smaller and larger than 5 μm separates those more likely to play a role in weather and climate (< 5 μm) from those less likely to do so (> 5 μm).

The meteorological role of particles depends on their optical and chemical characteristics as well as their sizes. Most important are the optical absorption and scattering of particles. Unfortunately, the lack of knowledge about these phenomena proves to be a vital missing link in predicting the effects of atmospheric particulates on climatic change, since the ratio of absorption to scattering determines whether a cloud of particles in the lower atmosphere warms or cools the air.

TABLE F-10 Estimated Global Direct and Converted Particle Production Due to Natural Phenomena

Source of Particles	Rate of Production by Particle Diameter, 10^6 metric tons/yr	
	>5 μm diam	< 5 μm diam
Direct Particle Production		
Sea salt	500	500
Windblown dust	250	250
Forest fires	30	5
Meteoric debris	10	0
Volcanoes[a]	?	25
TOTAL	790+	780
Particles Formed From Gases		
Sulfates	85	335
Hydrocarbons	0	75
Nitrates	15	60
TOTAL	100	470

SOURCE: Matthews *et al.* (1971).
[a] Volcanic emissions are highly variable from year to year.

TABLE F-11   Estimated Direct and Converted Particle Emissions From All Countries Due to Human Activities

Source of Particles	Rate of Production by Year and Particle Diameter, 10^6 metric tons/yr[a]		
	1968		2000
	>5 μm diam	<5 μm diam	<5 μm diam
Direct Particle Emissions			
Transportation	0.4	1.8	
Stationary sources (fuel combustion)	33.8	9.6	
Industrial processes	44.0	12.4	
Solid waste disposal	2.0	0.4	
Miscellaneous	23.4	5.4	
TOTAL	103.6	29.6	100
Particles Formed From Gases			
Converted sulfates	20	200	450
Converted nitrates	5	35	80
Converted hydrocarbons	0	15	50
TOTAL	25	250	580

SOURCE: Matthews *et al.* (1971).
[a] These emissions (for both 1968 and 2000) use the amount of emission control available in 1968.

There exist very few data that can shed light on global trends in atmospheric particulate loading. Most measurements of this kind are made at ground level within built-up areas and reflect merely local conditions. However, the available evidence suggests that many locations in temperate latitudes have experienced increasing particle concentrations since about the 1940's. On the other hand, south of about 30 °N, only stations near major cities or industrial areas show increased dust concentrations in recent decades; others remote from such centers show no change.

It is not possible to predict with certainty even the size of the ground-level temperature change that would accompany an increase in the concentration of atmospheric particles. The most obvious situation is one in which the particles would increase the amount of solar energy reflected back into space, so that the atmosphere is cooled. However, if the particles have an absorption to back-scattering ratio greater than a certain critical value, the lower atmosphere may be warmed by increasing particulate content. Very large particles can provide a "greenhouse" effect similar to that of CO_2; however, except for very heavy industrial pollution or at high altitude, the attenuation of solar radiation by particles will almost always exceed radiative effects at infrared wavelengths.

Stratospheric Effects

Between approximately 10 and 50 km above the earth's surface, in a region termed the stratosphere, the temperature of the earth's atmosphere increases with altitude. In this region air is buoyantly stable; that is, if a parcel is displaced above or below some initial altitude, it will tend to return to its original height. Consequently, vertical motions are strongly damped and the constituents of the air tend to be horizontally stratified.

While in the atmosphere as a whole chemical reactions do not strongly affect motions or temperatures, in the stratosphere the dominant heating results from absorption of solar energy by ozone. Consequently, the chemistry of the photosynthesis and decay of ozone crucially influences physical state of the stratosphere. Conversely, because motions in the stratosphere transport ozone between regions of differing photochemical activity, transport and chemistry are strongly coupled to one another, and neither may safely be discussed alone.

The stratosphere is important to man. The interface between the stratosphere and the greater bulk of the earth's atmosphere establishes a boundary condition that affects the vertical scales of weather in the troposphere. Because ozone is effectively opaque to solar wavelengths shorter than 3000 Å and because protoplasm is vulnerable to damage by exposures to these wavelengths, changes in the transport and chemistry of stratospheric ozone could influence the latitude distributions of various living species.

Somewhat surprisingly, these profound influences result from a very minor chemical constituent (the mixing fraction of ozone is rarely higher than 10^{-5}). Other species which may modify concentrations of ozone are effective at mixing fractions less than 10^{-9}. The influences of relatively minor chemical additions to the stratosphere are therefore potentially significant, a circumstance that is amplified by the long mixing times for transport downward across the tropopause (1–2 years) and from one stratospheric hemisphere to the other (2–3 years). All these considerations have recently stimulated increased concern over the possibilities of unintentional global modifications, particularly due to aircraft flying in the stratosphere, which might affect global weather patterns and human health.*

The following simple and qualitatively correct chemical model to account for stratospheric ozone was first given by Chapman:

$$O_2 + \text{solar light} \xrightarrow{J_2} O + O$$

$$O + O_2 + M \xrightarrow{k_3} O_3 + M$$

$$O_3 + \text{solar light} \xrightarrow{J_3} O_2 + O$$

$$O + O_3 \xrightarrow{k_2} O_2 + O_2 \ .$$

In the above, M is any air molecule (e.g., N_2 or O_2), k_3 and k_2 symbolize ordinary rate constants for the third and second order reactions, respectively, and J_2 and J_3 are effective photochemical rate constants resulting from wavelength integrals over the local solar flux distributions multiplied by the appropriate photodissociation cross sections. Due to self-shielding of the solar radiation by ozone and oxygen, J_2 and J_3 (and J_2/J_3) diminish with decreasing altitude. Chapman showed that an expression for the ozone concentration at high altitudes that is consistent with these reactions is

$$\frac{O_3}{O_2} \approx \frac{J_2 k_3 \, [M]}{(J_3 k_2)^{1/2}};$$

therefore

$$O_3 \sim (\text{function of altitude}) \times (\text{pressure})^{3/2}.$$

This formula successfully explains the observation that the high altitude scale height for ozone is about two-thirds that of the major molecular species, and that ozone concentrations first increase with decreasing altitude and then diminish rapidly (with J_2/J_3) below about 25 km. Quantitatively, however, this simplest mechanism tends to predict a total ozone inventory that is high by about a factor of 2 for the earth as a whole. We refer to this discrepancy as the *Chapman excess*.

To explain the Chapman excess, much effort has recently been spent in seeking additional chemical processes that might act to diminish the concentration of ozone in the earth's atmosphere. Several authors have

*The interested reader is referred to an extensive study on these questions which is currently under preparation by the Department of Transportation. Queries should be directed to Dr. Alan Grubecker, Director, Climatic Impact Assessment Program, Office of the Secretary, 400 Seventh St., S.W., Washington, D.C. 20590.

constructed chemical models that postulate reactions of ozone with hydroxyl (OH) and hydroperoxyl (HO$_2$) radicals which, with assumed rate constants, tend to ameliorate the Chapman excess. The resulting "wet photolysis" model has been used to estimate potential effects of supersonic transport (SST) traffic. The reaction,

$$HO_2 + O_3 \longrightarrow HO + O_2 + O_2,$$

for which no rate measurement was available, was "conservatively" guessed to have a rate coefficient near 10^{-16} cm^3 s^{-1}. With this assumption a regenerating water chain was postulated which could be shown to influence the steady-state expression for ozone concentration, so that

$$[O_3] \sim [H_2O]^{-1/3}.$$

Recent attempts to measure the reaction directly, however, yield an upper limit for the coefficient of less than 10^{-21} cm^3 s^{-1}. With this revised value the water chain cannot contribute appreciably, at least in the form originally postulated (Langley and McGrath, 1971).*

Quite recently Johnston (1971) has re-emphasized the potential role of nitrogen oxides in the stratospheric chemical cycle. Among many reactions which may plausibly affect the profile of ozone, most likely to be significant are

$$NO + O_3 \xrightarrow{k_f} NO_2 + O_2,$$
$$NO_2 + \text{solar light} \xrightarrow{J_4} NO + O,$$

and

$$NO_2 + O \xrightarrow{k_g} NO + O_2.$$

Including these and several other reactions into the Chapman scheme results in approximately a 10 percent computed diminution of the total ozone if α (the mixing fraction of nitrogen oxides) is 10^{-9}, and 30 percent if α is 10^{-8} (Figure F-13).

Unfortunately, good measurements of natural background concentration of nitrogen oxides in the stratosphere have not yet been reported. However, in the troposphere, at locations far removed from contaminating cities, α is about 3×10^{-9}. Measurements of the earth's ultraviolet fluorescence at altitudes near 75 km have been interpreted to suggest $\alpha \approx 5 \times 10^{-8}$. It has been suggested that oxidation of N$_2$O (which is a

---

*"Demore (1973) has recently given a value of 3×10^{-15} cm^3 sec^{-1} for the rate coefficient discussed in this paragraph, which suggests that water effects may indeed be important in the destruction of atmospheric ozone."

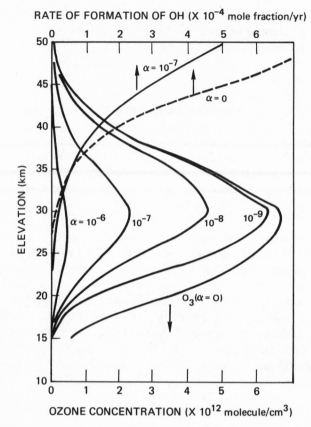

RATE OF FORMATION OF OH (X 10^{-4} mole fraction/yr)

FIGURE F-13   Computed ozone profiles for various nitrogen oxide mixing ratios α (from Johnston, 1971)

metabolic product and is present in the troposphere at mixing fractions near 10^{-6}) by metastable oxygen atoms may enhance in the stratosphere. Nitrogen dioxide absorption has been observed in the stratosphere at infrared wavelengths, by balloon borne spectrophotometers looking tangentially towards the setting sun. The resulting absorptions were roughly consistent with $\alpha \approx 10^{-8}$. Similar satellite-borne measurements are scheduled for a later Nimbus flight.

With regard to the problem of attempting to predict the atmospheric effects of the SST, estimates of air fleets, route structures, and engine emissions can be combined to estimate an addition to the natural α of about 10^{-8}. At present, however, the natural background and distribution of stratospheric nitrogen oxides must be regarded as unknown.

Nevertheless, pending good measurements, the decision matrix given in Table F-12 appears sensible.

Of course, in the not unlikely case that the natural value of α should turn out to be near to 10^{-8}, then all the matrix elements revert to an equivocal "maybe."

Perhaps of more immediate concern, is the suggestion that man's activities may already be affecting stratospheric chemistry by the following route. Methane and carbon monoxide consume hydroxyl radicals via the reactions.

$$CH_4 + OH \rightarrow CH_3 + H_2O$$

and

$$CO + OH \rightarrow CO_2 + H \quad .$$

These reactions are believed to be responsible for the principal sinks for the earth's methane and carbon monoxide and, in the latter case, to account for what has until quite recently been a puzzling paradox over the short residence time for CO in the atmosphere. Further reactions include

$$H + O_2 + M \rightarrow HO_2$$
$$HO_2 + NO \rightarrow NO_2 + OH,$$

which regenerates the hydroxyl radical. The nitrogen dioxide may photolyse at wavelengths less than 4600 Å, to produce ozone

$$NO_2 + h\nu \rightarrow NO + O$$
$$O + O_2 + M \rightarrow O_3 + M,$$

TABLE F-12 · Possible Effects of SST on Stratospheric Ozone

	Natural mixing fraction α of stratospheric nitrogen oxides significantly $<10^{-8}$	Natural mixing fraction α of stratospheric nitrogen oxides significantly $>10^{-8}$
"Chapman excess explained"	NO	YES
SST traffic should significantly affect global ozone	YES	NO

and ozone may photolyse at wavelengths less than 3300 Å to produce metastable oxygen atoms

$$O_3 + h\nu \rightarrow O_2 + O\ (^1D).$$

These in turn generate vibrationally excited hydroxyl radicals:

$$O(^1D) + H_2O \rightarrow OH + OH^+\ (\nu \leqslant 2)$$

where ν is the quantum number of the vibrational state. In still a further sequence, these again may attack ozone:

$$OH^+\ (\nu \geqslant 2) + O_3 \rightarrow O_2 + O_2 + H\ (\text{or } HO_2 + O_2).$$

Additionally, the hydrogen atom produced above, by the reaction of OH with CO, may also react quickly with O_3:

$$H + O_3 \rightarrow OH + O_2.$$

Clearly, all these interactions are complex, indeed, sufficiently so that we cannot deny the possibility that methane and carbon monoxide production, augmented by man's activities, may already have modified the natural stratosphere. More argumentation than measurement has been expended on this question. The measurements we have, which suggest that the global ozone column diminished somewhat during the decade of the 1960's, cannot yet be firmly ascribed to chemical causes. Nevertheless, a watchful attitude is clearly prudent, and we judge it within the charter of the EPA to be concerned over the possible effects of present and future chemical discharges into the atmosphere upon the earth's stratospheric ozone.

REFERENCES

Sources and Dispersal of Atmospheric Pollution

Engelmann, R.J. 1970. Scavenging Prediction Using Ratios of Concentrations in Air and Precipitation. In: *Precipitation Scavenging.* Proc. CONF. 700601. National Technical Information Service, Springfield, Va. pp. 475–485.

Holzworth, G.C. 1972. *Mixing Heights, Wind Speeds, and Potential for Urban Air Pollution Throughout the Contiguous United States.* Publ. No. AP-101. Environmental Protection Agency, Office of Air Programs, Rockville, Md. 118 pp.

Slade, D.H., ed. 1968. *Meteorology and Atomic Energy.* U.S. Atomic Energy Commission. Access No. TID-24190. National Technical Information Service, Springfield, Va. 450 pp.

Gas-to-Particle Conversion

Junge, C.E. 1963. *Air Chemistry and Radioactivity*. Academic Press, New York. 382 pp.

Whitby, K.T., B.Y.H. Liu, R.B. Husar, and N.J. Barsic. 1972. The Minnesota-Aerosol-Analyzing System used in the Los Angeles Smog Project. *J. Colloid Interface Sci.* 39:136–164.

Photochemical Reactions in the Atmosphere

Altshuller, A.P., W.A. Lonneman, F.D. Sutterfield, and S.L. Kopczynski. 1971. Hydrocarbon composition of the atmosphere of the Los Angeles basin—1967. *Environ. Sci. Technol.* 5:1009–1016.

Bates, D.R. and A. Witherspoon. 1952. The photo-chemistry of some minor constituents of the earth's atmosphere (CO_2, CO, CH_4, N_2O). *Mon. Not. R. Astron. Soc.* 112:101–124.

Herzberg, G. 1950. *Molecular Spectra and Molecular Structure*, Vol. I. Spectra of Diatomic Molecules, 2nd ed. Van Nostrand Reinhold, Princeton, N.J. 658 pp.

Inn, E.C.Y., and Y. Tanaka. 1953. Absorption coefficient of ozone in the ultraviolet and visible regions. *J. Opt. Soc. Am.* 43:870–873.

Junge, C.E. 1963. *Air Chemistry and Radioactivity*. Academic Press, New York. 382 pp.

Leighton, P.A. 1961. *Photochemistry of Air Pollution*. Academic Press, New York. 300 pp.

Levy H., II. 1972. Photochemistry of the lower troposphere. *Planet. Space Sci.* 20:919–935.

Robinson, E., and R.C. Robbins. 1968. Sources, Abundance, and Fate of Gaseous Atmospheric Pollutants. Publ. 4007. Amrican Petroleum Institute, Washington, D.C. 123 pp.

Seiler, W., and C. Junge. 1970. Carbon monoxide in the atmosphere. *J. Geophys. Res.* 75:2217–2226.

Stevens, C.M., L. Krout, D. Walling, A. Venters, A. Engelkermeir, and L.E. Ross. 1972. The isotopic composition of atmospheric carbon monoxide. *Earth Planet. Sci. Lett.* 16:147–165.

Weinstock, B. 1969. Carbon monoxide: Residence time in the atmosphere. *Science.* 166:224–225.

Weinstock, B., and H. Niki. 1972. Carbon monoxide balance in nature. *Science* 176:290–292.

Wofsy, S.C., J.C. McConnell, and M.B. McElroy. 1972. Atmospheric CH_4, CO and CO_2. *J. Geophys. Res.* 77:4477–4493.

Clouds and Precipitation

Biswas, K.R., R.K. Kapoor, K.K. Kanuga, and Bh.V. Ramana Murty. 1967. Cloud seeding experiment using common salt. *J. Appl. Meteorol.* 6:914–923.

Biswas, K.R., and A.S. Dennis. 1971. Formation of a rain shower by salt seeding. *J. Appl. Meteorol.* 10:780–784.

Frederick, R.H. 1970. Preliminary results of a study on precipitation by day-of-the-week over eastern United States. In *Preprints, Second National Conference on Weather Modification*. American Meteorological Society, Boston. pp. 209–214.

Hobbs, P.V., and J.D. Locatelli. 1969. Ice nuclei from a natural forest fire. *J. Appl. Meteorol.* 8:833–834.

Hobbs, P.V., L.F. Radke, and S.E. Shumway. 1970. Cloud condensation nuclei from industrial sources and their apparent influence on precipitation in Washington State. *J. Atmos. Sci.* 27:81–100.

Hobbs, P.V., and L.F. Radke. 1973. Redistribution of snowfall across a mountain range by artificial seeding: A case study. *Science* 181:1043–1045.

Huff, F.A., and S.A. Changnon, Jr. 1972. *Climatological Assessment of Urban Effects on Precipitation.* State Water Survey Contract Report No. 133. Illinois State Water Survey, Urbana. 237 pp.

Langer, G. 1968. Ice Nuclei Generated by Steel Mill Activity. In M. Neilburger and H.C. Chin, eds., *Proceedings of the First National Conference on Weather Modification.* American Meteorological Society, Boston. pp. 220–223.

Langer, G. 1970. A Study of Automobile Exhaust as a Source of Ice Nuclei. In *Preprints, Second National Conference on Weather Modification.* American Meteorological Society, Boston. pp. 242–243.

National Research Council. Committee on Atmospheric Sciences. 1973. *Weather and Climate Modification: Problems and Progress.* National Academy of Sciences, Washington, D.C. 258 pp.

Schaefer, V.J. 1966. Ice nuclei from automobile exhaust and iodine vapor. *Science* 154:1555–1557.

Warner, J. 1968. A reduction in rainfall associated with smoke from sugarcane fires—An inadvertent weather modification? *J. Appl. Meteorol.* 7:247–251.

Radiation Transfer

Herman, B.M., and S.R. Browning. 1965. A numerical solution for the equation of radiative transfer. *J. Atmos. Sci.* 22:559–566.

Schneider, S.H. 1972. Cloudiness as a global climatic feedback mechanism: The effects on the radiation balance and surface temperature of variations in cloudiness. *J. Atmos. Sci.* 29:1413–1422.

Try, P.D. 1972. An Investigation of the Influence of Aerosols on the Solar Radiation Field and the Heating of a Multiple Scattering Polluted Urban Atmosphere. Ph.D. Dissertation, University of Washington, Seattle.

Global Effects of Pollutants on Climate

Demore, W.B. 1973. Rate constants for the reactions of hydroxyl and hydroperoxyl radicals with ozone. *Science* 180:735–737.

Johnston, H. 1971. Reduction of stratospheric ozone by nitrogen oxide catalysts from supersonic transport exhaust. *Science* 173:517–522.

Keeling, C.D., A.E. Bainbridge, C.A. Ekdahl, P. Guenther, and J.F. S. Chin. (In preparation.) Atmospheric carbon dioxide variation at Mauna Loa Observatory, Hawaii, 1958–1970.

Langley, K.F., and W.D. McGrath. 1971. Ultra-violet photolysis of ozone in the presence of water vapor. *Planet. Space Sci.* 19:413–15.

Manabe, S., and R.T. Wetherwald. 1967. Thermal equilibrium of the atmosphere with a given distribution of relative humidity. *J. Atmos. Sci.* 24:241–259.

Matthews, W.H., W.H. Kellogg, and G.D. Robinson, eds. 1971. *Man's Impact on the Climate.* M.I.T. Press, Cambridge, Mass. 594 pp.

SUGGESTED READINGS

Wilson, C.L., and W.H. Matthews, eds. 1970. *Man's Impact on the Global Environment: Assessment and Recommendations for Action.* M.I.T. Press, Cambridge. 319 pp.

Wilson, C.L., and W.H. Matthews, eds. 1971. *Inadvertent Climate Modification.* M.I.T. Press, Cambridge. 308 pp.

G

Inanimate
Materials

Supplementary Material to Chapter XIX

TESTING METHODS FOR INANIMATE MATERIALS

Tests have been conducted on a variety of materials under various conditions over the years and consequently, established procedures for evaluating the effects of chemicals on inanimate materials are available. Numerous industries, professional organizations, and government agencies have made significant contributions toward the standardization of test methods.

The following abbreviations are used throughout this appendix.

AMHA— American Hotel and Motel Association, New York
ASTM— American Society for Testing and Materials
      1916 Race Street
      Philadelphia, Pennsylvania 19103
NACE— National Association of Corrosion Engineers
      2400 West Loop South
      Houston, Texas 77027
OCF — Owens-Corning Fiberglas Corporation
      Fiberglas Tower
      Toledo, Ohio 43601
PPG — PPG Industries, Inc.
      Fiber Glass Division
      One Gateway Center
      Pittsburgh, Pennsylvania 15222

TAPPI— Technical Association of the Pulp and Paper Industry
One Dunwoody Park
Atlanta, Georgia 30341

METALS

Standardized Methods

Source	Method	Title
ASTM Committee G-1	Forthcoming in 1974	Standard test for evaluating materials in the atmosphere
ASTM Committee B-8	B-537	Nickel–chrominum plated coatings
NACE	Standard TM-01-69	Laboratory corrosion testing of metals for the process industries
NACE	Standard TM-02	Method of conducting controlled velocity laboratory tests

References

Champion, F.A. 1964. *Corrosion Testing Procedures.* John Wiley and Sons, New York.
Department of Transportation. 1972. Hazardous Materials Regulations. Title 49, Code of Federal Regulations, Parts 170–180, 1972 Revision. Office of Hazardous Materials, U.S. Department of Transportation, Washington, D.C.

CONCRETE, MORTAR, AND STONE

Tests are currently available, although not necessarily standard, which can evaluate the effect of chemical substances. After periods of controlled exposure, concrete, mortar, or stone test specimens should be examined by a petrographer experienced in working with that material. Concrete petrographers are not numerous, but competent ones are to be found. Such examination is rapid and an excellent means of predicting the outcome with actual exposure.

Measurements of changes in length, volume, or resonance frequency of test specimens undergoing exposure are commonly employed in nondestructive test methods.

Part 10 of the ASTM *Book of Standards* describes several applicable procedures:

Source	Method	Title
ASTM	Recommended practice C-25	Chemical analysis of limestone, quick-lime and hydrated lime
ASTM	C-88	Test for soundness of aggregates by use of sodium sulfate or magnesium sulfate
ASTM	C-157	Test for length change of cement mortar and concrete
ASTM	C-215	Test for fundamental transverse, longitudinal and torsonial frequencies of concrete specimen
ASTM	C-597	Test for pulse frequency through concrete
ASTM	C-672	Test for scaling resistance of concrete surfaces exposed to deicing chemicals

WOOD

ASTM method D-143-52 (Reapproved 1972) is a standard method for testing clear specimens of timber, which appears in Part 16 of the ASTM *Book of Standards.*

PAPER

Source	Method	Title
TAPPI	T 403	Bursting strength
TAPPI	T 404	Tensile strength
TAPPI	T 423	Folding endurance

FIBER TEXTILES

Standardized Methods

Source	Method	Title
ASTM	D-76-67	Tensile strength
ASTM	D2256-69	Tensile strength
ASTM	D1445-67	Tensile strength
ASTM	D2529-69	Tensile strength

References

American Society for Testing and Materials. 1971. Part 24-25. ASTM *Book of Standards*. American Society for Testing and Materials, Philadelphia.

U.S. Department of Defense. 1968. (federal test methods) Standard No. 191, Textile Test Methods, December 31, 1968.

PLASTICS

Standardized Methods

Source	Method	Title
ASTM	D543	Test for resistance of plastics to chemical reagents
ASTM	C581	Test for chemical resistance of thermosetting resins used in glass fiber reinforced structures
ASTM	D756	Tests for resistance of plastics to accelerated service conditions
ASTM	D814	Test for permeability of vulcanized rubber to volatile liquids
ASTM	D1239	Test for resistance of plastic films to extraction by chemicals
ASTM	D1435	Rec. practice for outdoor weathering of plastics
ASTM	D2126	Test for resistance of rigid cellular plastics to simulated service conditions

References

American Society for Testing and Materials. 1958. *Simulated Service Testing in the Plastics Industry*. Special Technical Publication No. 375, American Society for Testing and Materials, Philadelphia.

Fenner, O.H. 1969. Chemical resistance of polymeric materials. Presented November 13, Plastic Design Institute, Symposium on Permanence of Polymeric Materials, Cherry Hill, New Jersey. (Address: Corporate Engineering, Monsanto Company, St. Louis, Missouri).

Kambour, R.P. 1967. The role of organic agents in the stress crazing and cracking of glassy polymers. General Electric Research and Development Center publication.

Lever, A.E. and J. Rhys. 1958. *The Properties and Testing of Plastic Materials*. Chemical Publishing Co., New York.

Modern Plastics Encyclopedia. 1969. Simplified explanations of common ASTM tests mentioned in the plastics properties chart, 1969–70. McGraw-Hill, New York. 46(10A).

GLASS

Flat Glass

It is the experience of the flat-glass industry that the only significant kind of environmental damage is associated with "staining" (etching) of the surface of stored glass caused by the deposition of moisture from the atmosphere. This usually occurs in unheated warehouses where a change in the weather can expose cold glass to warm, moist air. Certain volatile acidic (SO_2) or basic (NH_3) substances in contaminated air could be co-deposited with moisture under these circumstances. Although the staining of stored glass by these contaminants is not likely to be significant, a qualitative test could be devised by adapting the "cyclic humidity" test of H.E. Simpson (*Am. Ceramic Soc. Bull.* 30:41–45, 1951).

The industry has recently introduced glasses coated with thin layers of metal (Cr) or metal oxides (of Fe, Co, Ni). The thinness and intense coloration of these films means that they will be seriously affected in terms of appearance and function by any reagent that produces a significant degree of attack. Again, there is no standard test method, but optical measurements are obviously applicable.

Instruments for measuring haze and gloss are commercially available.

Containers

In the container industry, the "internal" environment is the only one that has been given any serious consideration as far as chemical attack is concerned. There is a standard autoclave test for leachability of the interior of containers used for sensitive products (ASTM C-225-68, Resistance of Glass Containers to Chemical Attack).

Optical Glass

The reader should consult the manufacturers of optical glass concerning the availability of test procedures.

Glass-Fiber Textiles

Source	Method	Title
AHMA	L24-1963	Performance requirements for institutional textiles

Glass-Fiber Textiles (Continued)

Source	Method	Title
ASTM	D 579	Ravel strip test method for determining breaking strength of fabric
ASTM	D-1175	Method of test for flex abrasion of fabric
OCF	DF509	Breaking strength, ravel strip method
OCF	DF511	Burst strength of fiberglass decorative fabrics
OCF	DF515	Test method to determine breaking strength retention after dynamic creasing
OCF	DF517	Method of test for determining properties of fiberglass draperies by the dynamic drapery tester
PPG	S 01 Aa	Test method to determine breaking strength retention after static folding

Glazed Ceramics

The reader should consult the manufacturers of glazed ceramic products concerning the availability of test procedures.

PERFORMANCE OF MATERIALS

Common inanimate materials in widespread use serving mankind in his daily environment include ferrous and nonferrous metals, glass, wood, paper, concrete, stone, plastics, and natural and synthetic fibers. Many species within these classes of materials, which are designed for special industrial services, are not included in this discussion because they are not associated with widespread usage in the environment.

The selection of a material for specific application depends upon its mechanical and physical properties, as well as its resistance to deterioration by the natural environment prevailing, which consists of

1. naturally occurring air atmospheres supporting human life, and
2. naturally occurring waters for both potable and industrial uses.

Effects on the expected performance of these materials from chemicals escaping into these environments are of potential concern. Many existing structures and objects could be adversely affected in utility, durability, and/or appearance by such exposure.

The extensive use of the materials considered here attests to their proven durability for the services intended. A summary of their performance characteristics in the most commonly encountered environments is presented in this section as a guide to predicting the possible effects of new chemicals.

Ferrous Metals

The effects of atmospheric contamination on ferrous metals are summarized in Table G-1. Table G-2 contains performance data for ferrous metals exposed to various liquids.

TABLE G-1   Effects of Atmospheric Exposure of Ferrous Metals

Metal	Exposure Conditions	Performance	Reference
Carbon steel[a]	NaCl in moist air	Protective film destroyed	b-e
	Sulfur oxides	Corrosion	
Alloy steels[a]	Atmospheric	Improved resistance over carbon steel	e
Zinc-coated steels	Acidic industrial atmosphere with frequent wetting	Formation of protective coating inhibited	
Aluminum-coated steels	Rural, industrial, and marine atmosphere	More resistant than zinc	f, g
	Industrial atmosphere contaminated with combinations of H_2S, CO_2, NH_3, SO_2, moisture, and dirt	Highly resistant to corrosion	
	Humid atmospheres containing $CaCl_2$, $FeCl_3$, $KMnO_4$, or NaF	Corrosion	

TABLE G-1 –*Continued*

Metal	Exposure Conditions	Performance	Reference
Nickel-coated steels	Indoor atmosphere	Resists tarnishing	*b*
	Outdoor atmosphere	Dull or tarnished surface	
	Industrial sulfurous atmosphere	Green or mottled gray tarnish	
	Rural atmosphere	Faint gray tarnish	
Nickel–chromium-coated steels	Atmospheric (auto bumpers)	No tarnishing	
Stainless steels			
12% chromium	Industrial atmosphere	Resists corrosion	*h*
15% chromium	Marine atmosphere	Slight pitting and rust staining	*h*
28% chromium	Marine atmosphere	Resists corrosion	*h*
Austenitic	Urban atmosphere, 26 years	Unaffected	*i*
	Industrial atmosphere containing Cl_2 and HCl		
AISI Types 304 & 316	Urban atmosphere	Resistant to attack	*j*
ASTM Types A606 Type 4 A202 Type 1 A588 Grade A	Contaminated atmospheres	Highly resistant	*k*

a For an extensive discussion of carbon steel, low-allow and alloy steels, see Schmitt (1960).
b American Society for Testing and Materials (1959).
c Guttman and Sereda (1968).
d Copson (1945).
e Schmitt (1960).
f Walton and King (1956).
g Anderson (1956).
h Schmitt and Mullen (1969).
i American Society for Metals (1961).
j American Society for Testing and Materials (1961).
k Schmitt and Gallagher (1969).

Nonferrous Metals

The performance of nonferrous metals when exposed to chemicals is summarized in Table G-3.

Glass

The term "glass" as used here applies to materials of the following types.

TABLE G-2 Performance of Ferrous Metals Exposed to Liquids

Material	Exposure Conditions	Performance
Carbon, alloy, and stainless steels	Alkaline solutions at moderate temperatures	Very resistant
	Hot concentrated alkalies	Corrosion and stress-cracking possible
	Organic solvents, dry	Unaffected
	Organic solvents in presence of water	Corrosion, especially with chlorinated solvents
Carbon and alloy steels	All acids	Some degree of attack
	Alkaline salts (carbonates, phosphates, and silicates)	Not readily attacked
	Neutral salts	Attacked
	Acid salts	Corrosion
Stainless steel	Halogen acids	Attacked
	Sulfuric acid	Attacked
	Other acids (nitric, phosphoric, acetic, formic, lactic, oxalic), moderate temperature	Highly resistant
	Halide salt solutions	Attacked under certain conditions
	Other salts	Excellent resistance
Zinc-coated steel	Acidic solutions (pH <6.0)	Rapid corrosion
	Strong alkalies (pH > 12.5)	Rapid corrosion
	Soaps	Resistant
	Mild alkalies	Resistant
	Washing powders	Resistant
Nickel–chromium-coated steel	Deicing salt	Adversely affected

Flat glass—Includes glass used primarily for weathertight, transparent glazing, as in commercial residential architecture, automobiles, and aircraft.

Containers—Includes bottles, tubing, pressed glassware, household glassware.

Optical glass—Includes spectacles and the refractive and reflective components of optical instruments.

Glass-fiber textiles—Includes only textiles that are exposed directly

TABLE G-3 Effects of Chemicals on Nonferrous Metals

Material	Exposure Conditions	Performance	Reference
Aluminum		See "Aluminum-coated" steel," Table G-1	
Copper and copper-base alloys	Rural, marine, and industrial atmospheres	Highly resistant to corrosion but subject to tarnishing	
	Drinking water	Highly resistant to corrosion	
	Household soaps and detergents	Highly resistant to corrosion	
Copper-base alloys	Ammonia and ammonia-base chemicals	Stress corrosion cracking	*a-d*
	Mercury and its compounds	Stress cracking	
Nickel–copper alloys	Natural fresh waters	Low corrosion rate	*a-i*
	Acids in fresh waters	Increased corrosion	
	Dilute alkalies	No adverse effect	
	Ammonia	No stress cracking	
	Neutral salts, low concentration	Little effect	
	Mercury and its compounds	Stress cracking	
Precious metals			
Silver	Breathable air	Tarnishing	
Gold, palladium, and platinum	Breathable air	No tarnishing	

a American Society for Testing and Materials (1971).
b Uhlig (1948).
c National Association of Corrosion Engineers (1974).
d LaQue and Copson (1963).
e International Nickel Co. no date, Bull. No. 1
f International Nickel Co. no date, Bull. No. 2
g International Nickel Co. no date, Bull. No. 3
h International Nickel Co. no date, Bull. No. 4
i International Nickel Co. no date, Bull. No. 5

to the environment, such as draperies. Textiles embedded in "plastic" are to be considered in connection with materials of that class.

Glazed ceramics—Includes "whiteware," glazed brick and tile, glass-ceramics.

Specifically excluded from this discussion are the following: unglazed brick and tile, such specialized optical materials as chalcogenide glasses, glasses used as encapsulants or active components of electronic devices, and glazes on metallic substrates.

All the glassy materials considered are based on silica as a major component; therefore, the chemical behavior of glasses approximates that of fused silica. Fused silica is well known for its chemical inertness; indeed, many applications of glasses in the chemical industry are based on this property. Silica is almost completely resistant to oxidizing agents, and to acids other than hydrofluoric, fluorosilicic, and fluoroboric.

Silica is less resistant to aqueous alkaline reagents; it is gradually corroded by hydroxides, carbonates, aqueous ammonia, and the like. Chemicals containing these substances or generating them upon hydrolysis or other chemical change may be destructive.

Silica is entirely resistant to organic compounds, although compounds containing fluorine, alkali and alkaline-earth metals, and amine nitrogen should be evaluated for the possible generation of corrosive products by oxidation, hydrolysis, photolysis, photooxidation, or other reactions suggested by their chemical structure.

One known class of organic compounds constitutes an exception to the above statement. The silicon ion is known to be chelated by phenolic compounds which present two phenol groups in an ortho position, such as o-catechol and pyrogallol. The reaction is very slow, however, and probably requires the presence of water. Other chelating agents for the silicon ion may exist that have not been identified. This chelation is not a major hazard, however, because the tetravalency and small diameter of the silicon ion makes its polymeric compounds very stable.

Most of the commercially utilized glasses are not pure silica, but contain various amounts of other oxides in a mutually dissolved state with silica. These diluents, in general, reduce the chemical durability below that of pure silica. The reduction is not serious unless the silica content falls below 70 percent by weight. Even below this level, chemical durability will be maintained if the diluent oxides include substantial amounts of those classified as "network formers," that is, Al_2O_3, ZrO_2, TiO_2, and, to a lesser extent, B_2O_3 and PbO. Glasses whose combined content of SiO_2 and Al_2O_3 is below 50 percent are rarely used in commerce. The following special considerations should be noted in the case of glasses containing diluent oxides.

• Multivalent and transition-metal oxide diluents are susceptible to the specialized solvent action of aqueous solutions containing chelating agents such as EDTA and phosphates. These agents are especially active under neutral or alkaline conditions.

- Glasses containing more than 10 percent B_2O_3 by weight are subject to a spontaneous phase separation that renders them leachable by acids.
- Optical glasses of the "flint" variety frequently contain large amounts of PbO, rare-earth oxides, and the like. The chemical durability of these glasses is marginal; it has been sacrificed in order to permit the attainment of the refractive index and refractive dispersion required in instruments. Such glasses are frequently susceptible to acids and to chemical chelating agents.

Table G-4 lists for several uses of glass the kinds of effects that are of greatest concern.

Concrete, Mortar, and Stone

The performance of concrete and stone under environmental exposure is usually expressed in terms of compressive strength and rigidity: For certain applications, however, appearance, smoothness, or resistance to wear by abrasion may be equally important. Resistance to chemical attack varies enormously as a function of raw materials and construction procedures. The most impermeable concretes have been found to be the most durable.

Concrete and stone are resistant to nearly all chemicals, if dry, but are not resistant to some chemical solutions or to alternate wetting and

TABLE G-4 Critical Effects of Chemicals on Glass

Type of Glass	Application	Critical Effect
Flat glass	Windows	Loss of transparency
Container glass	"Crystal glassware"	Deterioration of appearance
	Bottles	Contamination of contents due to corrosion and leaching on interior surfaces
	Lighting fixtures	Loss of transparency
Optical glass	Eyeglasses, instruments	Loss of transparency, changes in surface contours
Glass-fiber textiles		Loss of strength due to fiber breakage; breakage enhanced by deterioration of organic surface coatings
Glazed ceramics		Loss of gloss; leaching of toxic compounds into stored foodstuffs; exposure of porous substrate, especially in insulators

drying by such solutions (American Concrete Institute Committee, 1962; Woods, 1968; Kuenning, 1966; and American Concrete Institute Committee, 1966).

Concrete and mortars are chemically basic, having a pH of about 13; hence, they may be attacked by acid solutions having a pH less than 7. In general, good quality concrete performs well at pH values as low as 5.6. Such acids as fluorosilicic, tartaric, and oxalic, which form calcium salts of low solubility, are practically harmless to concrete. Considerable experience in acidic soils has demonstrated that the impermeability of a concrete is responsible for its success or failure.

Concrete is generally resistant to bases in less than a 10 percent solution. Some concrete aggregates are alkali-reactive, and their successful use requires special precautions. These aggregates, most often siliceous rocks of volcanic or other pyrogenic origin, will react with some potassium and sodium compounds, causing serious internal expansion evidenced by severe cracking of concrete structures.

Common salt, NaCl, is chemically harmless, but the chloride ion is a contributor to corrosion of reinforcing steel and, hence, is of serious concern to most concrete structures. Chlorides and nitrates of ammonia, magnesium, aluminum, and iron all attack concrete. Other salts, such as ammonium fluoride, which form insoluble compounds upon reaction with cement paste are not harmful to concrete.

Among the most detrimental chemicals to concrete are the sulfates, which—if allowed to permeate a portland cement concrete or mortar—will react with hydrated calcium aluminate forming an extremely expansive product which cracks and possibly destroys the concrete. The critical sulfate concentration above which damage may occur varies with the amount of calcium aluminate in the concrete. It ranges from 100 to 1000 ppm sulfate in solution, with 300 ppm not an unreasonable single value. If higher sulfate concentrations are anticipated, ASTM Type II or Type V cements can be used to raise the critical value to over 1000 ppm.

Sulfur dioxide from the combustion of fuels will react in the atmosphere to form sulfurous and sulfuric acids, which can etch concrete surfaces. Severe damage to limestone and marble monuments and statues has been attributed to attack by these air pollutants.

Natural Fibers

The materials to be considered under this classification are those fibers and textiles which are essentially cellulosic in nature, such as cotton, linen, hemp, jute, as well as the regenerated rayons; and the proteinaceous fibers, such as wool, mohair, cashmere, alpaca, and silk.

The production of cloth from animal and vegetable fibers is so old an art that we have no records of where or when it began. Textiles are relatively perishable, but in the dry climate of Egypt, for example, linen fabrics have been found in tombs believed to be almost 6000 years old. Thus these materials have had a long history of use, and a body of knowledge has been acquired as to their performance under a variety of use conditions.

Since textiles are important articles of commerce, standards and test methods have been devised for both the fibers themselves and the textiles produced from them. Technical associations especially concerned with these standards are the American Association of Textile Chemists and Colorists (American Association of Textile Chemists and Colorists, Issued annually) and the American Society for Testing and Materials (American Society for Testing and Materials, 1971). It is not believed that any new test procedures will need to be developed for assessing the impact of new chemicals on these materials.

Vegetable Fibers   All the vegetable fibers consist of more of less pure cellulose. Cellulose is composed of β-D-glucopyranose units linked together in straight chains by (1-4)-glycosidic bonds. In attempting to assess the action of a chemical on cellulose, once must consider its effect either on the glycosidic bond or on the glucopyranose unit.

The reactions which cellulose undergoes are relatively few and may be classified as follows (Othmer 1964).

- Hydrolysis by acids
- Depolymerization (alkaline oxidation for viscose production or controlled acid hydrolysis
- Oxidation (primary hydroxyl groups are oxidized to aldehyde or carboxyl groups, while secondary hydroxyl groups are oxidized to ketones, aldehyde, or carboxy groups; the formation of aldehyde or carboxyl groups by the oxidation of secondary hydroxyl groups involves bond cleavage)
- Substitution reactions involving the hydroxyl groups
- Graft addition reactions

Many of these reactions take place only under carefully controlled conditions which would not be encountered in the environment and will not be considered further.

Mineral acids degrade vegetable fibers, especially if allowed to dry. Dilute mineral acids at ordinary temperatures have little effect but, at high temperatures, destruction of the glycosidic bond is rapid.

Concentrated mineral acids can cause complete dissolution of cellulose, even when cold.

Volatile organic acids have little effect on cellulose; however, solutions of the nonvolatile organic acids, such as oxalic and citric, have a tendering action when their concentration increases on drying of the fabric.

Cotton is not normally attacked by alkalies. They are, in fact, used in finishing and processing to increase fiber strength. In the viscose process, however, a controlled depolymerization is brought about by air oxidation of alkali-treated cellulose.

Oxidizing agents, such as the hypochlorites and sodium and hydrogen peroxide, are used for bleaching the cellulosic fibers: They must be used with care since, in strong solutions, they can convert cellulose to oxycellulose with a consequent loss in tensile strength. Reducing agents, such as sodium hydrosulfite, are used in finishing processes and have little degradative effect on the fibers. Polar solvents, which can swell cellulose, will have about the same effect on vegetable fibers as water. Nonpolar solvents do not affect the strength of the vegetable fibers, and they are used in drycleaning.

Oils of vegetable, animal, or mineral origin have no effect on the strength of textile fibers and are often used in processing fabrics to impart lubricity, pliability, and softness. Neutral salts at ordinary temperatures have little effect on cellulosic fibers; however, complex ammonia and amine bases of copper are perhaps the best known solvents for cellulose.

Exposure of the vegetable fibers to polluted atmospheres can cause embrittlement if the pollutant is acidic or oxidative in nature.

Animal Fibers The animal fibers have a complex molecular structure and are essentially protein in character. Proteins are polymers of α-amino acids joined by amide linkages. These long polypeptide chains can be bound together by salt linkages between acidic and basic side chains of the amino acids, by covalent sulfur to sulfur bonds formed between cystine residues, and by hydrogen bonds between the $-CO-$ and $-NH-$ groups of neighboring peptides (Othmer, 1970a). Thus, degradation of the protein molecule can occur by the rupture of the peptide bond, rupture of the salt bridges due to acid or base, modification or rupture of the sulfur to sulfur bonds, and a decrease in hydrogen bonding by polar solvents.

Wool is much more resistant to dilute mineral acids than are the vegetable fibers, although even cold concentrated acids will decompose wool by breaking the peptide chain. Alkalies are injurious to wool.

Caustic soda in dilute solutions in the cold will completely disintegrate and dissolve wool fiber. Even sodium carbonate solutions should be used with caution.

Oxidizing agents—such as hydrogen peroxide and potassium permanganate—are used for bleaching silk and wool, but, again, caution must be used. The hypochlorites do not bleach wool, but give it a yellow tinge. Chlorine has been used in the production of unshrinkable woolen garments, but with some loss in wearing quality. Reducing agents attack wool at the disulfide groups. They are often used in processing fibers, but must be used with caution. The breaking of the disulfide crosslinkages can reduce the wet strength of the fiber by 90 percent, but almost all of the original strength can be restored by reforming the cross-linkages by oxidation.

With polar solvents, the wet strength of wool is lower than the dry strength but is regained on drying. Nonpolar solvents are without effect on wool, and many are used in dry cleaning.

Neutral salts are not very reactive with wool, with the exception of the heavy metal salts. Wool is very reactive toward iron, copper, chromium, and tin. When wool is boiled in solutions of these salts, they combine with the wool to form water-insoluble compounds.

Exposure of the animal fibers to polluted atmospheres will, in general, not be injurious to the fibers. Wool is amphoteric in nature so that small amounts of acids or bases can be neutralized by the fiber itself. Oxidizing atmospheres would be harmful.

Paper

Paper is produced from wood pulps prepared by two different processes, mechanical or chemical (Stamm and Harris, 1953). Groundwood pulp is produced by the wet abrasive action of a grindstone on the side-grain surface of logs. Chemical pulps are produced by a number of processes, but all involve the removal of lignin from the wood. Groundwood pulps are used for such paper products as newsprint in which strength and permanence are of little importance, while chemical pulps are used where strength and permanence are necessary.

Paper is made by beating, dispersing, felting, and drying the pulp. Beating consists of fibrillation, brushing of the fibers to increase their surface, softening them so that greater fiber-to-fiber bonding is obtained in the final sheet of paper, and perhaps forming a colloidal, mucilage-like surface on the fiber. The beaten pulp is then dispersed in a large amount of water to enhance felting and sheet formation on the paper machine, where the water is removed and the sheet dried.

Pulp additives are used to obtain certain properties in the final paper sheet. Sizing—usually rosin, paraffin or starch—is used to reduce the rate of penetration of liquids into the final product. Loading and filling agents, china clay, precipitated chalk, calcium sulfate, etc., are used to make the paper more opaque. For wet strength papers, various resins—such as the formaldehyde derivatives of phenol, urea, and melamine—are used.

The strength of paper is determined more by the bonding between fibers than the strength of the individual fibers themselves (Kallmes, 1970). Hydrogen bonding is thus the critical factor in paper strength.

Since hydrogen bonding is a most important factor in paper strength, water and all aqueous solutions are detrimental to paper quality (Byrd, 1971; Smith, 1965). All polar solvents that cause swelling of cellulose reduce paper strength. Neutral dry chemicals, in most cases, will be without effect, but hygroscopic salts are harmful. Acidic atmospheres will degrade paper by hydrolysis of cellulose.

Wood

Since wood is an important material in the building industry, data have been collected on the strength properties of commercially important species according to the test methods of the American Society of Testing and Materials (1972). Much of this information has been compiled in the *Wood Handbook* (U.S. Department of Agriculture, 1955).

Knowledge of the chemical composition of wood is necessary in order to estimate the effect of various chemicals on wood. The walls of wood cells are composed of three principal chemical materials: cellulose, hemicellulose, and lignin—all of which are polymeric (Othmer 1970b). In addition, there are small amounts of nonstructural materials—such as proteins, fats, waxes, starch, pectin, phenolics, terpenes, and ash—which are designated as extractives.

Cellulose represents the chief component of wood, constituting from 40 to 50 percent of the extractive-free wood. Since the strength properties of cellulose are related to a considerable extent to its molecular weight, any chemical which can reduce the degree of polymerization of the cellulose in wood will have a serious weakening effect on the strength of wood.

The hemicelluloses, which constitute from 15 to 25 percent of extractive-free wood, are low molecular weight polysaccharides. The hemicellulose molecule is essentially linear, but generally contains numerous and varied short side chains. In contrast to cellulose, the hemicelluloses are built up of a number of sugar residues, among which are D-xylose, D-mannose, D-glucose, D-galactose, L-arabinose, 4-*0*-methyl-D-glucuronic acid, D-galacturonic acid, and D-glucuronic acid. Generally, the hemicelluloses are more sensitive to chemicals than is cellulose.

Lignin is the component which gives the tree its rigidity. It is a complex, 3-dimensional polymer of phenyl-propane units and is present in wood in amounts of 20–35 percent. Unlike the polysaccharides, lignin cannot be hydrolyzed into its simple building blocks. It cannot be separated from the other wood components by neutral solvents. Lignin contains groups that are easily altered by the reagents used to isolate it so that there is a question as to the nature of lignin *in situ* as compared with isolated lignin. Lignin is more resistant to acids than are the polysaccharides, but more sensitive to oxidizing agents.

Most of the strength properties of wood increase with a decrease in moisture content below the fiber saturation point. The fiber saturation point of wood (about 30% for most woods) is that moisture content at which the fibers are completely saturated with water, but no water exists in the coarse, microscopically visible capillary structure. The increase in strength is due to secondary valence forces between the structural units. In the swollen condition, these valence forces are partially satisfied by water; but, as the water is removed, the valence forces between structural units mutually satisfy each other.

In considering the action of chemicals on wood, the permeability of the wood must be taken into account. Only the outer or sapwood portion of a tree takes part in the life process. The inner part of the sapwood in time becomes infiltrated with gums, resins, and other coloring matter and is converted to heartwood. In almost all cases, the heartwood is considerably more resistant than the sapwood to the passage of liquids and gases. This resistance probably is due to the clogging of fine interfiber communicating structures, such as the pits, by infiltrated material. Thus, the effects of short-term exposure of lumber to chemicals are apt to be confined to the surface.

The effects of various classes of chemicals on wood are summarized below.

- *Polar solvents*—Cause shrinking and swelling but have no permanent effect. If swelling occurs beyond the water-swollen dimensions of wood, weakening should be suspected.
- *Nonpolar solvents*—No effect on wood properties.

- *Oils, fats, waxes*—No effect.
- *Phenolic compounds*—Wood resistant to more complex phenols, but not to simple phenols.
- *Inorganic acids*—Wood resistant at low concentrations and ordinary temperatures, but not at higher concentrations or temperatures (Thompson 1969).
- *Organic acids*—Have little effect, with the exception of formic acid.
- *Alkalies*—Damage wood.
- *Neutral salts*—No effect.
- *Oxidizing agents*—If strong, have deleterious effect.
- *Reducing agents*—Other than bleaching, no effect under ordinary conditions.
- *Corrosive atmospheres*—In general, because of the low concentrations, only the surface affected, with little effect on strength properties.
- *Water*—In itself, little effect upon strength properties, but can be secondary effects due to decay by microorganisms.

Plastics

The resistance of the more common plastics to chemical attack is summarized in Table G-5.

Synthetic Fibers

The effects of chemicals on synthetic fibers are summarized in Table G-6.

Elastomers

The performance of elastomers is summarized in Table G-7.

Protective Coatings

Many architectural and industrial finishes have been developed as a result of the diversity of applications for which they are needed. The performance of a coating can be expressed in terms of its inherent weathering resistance, toughness, resiliency, continuity (non-porosity), and adhesion to the substrate surface. In general, the ability of a protective coating to withstand environmental exposure can be predicted if its resin system and the nature of the environment are known.

TABLE G-5   Performance of Plastics Exposed to Chemicals

Material	Resistant	Some Harmful Effects	Degraded
Thermoplastic resins in general	Weak acids, weak alkalies, salts		Strong concentrated inorganic acids; strong oxidizing agents; organic solvents
Polyolefins (polyethylene and polypropylene)	Solvents; food chemicals; alkalies; mineral acids; sea water	Chlorinated hydrocarbons; aliphatic hydrocarbons; aromatic hydrocarbons; some esters	Toluene; xylene; amylacetate; trichloroethylene; turpentine; and lubricating oils above 160 °F; surfactants (stress cracking)
Vinyl polymers	Acids; alkalies; strong inorganic acids; concentrated alkalies; aliphatic hydrocarbons; alcohols; inorganic salts		Esters; ketones; aromatic solvents
Epoxy resins	Water; sour crudes; salt water; strong alkalies; non-oxidizing acids; jet fuels; aliphatics; some aromatics		Strong oxidizing agents; chlorine; chlorinated solvents; most aromatic hydrocarbons
Phenolic resins	Most solvents; acids; aromatic hydrocarbons; aliphatic hydrocarbons; chlorinated solvents; alcohols; esters; ketones; weak alkalies		Strong alkalies; strong oxidizing agents
Polyesters	Non-oxidizing acids; corrosive salts; aliphatic solvents; aromatic compounds; chlorinated solvents	Weak bases; esters	Strong oxidizing agents; strong bases

TABLE G-6   Performance of Synthetic Fibers Exposed to Chemicals

Material	Resistant	Some Harmful Effects	Degraded
Polyacrylonitrile (orlon) and acrilonitrile-vinyl (Acrilan)	Acids; weak alkalies; organic solvents; oils; grease; most salts		Strong alkalies
Polyamide (nylon)	Alkalies; organic solvents; salts		Oxidizing agents; strong mineral acids; weak acids (hot)
Polyester (dacron)	Most acids; hydrofluoric acid; weak alkalies; organic compounds		Strong sulfuric acids; hot, concentrated alkalies
Polyolefins (polyethylene and polypropylene)	Most acids; alkalies	Aromatic solvents	Oxidizing acids
Vinyl chloride-vinyl acetate (vinyon)	Inorganic acids; alkalies		Some chlorinated hydrocarbons
Vinylidine chloride (Saran)	Acids; most alkalies		Ammonium hydroxide; esters; chlorinated hydrocarbons

TABLE G-7   Performance of Elastomers Exposed to Chemicals

Material	Resistant	Some Harmful Effects	Degraded
Natural rubber	Acids; alkalies	Oils; organic solvents	Ozone; oxygen
Styrenebutadiene rubbers (SBR)	Acids		Aliphatic, aromatic, and chlorinated solvents
Butyl rubber (HR)	Ozone; oils, acids; plasticizers		Aliphatic and aromatic hydrocarbons; halogenated solvents
Nitrile rubber	Oils; alcohols; aliphatic hydrocarbons; weak acids		Ketones; esters; aromatic solvents

TABLE G-7—*Continued*

Material	Resistant	Some Harmful Effects	Degraded
Polysulfide rubbers	Fuel oils; gasoline; kerosene; alcohols; glycols; dilute acids; salts		Concentrated acids; oxidizing acids
Neoprene rubber (CR)	Oils; atmospheric oxidants; aliphatic hydrocarbons; alcohols; ethylene glycol; freon; dilute mineral acids; concentrated sodium hydroxide; concentrated potassium hydroxide; inorganic salts		Chlorinated hydrocarbons; organic esters; aromatic hydrocarbons; phenol; cresol; ethylmethyl ketone; strong oxidizing agents
Acrylic rubbers	Sulfur-bearing oils	Acids	Water; alcohol; oxygenated solvents; alkalies
Chlorosulfonated polyethylene	Ozone; alcohol; esters; sodium hydroxide; dilute sulfuric acid; nitric acid; sodium hypochlorite; 85% phosphoric acid		Glacial acetic acid; acetone; concentrated sulfuric acid; aromatic solvents
Urethane elastomers	Aliphatic hydrocarbons; alcohol; ether	Aromatic hydrocarbons; some solvents (e.g., nitrobenzene, methyl chloride)	Acids; alkalies; hot water, steam
Fluoroelastomers	Aromatic hydrocarbons; aliphatic hydrocarbons; aromatic amines; chlorinated hydrocarbons; mineral acids; alkalies		Hydraulic fluids; concentrated nitric acid; ethyl acetate; many esters

REFERENCES

American Association of Textile Chemists and Colorists. (Issued annually.) *Textile Manual of the American Association of Textile Chemists and Colorists.* Research Triangle Park, N.C.

American Concrete Institute Committee 201. 1962. Durability of concrete in service. *J. Am. Concr. Inst.* 59:1771-1820.

American Concrete Institute Committee 515. 1966. Guide for the protection of concrete against chemical attack by means of coatings and other corrosion-resistant materials. *J. Am. Concr. Inst.* 63:1305-1392.

American Society for Metals. 1961. *Metals Handbook: Properties and Selection of Metals,* Vol. 1. American Society for Metals, Cleveland. 1300 pp.

American Society for Testing and Materials. 1959. Report of Sub-Group VII on Corrosiveness of Various Atmospheric Test Sites as Measured by Specimens of Steel and Zinc. Appendix 2. In *Proc. ASTM 59.* ASTM, Philadelphia.

American Society for Testing and Materials. 1961. Report of Inspection of Corrosion Resistant Steels in Architectural and Structural Applications. Appendix to Report of Committee A-10. In *Proc. ASTM 61.* ASTM, Philadelphia. pp. 188-194.

American Society for Testing and Materials. 1971. *Annual Book of ASTM Standards.* Parts 24, 25. ASTM, Philadelphia.

American Society for Testing and Materials. 1972. *Annual Book of ASTM Standards.* ASTM, Philadelphia.

Anderson, E.A. 1956. The atmospheric corrosion of rolled zinc. In *Symposium on Atmospheric Corrosion of Non-Ferrous Metals.* STP 175. ASTM, Philadelphia. pp. 126-133.

Byrd, V.L. 1971. The effects of humidity on paper. *Chem. 26/Pap. Process.* 7:30, 31, 34, 35.

Copson, H.R. 1945. A theory of the mechanisms of rusting of low-alloy steels in the atmosphere. In *Proc. ASTM 45.* ASTM, Philadelphia. pp. 554-580.

Guttman, H., and P.J. Sereda. 1968. Measurement of atmospheric factors affecting the corrosion of metals. In *Metal Corrosion in the Atmosphere.* STP 435. ASTM, Philadelphia. pp. 326-359.

International Nickel Co. (No date.) *Resistance of Nickel and High Nickel Alloys to Corrosion by Sulfuric Acid.* Corrosion Engineering Bull. No. 1. Publ. A-280. International Nickel Co., New York. 45 pp.

International Nickel Co. (No date.) *Corrosion Resistance of Nickel and Nickel-Containing Alloys in Caustic Soda and Other Alkalies.* Corrosion Engineering Bull. No. 2. Publ. 281. International Nickel Co., New York. 40 pp.

International Nickel Co. (No date.) *Resistance of Nickel and High Nickel Alloys to Corrosion by Hydrochloric Acid, Hydrogen Chloride and Chlorine.* Corrosion Engineering Bull. No. 3. Publ. A-279. International Nickel Co., New York. 31 pp.

International Nickel Co. (No date.) *Corrosion Resistance of Nickel-Containing Alloys in Phosphoric Acid.* Corrosion Engineering Bull. No. 4. Publ. A-415. International Nickel Co., New York. 40 pp.

International Nickel Co. (No date.) *Corrosion Resistance of Nickel-Containing Alloys in Hydrofluoric Acid, Hydrogen Fluoride and Fluorine.* Corrosion Engineering Bull. No. 5. Publ. A-443. International Nickel Co., New York. 36 pp.

Kallmes, O.J. 1970. Behavior of paper under strain. *Pap. Trade J.* 154:54-57.

Kuenning, W.H. 1966. Resistance of Portland cement mortar to chemical attack— A progress report. *Highw. Res. Rec.* 113:43-87.

LaQue, F.L., and H.R. Copson, eds. 1963. *Corrosion Resistance of Metals and Alloys,* 2nd ed. Reinhold Publ. Corp., New York. 712 pp.

National Association of Corrosion Engineers. 1974. *Corrosion Data Survey—Metal Section,* 5th ed. National Association of Corrosion Engineers, Houston. 312 pp.

Othmer, K. 1964. Cellulose. In *Encyclopedia of Chemical Technology,* 2nd ed. Vol. 4. John Wiley and Sons, Inc., New York. pp. 593–616.

Othmer, K. 1970a. Wool. In *Encyclopedia of Chemical Technology,* 2nd ed. Vol. 22. John Wiley and Sons, Inc., New York. pp. 387–418.

Othmer, K. 1970b. Wood. In *Encyclopedia of Chemical Technology,* 2nd ed. Vol. 22. John Wiley and Sons, Inc., New York. pp. 358–387.

Schmitt, R.J. 1960. The use of non-carbon steel and alloy steel in the chemical industry. In *Proceedings of a Short Course on Process Industry Corrosion.* National Association of Corrosion Engineers, Houston. pp. 31–60.

Schmitt, R.J., and W.P. Gallagher. 1969. Unpainted high-strength low alloy steel. *Mater. Prot.* 8:70–71.

Schmitt, R.J., and C.X. Mullen. 1969. Influence of chromium on the atmospheric corrosion behavior of steel. In *Stainless Steel for Architectural Use.* STP 454. ASTM, Philadelphia. pp. 124–136.

Smith, W.E. 1965. Determination of the relative bonded area of handsheets by direct-current electrical conductivity. *TAPPI* 48:476–480.

Stamm, A.J., and E.E. Harris. 1953. Chapter 10. In *Chemical Processing of Wood.* Chemical Publ. Co., New York.

Thompson, W.S. 1969. *Effects of Chemicals, Chemical Atmospheres, and Contact with Metals on Southern Pine Wood: A Review.* Res. Rep. No. 6. Forest Products Utilization Laboratory, Mississippi State University, State College. 33 pp.

Uhlig, H.E., ed. 1948. *Corrosion Handbook.* John Wiley and Sons, Inc., New York, 1188 pp.

U.S. Department of Agriculture. 1955. Strength values of clear wood and related factors. In *Wood Handbook.* Agric. Handbook No. 72. U.S. Government Printing Office, Washington, D.C. pp. 67–103.

Walton, C.J., and W. King. 1956. Resistance of aluminum-base alloys to 20 year atmospheric exposure. In *Symposium on Atmospheric Corrosion of Non-Ferrous Metals.* STP 175. ASTM, Philadelphia. pp. 21–44.

Woods, H. 1968. *Durability in Concrete Construction.* ACI Monogr. No. 4. American Concrete Institute, Detroit. 190 pp.

SUGGESTED READINGS

American Society for Testing and Materials. 1968. *Metal Corrosion in the Atmosphere.* STP 435. ASTM, Philadelphia.

Anaconda American Brass Co. 1962. *Corrosion Resistance of Copper Metal.* Publ. B-36. Anaconda American Brass Co., Waterbury, Conn.

Komp, M.E., and R.J. Schmitt. 1966. Selection and application of stainless steel for corrosive environments. In *Metallurgical Social Conference.* Vol. 40. Gordon Breach Publ. Co., New York. pp. 45–88.

List of Participants

COMMITTEE FOR THE WORKING CONFERENCE ON PRINCIPLES OF PROTOCOLS FOR EVALUATING CHEMICALS IN THE ENVIRONMENT

Dr. Norton Nelson, New York University Medical Center, New York, New York, *Chairman*

Dr. John Cairns, Jr., Virginia Polytechnic Institute and State University, Blacksburg, Virginia

Dr. Theodore L. Cairns, E. I. duPont de Nemours & Co., Wilmington, Delaware

Dr. Lyle D. Calvin, Oregon State University, Corvallis, Oregon

Bertram D. Dinman, M.D., The University of Michigan, Ann Arbor, Michigan

Dr. William H. Drury, Jr., Massachusetts Audubon Society, Lincoln, Massachusetts

Dr. Hans L. Falk, National Institute of Environmental Health Sciences, Research Triangle Park, North Carolina

Dr. Virgil H. Freed, Oregon State University, Corvallis, Oregon

Dr. Edward D. Goldberg, Scripps Institution of Oceanography, La Jolla, California

Dr. Francis A. Gunther, University of California, Riverside, California

Dr. Roy W. Hann, Jr., Texas A&M University, College Station, Texas

Dr. Peter V. Hobbs, University of Washington, Seattle, Washington

Mr. J. Anthony Keith, Canadian Wildlife Service, Ottawa, Ontario, Canada

Dr. Ian C. T. Nisbet, Massachusetts Audubon Society, Lincoln, Massachusetts

Harold M. Peck, M.D., Merck Institute for Therapeutic Research, West Point, Pennsylvania

Dr. Adel F. Sarofim, Massachusetts Institute of Technology, Cambridge, Massachusetts

Mr. Robert J. Schmitt, U.S. Steel Corporation, Monroeville, Pennsylvania

Dr. George Sprugel, Jr., Illinois Natural History Survey, Urbana, Illinois

Dr. Herbert E. Stokinger, National Institute for Occupational Safety and Health, Cincinnati, Ohio

Dr. Bernard Weiss, University of Rochester, Rochester, New York

Dr. Carroll L. Wilson, Massachusetts Institute of Technology, Cambridge, Massachusetts

James G. Wilson, M.D., The Children's Hospital Research Foundation, Cincinnati, Ohio

NAS-NRC STAFF

Dr. Charles R. Malone, Staff Officer, Environmental Studies Board, NAS-NAE

Mr. Ralph C. Wands, Director, Advisory Center on Toxicology, NRC

Dr. J. Charles Baummer, Jr., Staff Officer, Environmental Studies Board, NAS-NAE

Dr. David W. Fassett, Consultant, Advisory Center on Toxicology

EPA LIAISON

Dr. Kenneth Bridbord, Office of Research and Monitoring, Washington, D.C.

Dr. John L. Buckley, Office of Research, Washington, D.C.

Dr. Alphonse F. Forziati, Office of Toxic Substances, Washington, D.C.

Panel on Acute Toxicity

Harold M. Peck, M.D., Merck Institute for Therapeutic Research, West Point, Pennsylvania, *Chairman*

Dr. John P. Frawley, Hercules Powder Company, Wilmington, Delaware

Dr. Robert Hehir, Food and Drug Administration, Washington, D.C.

Dr. Edward D. Palmes, New York University Medical Center, New York, New York

Dr. Robert J. Weir, Jr., Litton Bionetics, Inc., Bethesda, Maryland

Panel on Chronic Toxicity

Bertram D. Dinman, M.D., The University of Michigan, Ann Arbor, Michigan, *Chairman*

Dr. Joseph F. Borzelleca, Virginia Commonwealth University, Richmond, Virginia

Joseph C. Calandra, M.D., Industrial Bio-Test Laboratories, Inc., Northbrook, Illinois

Dr. Julius M. Coon, Thomas Jefferson University, Philadelphia, Pennsylvania

Dr. Herbert E. Stokinger, National Institute for Occupational Safety and Health, Cincinnati, Ohio

Panel on Carcinogenesis

Dr. Hans L. Falk, National Institute of Environmental Health Sciences, Research Triangle Park, North Carolina, *Chairman*
Dr. Leila Diamond, Wistar Institute, Philadelphia, Pennsylvania
Dr. Leo Friedman, Food and Drug Administration, Washington, D.C.
Dr. Katherine L. Sydnor, University of Kentucky, Lexington, Kentucky
Dr. Elizabeth Weisburger, National Institutes of Health, Bethesda, Maryland

Panel on Reproduction

James Wilson, M.D., The Children's Hospital Research Foundation, Cincinnati, Ohio, *Chairman*
Dr. Robert L. Brent, Jefferson Medical College, Philadelphia, Pennsylvania
Dr. W. Gary Flamm, Food and Drug Administration, Washington, D.C.
Dr. Warren W. Nichols, Institute for Medical Research, Camden, New Jersey
Dr. Jerry Rice, National Institutes of Health, Bethesda, Maryland
Dr. Hilton A. Salhanick, School of Public Health, Harvard University, Boston, Massachusetts
Dr. Joan Spyker, University of Virginia Medical School, Charlottesville, Virginia
Dr. Fred de Serres, National Institute of Environmental Health Sciences, Research Triangle Park, North Carolina

Panel on Behavioral Toxicology

Dr. Bernard Weiss, University of Rochester Medical Center, Rochester, New York, *Chairman*
Dr. Josef Brozek, Lehigh University, Bethlehem, Pennsylvania
Dr. Harley Hanson, Merck, Sharp and Dohme, West Point, Pennsylvania
Dr. Russell C. Leaf, Rutgers University, New Brunswick, New Jersey
Dr. Nancy K. Mello, National Institute of Mental Health, Washington, D.C.
Dr. Joan M. Spyker, University of Virginia Medical School, Charlottesville, Virginia

Panel on Environmental Toxicology

Dr. John Cairns, Jr., Virginia Polytechnic Institute and State University, Blacksburg, Virginia, *Chairman*
Professor Robert Lee Metcalf, University of Illinois, Urbana, Illinois
Dr. David B. Peakall, Cornell University, Ithaca, New York
Dr. George Sprugel, Jr., Illinois Natural History Survey, Urbana, Illinois
Dr. Gordon T. Goodman, University of London, London, England

Panel on Simulated Systems

Dr. Ian C.T. Nisbet, Massachusetts Audubon Society, Lincoln, Massachusetts, *Chairman*

Dr. Carol W. Chen, Tetra Tech, Inc., Lafayette, California
Professor Simon Levin, Cornell University, Ithaca, New York

Panel on Field Studies of Populations

Mr. J. Anthony Keith, Canadian Wildlife Service, Ottawa, Ontario, Canada, *Chairman*
Dr. Gordon T. Goodman, University of London, London, England
Dr. Robert W. Risebrough, Canadian Wildlife Service, Ottawa, Ontario, Canada
Dr. Ray F. Smith, University of California, Berkeley, California

Panel on Field Studies of Ecosystems

Dr. Roy W. Hann, Jr., Texas A&M University, College Station, Texas, *Chairman*
Dr. Martin Alexander, Cornell University, Ithaca, New York
Dr. John Cairns, Jr., Virginia Polytechnic Institute and State University, Blacksburg,
Virginia
Dr. Bostwick H. Ketchum, Woods Hole Oceanographic Institution, Woods Hole,
Massachusetts

Panel on Atmosphere

Dr. Peter V. Hobbs, University of Washington, Seattle, Washington, *Chairman*
Dr. Halstead Harrison, University of Washington, Seattle, Washington
Dr. Lester Machta, National Oceanic and Atmospheric Administration, Silver
Spring, Maryland
Dr. Hiromi Niki, Ford Motor Company, Dearborn, Michigan
Professor Elmer Robinson, Washington State University, Pullman, Washington

Panel on Inanimates

Mr. Robert J. Schmitt, U.S. Steel Corporation, Monroeville, Pennsylvania, *Chairman*
Mr. Fred M. Ernsberger, PPG Industries, Pittsburgh, Pennsylvania
Mr. Otto H. Fenner, Monsanto Chemical Company, St. Louis, Missouri
Dr. George J. Hajny, U.S. Forest Service, Madison, Wisconsin
Dr. Charles F. Scholer, Purdue University, Lafayette, Indiana
Mr. E.A. Tice, International Nickel Company, New York, New York

Panel on Estimation of Exposure Levels

Dr. Edward D. Goldberg, Scripps Institution of Oceanography, La Jolla, California,
Co-Chairman
Dr. Adel F. Sarofim, Massachusetts Institute of Technology, Cambridge, Massachu-
setts, *Co-Chairman*
Dr. Carroll L. Wilson, Massachusetts Institute of Technology, Cambridge, Massachu-
setts, *Co-Chairman*

Professor John Brewer, University of California, Davis, California
Dr. Hugo B. Fischer, University of California, Berkeley, California
Dr. Sheldon Friedlander, California Institute of Technology, Pasadena, California
Dr. Rizwanul Haque, Oregon State University, Corvallis, Oregon
Dr. Sheldon M. Lambert, Shell Chemical Company, Houston, Texas
Dr. Frederick T. Mackenzie, Northwestern University, Evanston, Illinois
Dr. William H. Matthews, Massachusetts Institute of Technology, Cambridge, Massachusetts
Dr. John Wood, University of Illinois, Urbana, Illinois

Panel on Benefits

Dr. Theodore L. Cairns, E.I. duPont de Nemours & Co., Wilmington, Delaware, *Chairman*
Dr. Henry E. Baumgarten, The University of Nebraska, Lincoln, Nebraska
Dr. Milton Harris, Washington, D.C.
Dr. Glenn E. Ullyot, Smith Kline & French Laboratories, Philadelphia, Pennsylvania

Panel on Analysis and Monitoring

Dr. Virgil H. Freed, Oregon State University, Corvallis, Oregon, *Co-Chairman*
Dr. Francis A. Gunther, University of California, Riverside, California, *Co-Chairman*
Mr. Roger C. Blinn, American Cyanamid Company, Princeton, New Jersey
Mr. Charles Dunn, Hercules, Inc., Wilmington, Delaware
Mr. Herman Feltz, U.S. Geological Survey, Arlington, Virginia
Dr. Don W. Hayne, North Carolina State University, Raleigh, North Carolina
Dr. Alan Isensee, U.S. Department of Agriculture, Beltsville, Maryland
Mr. Herbert B. Mendietta, U.S. Geological Survey, Austin, Texas.

Panel on Statistics

Dr. Lyle D. Calvin, Oregon State University, Corvallis, Oregon, *Chairman*
Professor Douglas S. Robson, Cornell University, Ithaca, New York

Panel on Episodic Exposures

Dr. Roy W. Hann, Jr., Texas A&M University, College Station, Texas, *Chairman*
Dr. John Cairns, Jr., Virginia Polytechnic Institute and State University, Blacksburg, Virginia

Observers

Dr. Kenneth C. Back, Wright-Patterson Air Force Base, Ohio
Dr. Paul E. Brubaker, National Environmental Research Center, Research Triangle Park, North Carolina
Dr. William S. Brungs, National Water Quality Laboratory, Duluth, Minnesota
Dr. Kirby Campbell, National Environmental Research Center, Cincinnati, Ohio
Dr. David Coffin, National Environmental Research Center, Research Triangle Park, North Carolina
Mr. Joseph J. Cummings, Environmental Protection Agency, Washington, D.C.
Dr. Homer E. Fairchild, Environmental Protection Agency, Washington, D.C.
Dr. Farley Fisher, Environmental Protection Agency, Washington, D.C.
Dr. David Gaylor, National Center for Toxicological Research, Jefferson, Arkansas
Dr. George M. Goldstein, National Environmental Research Center, Research Triangle Park, North Carolina
Dr. Douglas Grahn, Atomic Energy Commission, Washington, D.C.
Dr. Elmer B. Harvey, Atomic Energy Commission, Washington, D.C.
Dr. Harry W. Hays, U.S. Department of Agriculture, Beltsville, Maryland
Dr. Walter W. Heck, National Environmental Research Center, Research Triangle Park, North Carolina
Lt. Cdr. Thomas Hill, National Naval Medical Center, Bethesda, Maryland
Dr. I. Hoffman, National Research Council of Canada, Ottawa, Ontario, Canada

---

In many instances, these participants contributed substantially to the preparation of the report.

Dr. Robert J.M. Horton, National Environmental Research Center, Research Triangle Park, North Carolina

Dr. F. Gordon Hueter, National Environmental Research Center, Research Triangle Park, North Carolina

Mr. Victor W. Lambou, Environmental Protection Agency, Washington, D.C.

Miss Jane Lewis, Department of Commerce, Washington, D.C.

Dr. Bernard P. McNamara, U.S. Army Materiel Command, Edgewood Arsenal, Maryland

Dr. Calvin M. Menzie, Department of the Interior, Washington, D.C.

Dr. John A. Moore, National Institute of Environmental Health Sciences, Research Triangle Park, North Carolina

Dr. Donald I. Mount, National Water Quality Laboratory, Duluth, Minnesota

Dr. Vaun A. Newill, Executive Office of the President, Washington, D.C.

Dr. Michael J. Prival, Environmental Protection Agency, Washington, D.C.

Dr. William G. Roessler, Environmental Protection Agency, Washington, D.C.

Dr. Lawrence M. Roslinski, Environmental Protection Agency, Washington, D.C.

Brig. Gen. F.G. Schafer, USAF, Brooks Air Force Base, Texas

Dr. Herbert Schumacher, National Center for Toxicological Research, Jefferson, Arkansas

Dr. Charles B. Smith, Department of Transportation, Washington, D.C.

Lt. Col. Marshall Steinberg, U.S. Army Environmental Hygiene Agency, Aberdeen Proving Ground, Maryland

Dr. Robert G. Tardiff, National Environmental Research Center, Cincinnati, Ohio

Dr. C. Hugh Thompson, Environmental Protection Agency, Arlington, Virginia

Dr. Jack Thompson, National Environmental Research Center, Research Triangle Park, North Carolina

Dr. Herbert L. Wiser, Environmental Protection Agency, Washington, D.C.

ATTENDING IN PERSONAL CAPACITY

Dr. Arne Jernelov, World Health Organization, Copenhagen, Denmark

Dr. V.B. Vouk, World Health Organization, Geneva, Switzerland